T0366991

TEACHING DEMENTIA CARE

TEACHING DEMENTIA CARE

Skill and Understanding

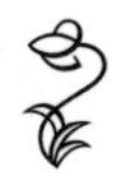

NANCY L. MACE

with

DOROTHY H. COONS & SHELLY E. WEAVERDYCK

THE JOHNS HOPKINS UNIVERSITY PRESS
Baltimore & London

Printed in the United States of America on acid-free paper
2 4 6 8 9 7 5 3 1

The Johns Hopkins University Press
2715 North Charles Street
Baltimore, Maryland 21218-4363
www.press.jhu.edu

Library of Congress Cataloging-in-Publication Data

Mace, Nancy L.
Teaching dementia care : skill and understanding / Nancy L. Mace with Dorothy H. Coons and Shelly E. Weaverdyck.
p. ; cm.
Includes bibliograpical references and index.
ISBN 0-8018-8042-4 (hardcover : alk. paper)—ISBN 0-8018-8043-2 (pbk. : alk. paper)
1. Dementia—Patients—Care—Study and teaching. 2. Dementia—Patients—Care. 3. Nursing—Study and teaching.
[DNLM: 1. Dementia—nursing. 2. Education, Nursing—methods. 3. Teaching—methods. WY 152 M141t 2005] I. Coons, Dorothy H. II. Weaverdyck, Shelly. III. Title.
RC521.M325 2005
616.8′3—dc22 2004012461

A catalog record for this book is available from the British Library.

TO

LAURA J. REIF, PH.D.,

&

RICHARD A. LANNON, M.D.,

FOR THEIR FRIENDSHIP & ENCOURAGEMENT

CONTENTS

ACKNOWLEDGMENTS

I am indebted to my collaborators, Dorothy Coons and Shelly Weaverdyck, who contributed their expertise and devoted many months to editing a partially written manuscript. Without their dedication, the manuscript would not have been published.

This book is the culmination of what I have learned in my career in dementia care. I am indebted to every person I encountered. That learning began with the many family members of people with dementia I have known, worked with in the Alzheimer disease associations in the United States and abroad, and who have called, written, or talked with me.

I have learned from people with dementia who have spoken to me both verbally and nonverbally, but always loud and clear.

This book would not have been possible without the enormous contribution of direct care providers: nursing assistants, activity directors, and many others. Their expertise and their love of their work and the people they care for continue to move and impress me. As one caregiver stated, "We love them and we try to understand them."

I have learned from the professionals who work with people with dementia: physicians, nurses, social workers, physical and occupational therapists, and administrators. These are the people in the middle who provide good-quality care despite a long list of limitations.

It would not be possible to write a sensible text about care without an understanding of policy issues. I am indebted to the staff of the (then) Health Care Financing Administration; the Alzheimer's Association; the team who put together the Resident Assessment Instrument; and state and federal surveyors, legislators, government leaders, and lobbyists in this country and abroad. I have learned from all my colleagues with whom I have shared panels, planning committees, and state or local Alzheimer planning organizations. This text has benefited from the work of the many researchers who have shared their knowledge and ideas.

I wish to thank the personnel of those special Alzheimer care units in the United States, Canada, Europe, Australia, New Zealand, and Japan who developed remarkable programs and shared the range of their knowledge in great depth. They were generous hosts who welcomed me to their country or region. In the early 1980s innovative providers recognized that ambulatory people with dementia needed an alternative to traditional home care or nursing home care. They designed special residential, nursing home, home care, and day care programs. Most of the people involved in these programs were unaware of the efforts of their colleagues in other places. There were no guidelines, few regulations, and no models of best care. I visited many of these programs, and much of what this text contains arises from the insights I gained from the programs and their excellent staff. From them I learned that people with dementia with a history of serious behavioral problems could be cared for in ways that significantly reduced these problems. I am grateful to these programs for permitting me to inquire into their methods, staffing costs, and administrative issues. Programs everywhere have trusted me with their special knowledge, dreams, visions, materials, and even problems. Without such generosity, this book would not be possible.

A very special thanks is due to my editor, Wendy Harris. This book was a long time in the making, and she has been patient and supportive. She read and edited many drafts of the manuscript and truly kept me going. An author could have no more loyal supporter. My copy editor, Grace Carino, remained faithful to the text and was a pleasure to work with.

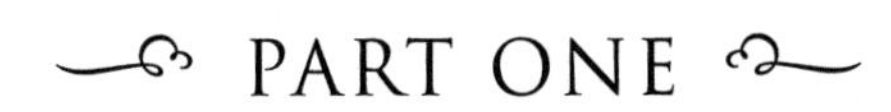

PART ONE

GETTING STARTED

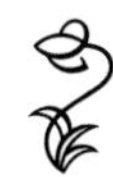

CHAPTER I

LAYING THE GROUNDWORK FOR CHANGE

Dementia afflicts millions of Americans, and the economic and emotional costs of care for individuals with the disorder are astronomical. Unlike most other chronic and long-term illnesses, dementia primarily affects the brain. Memory loss is irreversible, depression is common, and behavioral symptoms such as screaming, searching for someone, overreacting to stress, and resisting care are evidence of the distress it causes. Dementia changes the person's understanding of the need for care, devastates relationships, and results in behaviors that are difficult for caregivers to understand and manage.

People with dementia are usually cared for by family members for most of their illness, and it has been well documented that care overwhelms and exhausts family members. Many of those with dementia eventually need formal care—home care, adult day care, residential care, or nursing home care. The majority of direct care in formal settings is provided by nonprofessional staff members—nursing aides, unlicensed homemakers, and nursing assistants—under the supervision of nurses, social workers, and other professionals. The behavioral symptoms of dementia also challenge formal care systems. Clients resist being bathed, strike out at care providers, elope from the care setting, and show other behavioral symptoms that create burdens for the staff and increase costs.

Both family members and the formal care system are pushing to find ways to improve the quality of life for those with dementia. Most care providers train their staff in dementia care, and a wide range of educational materials are available. Yet too often staff members are unable to implement newly learned skills in daily practice in the workplace. Thus, the suffering and distress people with dementia experience continue, and frustrated staff members conclude that, even with training, nothing much can be done.

There are many reasons why current approaches to staff training have failed to alleviate clients' suffering and distress. First, caring for people with dementia is challenging: the best-trained people with the best intuitive skills are sometimes unable to reach and comfort people with dementia. Second, good dementia care can be costly. Third, there is a lack of qualified nursing staff members, trained nursing aides, geriatricians, and mental health professionals. These are major obstacles to ideal care, and no training program alone can overcome them, although good training can help to compensate for them. However, there are other reasons why training fails to alter the quality of care provided. Addressing these will result in change, despite the limitations just mentioned.

Some home care programs, adult day care centers, residential care facilities, and nursing homes have demonstrated dramatic changes in their clients' behavioral symptoms and apparent quality of life. These model programs show that significant improvement is possible even when they have significant budget and staffing limitations.

To improve the quality of life for people with dementia, training must do more than just provide facts and recommendations for treating symptoms. Despite the limitations in resources, training must assist direct care providers in changing their behavior, not just their knowledge base. The goal of this book is to address this gap between the available knowledge base and the care actually provided, thus opening the door to learning that works in the workplace.

The Teaching Process

Learning is a collaboration between teacher and student. It guides the teacher to reinforce positive experiences and to help the students gain confidence in their abilities. The training supports the dignity, self-esteem, and personhood of the teacher, supervisors, direct care staff members, clients, and families.

The *process* of teaching—how students are taught—is essential to their success in transferring skills to their job. This book guides the teacher in the use of didactic and active teaching methods, such as role play as a problem-solving tool and humor in caregiving. The process respects students' self-esteem, allows learning at the pace of the group, and adapts to the demands of the setting and the clients' needs. Because learning must be transferred into real settings with real limitations, each lesson discusses for the teacher possible problems and suggests ways to respond to them.

The teaching materials and the process by which they are taught must ensure that the students "buy into" the course. This course begins with an exercise that encourages student commitment. Many such exercises and clinical experiences support students' investment in the training.

This book emphasizes the use of clinical experiences in which students can discuss the application of new learning, plan ways to implement it, and modify what is taught to fit the workplace. They are then encouraged to try small, supervised interventions in the workplace and to evaluate their success in the classroom. Without planning and trying new knowledge in the workplace, very little will survive the eventual application of training to care.

Often staff members do not think that new approaches will work or assume that they will be too time consuming. Enabling students and staff in training to try out new approaches in the safety of the learning setting and with only one or two individuals encourages them to use the new approach.

External obstacles—the setting, other staff members, management policies—can interfere with the application of new skills. Clinical experience allows the student to identify obstacles and to explore in the classroom ways to circumvent them.

Long-term care settings tend to be rigid yet demand that staff members learn to work within changing circumstances and with a wide variation in clients' behavioral symptoms and levels of function. The teacher is guided to assist the student in devising day-by-day problem-solving approaches to meet this need. Teamwork is important in such settings, but staff must experience (rather than being told) that teamwork saves time. The classroom is used to allow the trainee to experience teamwork.

Students and staff are adults with knowledge, opinions, and a sense of optimism or defeat. They know their setting and their co-workers and often have commonsense ideas for change. A chapter on teaching adults addresses ways to respond to classroom challenges.

The Role of Management

Management plays an essential role in training. Depending on the structure of the organization, management may include the administrator, senior or supervisory staff members, and people from corporate headquarters. It includes anyone with the responsibility to ensure that training and policy are in accordance. It is the task of management to select materials and a teacher to meet the needs of the facility, and it is management's responsibility to ensure that learning is applied in the workplace.

A common error that staff and management make is to expect dramatic changes in their clients right away and to plan larger interventions than can be implemented. This book emphasizes the findings of successful programs: small, simple interventions are most effective—and most possible. Because staff members may not recognize the subtle gains in their clients, the book teaches them what to look for.

Considerable advance planning by management is necessary to ensure that a maximal amount of what is learned is applied in client care. Following are a number of essential tasks.

Set Goals

Goals define what you want to accomplish and allow you to evaluate whether you did so. The goals for the training program will shape the topics selected, the teaching methods used, the methods used to transfer skills to the workplace, and the evaluation. Characteristically, when goals are clear, more learning is achieved, and new skills are better retained and applied.

Set goals that your program and your staff can reach. Success encourages everyone to continue. Tell participants your goals for the training, and invite them to define their own goals.

Understand the Process of Change

Changing existing behaviors is more difficult to accomplish and to sustain over time than is simply teaching new material. If you train staff members to use new behaviors toward people with dementia, both they and the facility must be open to change.

Recognize the areas in which your facility can and cannot support changes in staff behavior. Recognize when the staff might be given conflicting messages (for example, you say "Take time with each person," but budget demands reducing staff). Plan how to consistently reward desired behavioral changes.

People with dementia will respond well to even small positive changes in care. The sum of many small positive changes may be more beneficial than major, expensive changes. Many facilities can make these small changes without extensive investment. These often are changes in staff attitude and facility flexibility.

Successful change is usually accomplished slowly. Make a three-month, six-month, and year-long plan for an ongoing process of change—and training. Include in this plan opportunities for staff members to test new ideas with one or two people. Write in plans for reinforcing new learning. Be able to point out to the staff what goals have been met.

Support the Staff

A facility's staff is more important than its physical plant.

The task of giving individualized, affectionate care to severely ill people places heavy psychological demands on the staff. The staff must not be subjected to unnecessary on-the-job stress or fear of recrimination. They cannot be subjected to routine physical abuse from clients or to criticism from supervisors or family members. They will need extra support when the demands of caregiving are emotionally draining. They require—and deserve—respect.

Teamwork across ranks and disciplines has been shown to be more successful than hierarchical management for the care of people with dementia. The staff members require clear direction from management if they are to be willing to change their routines, spend more time at tasks, or risk change.

Satisfying, positive feelings regarding work must be more common than negative feelings. Achieving this kind of staff environment requires strong, directed leadership and a willingness to take planned risks.

Plan the Training to Fit Your Needs

The materials in this book give management and the teacher flexibility in what will be taught. This makes it a little more time-consuming to use but much more successful than "canned" materials. Consider: Must modifications be made to the program or to the materials to ensure a good fit? Are goals of the training compatible with the long- and short-term goals of the organization? Are the new skills being taught compatible with the planned budget? with staff limitations? Do they fit agency policy? the expectations of the local regulators? the layout of the building?

Know What Is Being Taught and Be Prepared to Support Changes

Even obvious statements such as "Treat people with dignity" or "Understand that they don't remember" must be implemented by changes in staff behavior. Each program is unique in the amount and type of change it can support. Teaching the staff care strategies they cannot implement discourages them from making any changes and blocks the learning process. Management must work closely with the teacher to match the lessons to the kind of care each program wants and can implement. You may choose to teach skills that will be implemented gradually over months.

Nursing home and residential care services are by nature inflexible, and long-term care is made particularly so by regulations, limited funding, and other outside forces. Therefore, management must negotiate for and support as much flexibility as the system will allow to enable staff success.

This course asks staff being trained to work

within available resources. Administrators have found that discussing these issues with students helps build bridges toward possible interventions.

Facilitate Cooperation between Departments

Training almost always requires cooperation from other departments—support from medicine, flexibility from dietary, tolerance of odd behaviors from maintenance, and so on (Exhibit I.1). Contractors and consultants will also be affected. Identify these needs and negotiate them with each department. Resistance to change and competition for influence and resources are natural and will demand your leadership skills.

Make Yourself Available

The active involvement of leadership spells out the value placed on staff training. Management should be present at the opening of the courses and to hand out the diplomas at the end. Direct care staff members have an intimate knowledge of clients and the physical plant that facilitates creative solutions. Listen to them. In the process of training, students will raise issues that they believe should be changed. Discussion will often lead to innovative improvements in care.

Make the Learning Environment Congenial

More learning takes place in a comfortable setting with good light, snacks, and regular breaks. This environment also emphasizes the value placed on learning (Exhibit I.2). Avoid interrupting classes, and plan adequate coverage so that those being trained and the teacher can participate in learning without interruption.

Remember: New Skills Are Fragile

Staff members with new skills must begin to use them quickly and receive reinforcement from supervisors

Exhibit I.1. Working with Medical Professionals

The physician's job description: The physician has education in dementia care and geriatrics and stays abreast of these rapidly growing fields. He or she sees patients regularly and promptly when change occurs. He works easily and communicates openly with the staff as team members.

The role of the community physician: During the admission process, explain to families that the individual's medical care is an integral part of your care package. Ask them to discuss the following with the client's physician:

- What formal training in geriatrics and dementia care has the physician obtained? Will the physician be attending seminars in this area?
- How quickly can the physician respond to calls from the staff?
- Can the physician see the patient as often as needed?
- Where will the physician see the patient?
- Will the physician talk with all relevant caregivers, including certified nurse assistants, to learn about patient function and to advise on interventions?
- What is the physician's position on the use of psychoactive drugs to manage behavioral symptoms of dementia, and what training has the physician had in their use?

Options: There may be no physicians in your community with training in geriatrics or dementia or who are readily available. Hire or contract with a geriatric nurse practitioner. Ask your medical director to discuss the facility's needs with private physicians. Join with others to give the physician in question a scholarship to a medical seminar in dementia or geriatrics. Communicate your concerns to the state medical board or the state surveyor's office. Both hold the physician responsible for the patient's medical care.

Exhibit I.2. Communicating the Importance of Learning: Dos and Don'ts

Do your homework to smooth the way.
Do let others know you support this training.
Do be present for the first class.
Do help staff in training overcome obstacles to good care.
Do let staff in training try out ideas.
Do treat staff in training the way you want your clients to be treated.
Do let your staff members know you are supporting them.
Do invest in people before plant.
Do maintain a sense of humor.
Do support the use of trial and error.
Do participate in celebration of completion.

Don't pull staff in training from class.
Don't cancel classes or use them for staff meetings.
Don't push people.
Don't blame people when new interventions don't work out.
Don't contradict the training by your expectations in the workplace.
Don't rotate staff members.
Don't expect your teacher to teach and to carry a full-time work load.

and peers. Faced with the pressures of the job, newly trained staff members tend to return to old habits quickly (rushing rather than working at the resident's pace, focusing on completing tasks rather than on quality of life). Staff members who have not had the new training add to the pressure to do things the old way (for example, feeling that "you're playing with the resident while I have to do the dirty work"). The expectations of the facility, management, regulators, and even families can prevent change. Newly trained staff members may not be sufficiently confident of their new skills to teach others.

Management must address this dilemma. It is important to plan the sequence of training for the greatest impact. Try training a group of staff members who can begin immediately in a setting where they will encounter limited resistance from others. Train people who will be best able to sustain their knowledge until the rest of the staff members are trained. Train a strong supervisor for this group. Provide brief "confidence booster" meetings for newly trained staff members. Train all supervisory staff so that they can support and lead the others, or train the natural peer leaders who otherwise might sabotage the training. Train as many people who work together as possible—for example, all one shift on one unit. There are significant advantages to training supervisors, activity staff, shift clerks, and nurses in the same group as aides.

Cooperation is improved when the training program is introduced to the entire facility or section at once through short in-service sessions. Provide a short orientation for those not in direct care.

Most systems subtly reward task-based work instead of client-based work. When task-based pressures remain in effect, newly trained staff members will gradually revert to routines in which they rush through the job and postpone or overlook client needs. The demands of hands-on care are so great that it is difficult for anyone to escape this.

Certain changes, such as increased flexibility or blurring of roles, may make staff members anxious. Accomplish change gradually through brief discussions at staff meetings or in-service programs and positive feedback. Change that seems threatening or that makes management and other supervisors uncomfortable can be first tried with just one client.

Provide Feedback and Evaluate

Positive feedback from management emphasizes the value placed on the application of new skills. Make a habit of noticing and pointing out small changes.

The evaluation process provides feedback to management, the teacher, and the trainees (see Chapter IV). It can reveal changes you did not anticipate. Use the findings of your evaluation in marketing, with families, with everyone whom you have asked to support new skills, with surveyors to justify your program (Exhibit I.3), and with the staff, to show how well they are doing. Use evaluations to plan subsequent training.

It's tempting to skip evaluations once the class is over and everyone is caught up in work, but there is no better tool for demonstrating that the time, effort, and money were well spent and to plan for further training, remodeling, or staff deployment.

Evaluation can be informal. The final lesson in this course asks the student to make a plan for implementing new skills. Follow up this plan at three months, six months, or a year. Ask to what extent the plan was carried out; what more needs to be done; what gains have been observed.

How to Use These Materials

This book is written for trainers. It is complete and can stand alone. However, it is also recommended for use by planners and administrators and as a text in gerontological courses. Key points for administrators and planners are indicated.

This section presents a preparation plan for educators who will be training staff people in a direct care setting. This book can be used to teach an introductory course and a core course of 24 to 30 hours. Additional materials are provided for special audiences and follow-up classes. The instructor has the option of breaking the material into shorter courses, adapting the content for the target audience, and selecting the teaching methods to be used.

This book contains a substantial amount of material. You will not use all of it in the beginning. Perhaps you will never need all of the material now in your hands.

Use this material in the following ways:

1. To enable you to plan a course that meets the specific needs of your program
   - You will use only what you need.
   - You will not lose key information.
2. To provide additional materials for special groups or for follow-up courses or later in-service training
3. To provide additional reference material

Exhibit I.3. Working with Surveyors to Make Change

The relationship between surveyors and facilities sometimes works well. Sometimes, however, it is fraught with misinformation, denial, and failure to communicate compounded by politics at the state level. There are good reasons why surveyors make narrow and seemingly ridiculous decisions. The multiple building codes and jurisdictions are good reasons why owners and architects become frustrated.

An honest and extended dialogue among all parties is the only way to address this problem. For those facilities that find that their ability to provide good dementia care is restricted, the following suggestions may help:

- Understand why the regulatory agencies act as they do.
- Avoid an adversarial stance. Relationships with regulators may be best initiated by an organization or at the state level.
- Let your staff members know you are supporting them. Even if you are turned down by regulators, support is important to the staff.
- Be in good standing.
- Seek to make a change with only a few clients, and state your reason for doing so.
- Document that you have tried other interventions first.
- Write up your plan.
- Include how you will evaluate the intervention and when it will terminate.
- Document what happened.

This structure allows the surveyor to justify his decision to his supervisors.

4. To allow you to identify the materials that are right for your group without spending time wading through what you don't need
5. To train students in academic settings. In such settings, the educator will use the book as a text, supplemental text, or reference.

This chapter will walk you step by step through customizing a training course that will meet the needs of your program. Write down your plans as you go through it; when you have completed the chapter, you will have completed a course plan and be ready to begin teaching.

The Organization of This Book

This book is divided into three parts. Part One (Chapters I through III) provides information about successful training programs for management and educators. Read this material before beginning to teach.

Chapter I. Introduction	General information about this course for administrators and for the educator
Chapter II. Teaching Techniques That Work	Information for the educator: How to make your teaching most effective
Chapter III. Teaching Adult Students	For the educator: A positive approach to the challenges that can arise in the classroom

The twelve lessons in Part Two are the heart of the book: they contain what is currently known about good dementia care. They may be used in their entirety as the substance of a comprehensive course, or they may be adapted or customized as needed for shorter sessions, in-service training, or academic courses. The lessons include group discussions and clinical experience exercises written for staff members who work together in a care setting. The educator using this book as a course text will omit these or recommend that the student use them in his or her own clinical training. The lessons also include overheads/handouts for direct care providers and teaching notes to accompany them. The teacher should feel free to reproduce, with attribution, the overheads/handouts. Remember that these teaching aids are not complete discussions and must be used in conjunction with the text. Many are examples or suggestions and do not include all options. Readers who wish to download the overheads/handouts in PDF format for use in electronic presentations (e.g., PowerPoint) should visit the World Wide Web at http://extras.press.jhu.edu/dementia_care/. At the prompt, please enter the following:

user name: dementia
password: Alois

Each lesson is divided into sections. This allows you to select the subjects that meet the needs of your group. If you are teaching direct care providers, follow the plan for either the introductory course or the core course.

Exhibits I.4 and I.5 recommend sections for an introductory course and for a core course, respectively. You may want to

a. teach the introductory course only;
b. teach the core course; or
c. teach the introductory course and follow up with additional sections from the core course as in-service training over time. If you are using the material for supplemental in-service lessons, use sections that you have not already used in the introductory or core course.

Exhibit I.6 identifies the sections targeted to special audiences (people responsible for diagnosis, assessment, referral, and treatment or activity professionals). You will want to provide this material to these professionals as reading or as group workshops.

Some lessons include sections labeled "select appropriate information." Rather than teach the entire section as part of your introductory or core course, select those parts of the section that are most appropriate for your group. This allows you to limit the amount of material (and time) taught and focus on what is most important to your group.

You can use this book to teach in an academic setting. If you are teaching academic students, select the topics most appropriate for your students or assign the text as reading. An ideal way to use this material is to ask academic students to use sections in their clinical training or to work through the course as a group.

Before you select the material you will teach, read

Exhibit I.4. Contents of the Introductory Course

The introductory course consists of sections taken from Lessons 1–6 and 12. Lesson 12 is a key part of the course.

Lesson 1. Helping the Person by Understanding the Problem
- Section 1.1. The Voice of the Person with Dementia: required
- Section 1.2. Establishing Student Goals: optional
- Section 1.3. Recognizing Terms and Differences: select appropriate information

Lesson 2. Helping the Person by Understanding How the Brain Affects Behavior
- Section 2.1. Understanding the Role of Brain Damage: required
- Section 2.2. Recognizing the Capacities That People with Dementia Commonly Retain: required
- Section 2.3. The Interplay of Personality, Life Experience, and Cognitive Losses: use a few examples

Lesson 3. Facilitating Function by Treating Excess Disability
- Section 3.1. The Importance of Treating Excess Disability: required
- Section 3.2. Illness, Pain, Reactions to Medication, Sensory Deficits, and Dizziness: optional

Lesson 4. Facilitating Function by Treating Stress
- Section 4.1. The Role of Stress in Behavioral Symptoms: required
- Section 4.2. Alleviating Symptoms of Stress: select a few items
- Section 4.3. Responding to a Catastrophic Reaction: required
- Section 4.4. The Need for Stimulation and the Difference between Stress and Stimulation: optional

Lesson 5. Applying Skills in Activities of Daily Living
- Section 5.1. The Importance of Individualized Care and the Application of New Knowledge: required
- Section 5.2. Implementing What You Have Learned about Activities of Daily Living: required
- Section 5.3. Using Individualized, Social, and Emotional Contexts of Care: use for suggestions

Lesson 6. Helping the Person by Enriching Communication
- Section 6.1. Verbal and Nonverbal Communication: required
- Section 6.2. Avoiding Patronizing Behavior: required

Lesson 12. A Plan and a Celebration
- Section 12.1. Making a Plan: recommended
- Section 12.2. Celebrating New Skills: required

the first page or two of each lesson. This provides you with a summary of the topics in the lesson.

We recommend that you review all the lessons before beginning to teach. This will provide you with background information that you may want to include for your group.

Each lesson and section build on the previous lessons. For example, students must understand how the disease affects behavior (Lesson 2) before they can effectively learn communication skills (Lesson 6).

We recommend that you teach the material in the order in which it is presented. Do not skip directly to lessons about areas in which you are having trouble or use these as in-services if you have not taught the introductory course. For example, many programs see their biggest need to be managing behavioral symptoms. If you skip directly to Lesson 11, your students will not have the skills to understand the material. Management of behavioral symptoms is discussed in every lesson, so by the time you reach Lesson 11, your students will already be skilled in managing behavioral symptoms.

Part Three (Chapters IV through VI) provides additional information about evaluating the training, making charting effective, and using assessment instruments in clinical care.

Exhibit I.5. Contents of the Core Course

The core course includes all the material in the introductory course plus additional sections from all 12 lessons. You may teach the introductory course first and add sections from the core course later.

Lesson 1. Helping the Person by Understanding the Problem
- Section 1.1. The Voice of the Person with Dementia: required
- Section 1.2. Establishing Student Goals: optional
- Section 1.3. Recognizing Terms and Differences: required

Lesson 2. Helping the Person by Understanding How the Brain Affects Behavior
- Section 2.1. Understanding the Role of Brain Damage: required
- Section 2.2. Recognizing the Capacities That People with Dementia Commonly Retain: required
- Section 2.3. The Interplay of Personality, Life Experience, and Cognitive Losses: use a few examples
- Section 2.4. Abilities Commonly Impaired in Dementia: required, use only some items

Lesson 3. Facilitating Function by Treating Excess Disability
- Section 3.1.The Importance of Treating Excess Disability: required
- Section 3.2. Illness, Pain, Reactions to Medication, Sensory Deficits, and Dizziness: required
- Section 3.3. Factors That Influence Excess Disability in People with Dementia: required

Lesson 4. Facilitating Function by Treating Stress
- Section 4.1. The Role of Stress in Behavioral Symptoms: required
- Section 4.2. Alleviating Symptoms of Stress: required
- Section 4.3. Responding to a Catastrophic Reaction: required
- Section 4.4. The Need for Stimulation and the Difference between Stress and Stimulation: required

Lesson 5. Applying Skills in Activities of Daily Living
- Section 5.1. The Importance of Individualized Care and the Application of New Knowledge: required
- Section 5.2. Implementing What You Have Learned about Activities of Daily Living: required
- Section 5.3. Using Individualized, Social, and Emotional Contexts of Care: use for suggestions

Lesson 6. Helping the Person by Enriching Communication
- Section 6.1. Verbal and Nonverbal Communication: required
- Section 6.2. Avoiding Patronizing Behavior: required

Lesson 7. Helping the Person by Sustaining Relationships
- Section 7.1. Family Relationships: optional
- Section 7.2. Friendships with Staff Members: optional
- Section 7.3. Friendships between People with Dementia: optional

Lesson 8. Caring for the Person by Meeting Emotional Needs
- Section 8.1. Emotional Needs: optional
- Section 8.2. The Changing Profiles as Impairment Increases: optional

Lesson 9. Helping the Person by Addressing Mood
- Section 9.1. Helping People Who Are Depressed: required

Lesson 10. Restoring Enjoyment through Activities
- Section 10.1. Making Your Program Work Better: required

Lesson 11. Thinking Through Challenging Behaviors
- Section 11.1. Facts about Behavioral Symptoms in Dementia: optional
- Section 11.2. Strategies for Intervention: required
- Section 11.3. Addressing Wandering: required

Lesson 12. A Plan and a Celebration
- Section 12.1. Making a Plan: required
- Section 12.2. Celebrating New Skills: required

Exhibit I.6. Sections for Special Groups

Individuals using these sections must also read or participate in the core course, including the optional sections.

Lesson 1. Helping the Person by Understanding the Problem
- Section 1.4. Information about Diagnosis and Evaluation
  - People responsible for diagnosis, assessment, referral, and treatment

Lesson 3. Facilitating Function by Treating Excess Disability
- Section 3.4. Information about Excess Disability and Delirium
  - People responsible for diagnosis, assessment, referral, and treatment

Lesson 5. Applying Skills in Activities of Daily Living
- Section 5.4. Suggested Interventions for Specific Activities of Daily Living
  - People responsible for diagnosis, assessment, referral, and treatment

Lesson 6. Helping the Person by Enriching Communication
- Section 6.3. Information about Assessing Communication
  - People responsible for diagnosis, assessment, referral, and treatment

Lesson 9. Helping the Person by Addressing Mood
- Entire lesson, including Section 9.2. Information about Depression and Other Psychiatric Symptoms
  - People responsible for diagnosis, assessment, referral, and treatment

Lesson 10. Restoring Enjoyment through Activities
- Section 10.1. Making Your Program Work Better
  - Core course: required, activity directors
- Section 10.2. Activities and Ideas
  - Activity staff

Lesson 11. Thinking Through Challenging Behaviors
- Section 11.1. Facts about Behavioral Symptoms in Dementia
  - People responsible for diagnosis, assessment, referral, and treatment
  - Administration and policy staff, recommended
- Section 11.4. Information about Sexual Behaviors
  - People responsible for diagnosis, assessment, referral, and treatment
- Section 11.5. Behavioral Symptoms in the Acute Care Setting
  - Staff in acute care settings

Chapter IV. Evaluating Your Training	Evaluation is important for both the program and the staff to determine whether their investment of time and effort has been useful. Several approaches to evaluation are discussed.
Chapter V. Making the Best Use of Charting and Information-Based Systems	If new skills are to be implemented in the workplace, information about client status must be transferred efficiently. Several approaches are discussed.
Chapter VI. Using Assessment Instruments	Step-by-step techniques for interviewing clients and for conducting the Mini-Mental State Examination (MMSE) are discussed. Use of the MMSE as an estimate of the client's spared and impaired functions in daily life is discussed. A brief discussion of staging instruments and the Minimum Data Set are included.

The Organization of the Lessons

The text for the lessons is long and potentially confusing. We outline here the organization of the lessons and how to use that organization effectively. Once you understand this, you will find that using the material is simple.

Much of the material in the lessons is presented in short, one- or two-sentence paragraphs, similar to a bulleted list. These are *notes,* not a complete lecture. They are brief ideas that you will want to expand on. Use this material as an outline and put the lecture or discussion into your own words. This material expands on the text of the overheads/handouts.

Use items 1–6 to plan and organize your lesson. This material is for the teacher's use only.

1. Lesson and Section Summaries	A quick glance at these tells you what the lesson and each section are about.
2. Using the Sections	These lines identify the sections for introductory course, core course, and special audiences.
3. Problems You May Have in Implementing This Lesson	In the best of all worlds, this section would not be needed. In reality, resources may not be available, the staff may not be ready for the material, and so on. It is important that educators be aware of possible obstacles to teaching so that they can modify their approach accordingly.
4. Objective	Every section lists the objective of the section. Use this statement of objectives when you apply for course credit or Continuing Education Units.
5. Background	Many sections provide background information for the educator. This information will not be taught to direct care providers.
6. Information and Instructions for the Teacher	Every section provides suggestions for how to use the material. Part of this is presented at the beginning of the lesson, and additional suggestions are inserted in the body of the lesson. This includes ideas such as when to use discussion, what questions you might ask, and how to help the student identify with the issue.

Present items 7–10 to your students. These include lecture, discussion, ways to help the clients, clinical experiences, and overheads/handouts.

7. Lecture/Discussion Notes to Be Presented to the Class	This is the information you provide to the class. It identifies the points at which overheads/handouts are to be used and discusses each one. It includes lecture notes and suggestions for discussion. It is most effectively used when you present it in your own words rather than reading the text to your class.
8. Exercises	The exercises will help your students think through the material you are teaching. Using them reinforces new learning. Exercises help to break up long stretches of lecture. Many of the exercises are discussions that help the students plan how they will implement care.
9. How We Help	This describes specific interventions direct care providers can apply to the issues discussed.
10. Clinical Experience	Most sections provide directions for a clinical experience. If the student is to transfer learning to the workplace, trying ideas in a clinical setting is essential. Instructions for the clinical experience component are on pp. 27–29.
11. Overheads/ Handouts	Instructions for the use of these are on p. 25.

Exhibit I.7. Setting the Goals of the Training

Why Set Goals?

1. Goals define the course and clarify what will and will not be done. This is important for marketing and to share with families.
2. The provider will not want to waste money on training unless it is clear that the training goals are goals of the provider agency.
3. Goals tell students what to expect from the course.
4. When varied parties have an interest in outcome, stated goals reduce the risk of dissatisfaction over the outcome or of sabotage. Participating in the drafting of goals gives invested parties an opportunity for input and compromise.
5. Goals tell the staff members who will not be trained what is going on and where they stand.
6. Goals are used to evaluate the outcome of the training.

How to Set Goals

Well-thought-out goals will lead you step by step through the rest of the planning, whereas vague goals prove a hindrance. Taking the time to plan goals usually results in satisfaction at the end.

1. Involve all affected parties in goal setting: management, department heads, and others who will be asked to support training.
2. Consider the full range of goals: patient quality of life, staff satisfaction, consumer satisfaction, regulation, marketing, profit, and so on. Write them down. When you have completed your plan for the course, review it to confirm that it will achieve these goals.
3. Be specific but allow flexibility. Avoid goals that are too general (everybody will know more about Alzheimer disease) or too rigid (27 of our 50 residents will stop waking at night).
4. Set both long-term and short-term goals for easy as well as more difficult goals. This allows successes and limits discouragement.
5. Review your goals often as you plan your course. Make sure your plan will deliver.
6. Be realistic. At this point, your goal making is confidential.

In the first lesson an optional exercise asks students to state their own goals for the course. You have the option of sharing management goals with them. This give-and-take helps the student know what is expected and feel that she will accomplish things that she values in the classroom.

Defining Your Needs

Begin by answering the following questions. Involve administrators and others who have an investment in the training.

1. How does this training fit with your mission and philosophy?
2. What are your primary goals in offering this course at this time? (See Exhibit I.7.)
3. What support can the administration offer? Budget, time, and space are the most important factors, but there are many other ways in which the administration lends support to (or ignores) a program. Can relief staff members be employed? Will students be paid while in the classroom? Are there time and money for the teacher's planning and teaching?
4. What management support is available for applying learning in the work setting? Staff members must be encouraged to apply what they learn in their daily work. Often this calls for changes in procedures and scheduling.
5. Whom do you want to train first? in subsequent classes? (See Exhibit I.8.)
6. What skills/interests does your target group of students have? What are their weaknesses?

Exhibit I.8. Selecting the Right People to Train

The primary audience for this book is the people who provide the direct care for persons with dementia and their supervisors: certified nursing assistants (CNAs), nurses, social workers, activity directors, physical and occupational therapists. Other audiences include college students, planners, educators, and others who work in fields related to the care of persons with dementia.

For training to be effective, both supervisors and staff must be trained. The supervisor must be able to facilitate the transfer of skills from the classroom to the workplace and not unwittingly impede this. When supervisors are trained and care staff members are not, care staff will lack skills in immediate problem solving. Care staff may resist change, and practical application of hands-on skills may be lost.

Teach supervisors and direct care staff together. People who work together must learn together and solve the problems of the real world together. Prior background is not as important to the learner as a shared perspective on care.

The interactive format allows the more sophisticated learner to move at his own pace. Advanced material is provided as well. Jargon terms are avoided, and the text is written in a clear, straightforward style that is accessible to anyone. Your program will benefit if administration, management, supervisors, direct care staff, and non–direct care staff (such as maintenance and housekeeping) receive some training. The introductory course will be useful for training these groups.

What Percentage of the Direct Care Staff Should Be Trained?

When a small group of direct care providers are trained and then return to the job, their new skills can be overwhelmed if their colleagues take the position that "this is how we have always done it." (The opposite, that the newly trained will teach their colleagues, rarely works.)

One-half to two-thirds of direct care staff will need to be fully trained in order to sustain significant change, yet many programs will find that it is not possible to train all staff members at once. There are many ways to bridge this, and each strategy has strengths and weaknesses.

1. The introductory course helps staff members who did not receive the full training.
2. Train all supervisors and as many care providers as possible.
3. Train a few staff members, and follow up by training everybody in small groups over time.
4. Avoid increasing group size, using only short courses, or skipping around through the material.

Whatever training you can afford and implement will have a positive impact on care. Plan for turnover: new people will need the training. Focus management's attention on strategies to retain staff members as well.

Note matters such as "already knowledgeable" or "resistant."

7. How many people will you teach at one time? (See Exhibit I.9.)
8. How many classroom hours can you commit to this now? in the future? when? (See Exhibit I.10.)
9. Who will teach this course? What skills/interests does the instructor have?
10. You will find yourself facing trade-offs as you plan: budget versus number of people to be trained; space and time versus in-depth training, and so on. The exhibits are designed to help you consider the pros and cons of these decisions.

Planning the Course Content

You are now ready to select the materials to teach in your course. Identify the sections that you will need to provide the course content. List your final selection of materials. Use Exhibit I.11 to record the groups

Exhibit I.9. Planning the Class Size

Will you train everyone in a dementia program at once, or will you train only some? To obtain the greatest impact, how many staff members should you train?

There is a close relationship between the amount of new learning applied in the workplace and the group size and course length. Students learn more and implement more of what they learn when taught in small groups. (This finding is so dramatic and universal that it leads to major political battles over the size of classrooms in the public schools. It is equally relevant in training staff members.)

The group size determines the teaching methods you will be able to use, and these, in turn, determine the amount and kind of learning possible.

Small-group teaching methods (discussion, asking questions, testing new ideas, role playing, feedback, case examples, team learning) allow the student to internalize new knowledge rapidly. Small groups allow the students to find solutions that will work in their situation.

Groups of about 15 are most successful in dementia training. As the group size increases, the time for each person to participate in discussion, exercises, and review is reduced. Also, as the group size increases, the instructor is increasingly limited to lecture, video, and written materials—nonparticipatory methods that do not encourage staff members to assimilate what they are learning.

Larger groups reach more people at less cost. The trade-off is less new knowledge put into action. Large groups are an excellent way to introduce new directions and to get everyone excited and interested. They are also useful as a means of letting non–direct care staff members know what is going on or to expose everyone to a dynamic speaker.

Although college students are trained in large groups and professionals may be accustomed to learning in this way, they, too, will benefit from small groups when skills and problem solving are emphasized.

You must decide on your group size before planning your course because size influences teaching methods. Factors such as release time and room size, though important, should not drive your decision. Determine what kind of learning you want to achieve and work from there. Once you have set a group size, do not agree to "slip in just one more." In groups of 20 or fewer, each additional person has an impact on learning.

you will be training, the class size, and the course length.

Perhaps your students have already had training in some areas. Your students' care skills will improve most if you teach the material again from this book. The book asks the student to apply new knowledge in ways that are realistic in the setting, and therefore caregiving methods can be taught best by consistent use of these materials. Encourage students to discuss what they already know and put it in the framework of these materials. This reinforces their knowledge. For the same reason, do not add materials from other courses. The object is to teach well, not to teach everything.

The teacher may be tempted to skip some of the exercises that are time consuming and that require small groups and to teach more facts instead. But discussion, clinical experience, and other small-group techniques allow the student to try new approaches. Students are encouraged to try an intervention with one person for a short period. Without this component, staff members who feel under pressure will revert to old habits.

Using the Material in Different Settings

The materials can be used by home care staff, day care staff, residential care staff, college students, policy makers, nursing home staff, acute care staff, or other audiences. Examples and case examples are set in different environments. In most cases, you will need to do little more than change the words for different audiences. Exercises ask students to figure out how to apply new learning in their particular situation.

Exhibit I.10. Planning the Course Length

The relationship between the amount of learning that occurs and course length is based not on the amount of information presented to the student but on the process of change that must mature within the student. There is no alternative to allowing time for that process to take place. This manual allows you to select a course length that meets your needs, budget, and goals.

Course Length	Goals	Comments
2–4 hours	Get people excited. Inform people about a longer course. Teach a few basics. Promote your program.	Will result in minimal change in caregiving.
6–12 hours	Provide a core set of tools for already knowledgeable professionals. Train staff members who will not receive full training. Train housekeeping, grounds, maintenance staffs, some clergy, volunteers.	A good start, but will not result in major, lasting behavioral changes.
14–20 hours	Provide solid, basic training. Supplement with in-service training.	A good compromise.
24–30 hours	Effectively enables the staff to provide better and more efficient care with improved patient outcomes.	Allow more time if problems arise.

Exhibit I.11. Worksheet: Determine Whom You Will Teach and Establish the Group Size

Group to Be Trained	Class Size	Course Length	Topics	Follow-up
First group				
Second group				

Exhibit I.12. Worksheet: Selecting the Course Site and Class Times

Site Check-off List

Can the students hear and see you?
Is there plenty of space for you to walk around?
Is audiovisual equipment available? Does it work?
Is the room temperature comfortable? Discomfort limits learning.
Must people listen over background noise?
Can you control interruptions?
Are the chairs comfortable?
Is there a table for students to write on? for supplies?
Is the room bright, well lit, without glare?
Are there toilets nearby?
What snacks will you be serving? Where are they?

Class Time Check-off List

Is the space available?
Will students be rested at this time?
Is transportation available for students at appropriate times?
Are your times consistent?
Check for conflicting holidays, festivals, exams.

You may be teaching people from different settings. You can handle these in the same classroom, although having many people from different settings limits team building.

Scheduling Class Time and Selecting a Site

As long as you plan in hour-long blocks, you can arrange the classes to suit the needs of your program: from 4 six-hour days in succession to 24 one-hour sessions once a month or anything in between. Never teach more than six hours at a time; for long sessions, use team teaching and vary the methods.

If you teach your groups more than one section of material at a time, assign clinical experience for only one section.

Consider planning different blocks of time. You may begin with a twelve-hour intensive and then offer the remaining materials as one-hour in-service sessions. Or you may follow up with a six-hour, weekend intensive course. Avoid splitting two closely related topics by a long time period.

Will this class schedule fit into staff work schedules and release time? Programs often schedule classes to follow the end of the first shift so that students from both first and second shifts can attend. The first shift will be tired. Avoid teaching right after lunch, when people are drowsy. Never schedule class to coincide with the staff's free time; this builds resentment. Be sure that you have a strong system to cover while staff members are in class. A guaranteed way to reduce learning is to call a staff member out or have someone interrupt the class to ask how to do something.

Use Exhibit I.12 to select a course site and schedule class times.

Write your teaching calendar on Exhibit I.13, and check to see that it is consistent. This creates the course schedule, which you will post. Students must know their schedule well in advance. This will reduce complaints that they "can't make" a class.

Preparing a Learning Environment

The classroom itself can have a major impact on whether people learn. You have probably had the experience of sitting on an uncomfortable chair in a stuffy, poorly lit room watching cluttered slides and trying to hear a lecturer who mutters. Yet when it comes time to prepare our own classroom, we often

Exhibit I.13. Worksheet: Course Plan

Date, Day, Time	Topic	Place, Room Number

(If not the usual day and time, note this clearly.)
Post this schedule at least two weeks before the first class, include it in the first class handouts, and discuss it, at least briefly, in the first class.

cut corners and figure that "it will do." Comfort is not a luxury: it pays back in additional learning. Comfort does not put people to sleep: stuffy, crowded, and poorly lit rooms put people to sleep. There is an old saying that "the mind can absorb only what the seat can endure." Discomfort and poor environments waste money and class time.

Check your classroom and equipment before each class. Be sure you know how to operate all equipment before you start.

Do not permit interruptions in your classroom. Discuss in advance with management the financial cost of time wasted on interruptions. Every time your group is interrupted, time is lost getting the discussion or ideas back on track. Interruptions are particularly costly because they prevent you from building teamwork. If you must carry a beeper or cell phone, switch it off or to vibrate during the class.

Making Final Preparations

Draft certificates and apply for continuing education credits. Use the course plan you have just developed and the objectives for each chapter you will be teaching. Plan other reward systems that you will offer.

Plan promotional and marketing material. Be sure to emphasize the quality of staff training in marketing your program.

Review your first class to be sure that you have developed all the materials you will need.

Terms Used in This Book

Student and *staff member* are used interchangeably to refer to those participating in the course. When the text refers to those not participating in the course, it states this.

Direct care staff refers to all staff members who provide direct care to people with dementia. This is often nursing assistants, but nurses and others also provide direct care.

Group care refers to all settings in which groups of people with dementia are served. This includes day care, nursing homes, residential care, and boarding care.

Person with dementia is used instead of a "demented person," just as we would not refer to a "cancered person." Those who have an illness are people first; their diagnosis comes second.

Clients refers to people with dementia.

CHAPTER II

TEACHING TECHNIQUES THAT WORK

Kahlil Gibran ([1923] 1970, p. 56) describes the philosophy of teaching we use in this manual: "The teacher . . . gives not of his wisdom but rather of his faith and his lovingness. If he is indeed wise, he does not bid you enter the house of his wisdom, but rather leads you to the threshold of your own mind."

Few rewards are as wonderful as helping people learn new material and become excited about it. The techniques outlined here will help you to do that. Because so many options are available to teachers, you can fit your strategy to the content you plan to teach and to the needs of the students. Have fun!

Rethinking the Learning Process

What is learning all about? What makes people learn? Are certain approaches more successful than others in helping people to learn? Are facts and skills taught in different ways?

This chapter answers these questions for you and ensures that your students learn as much as possible in the time they will be in the classroom.

This training material makes a distinction between learning facts (e.g., Alzheimer's is a disease) and changing behaviors, which results in more successful care. The methods described below are designed to help you help the student translate fact into behavior change.

It is sometimes said that students don't want to learn or don't have much learning capacity. Most adults will learn if the teacher can hit on the right motivation and teaching skills. Think of teaching as a sales job: your goal is to sell these ideas to whatever customers you get. When you teach as if you are sharing with others something you passionately believe in, people will want to buy it.

Teaching in itself is a skill. Specialists in human behavior and education have designed good teaching practices that will increase the amount of material your students use. This applied learning (behavior change) is more difficult to achieve than simply getting students to memorize new material and pass a test on it. We may tell a student to approach people with respect, or we may show films on how to calm down a resistant person, but will your students actually successfully *use* this information? You may have already observed that telling staff members to do these things, even telling them why they must do these things, may have minimal effect. The object of this course is to motivate the student to "buy into" these concepts so that the student spontaneously begins to implement them and thinks they are important.

Most people can remember large, stuffy classrooms in which the teacher droned on tiresomely. Nurses often report horror stories of clinical training in which the nurse educator belittled and berated the students. If a student learns anything under these circumstances, it is to the student's credit, not the teacher's. The adult learners in your classroom will learn so little under such circumstances that it is probably not worth the time to teach. Nevertheless, teachers often fall back on these role models for want of better ones. This chapter will show you how to avoid the pitfalls of this kind of teaching.

Do not permit interruptions, and never take your own beeper into the classroom. Teaching is hard work: you cannot do it well with distractions. It is often difficult to eliminate distractions. Talk with management about the cost of distractions before the course begins. Take care of yourself. Your fatigue will be apparent to your class and makes students less excited about what they are learning.

Instead of leaving during breaks, circulate among your group. This gives people a chance to ask questions they are hesitant to ask in the classroom. You may hear concerns about implementing learning. Of course, you will also hear about personal concerns not relevant to the course and about the doings of certain soap opera characters.

Never replace classes with staff meetings. Do not "pull" a staff member from class. Plan staff schedules and coverage so that the staff can reliably attend the courses.

Stay on time. Do not hold people after class even if they want to stay. This works once but gradually becomes a burden.

Provide breaks and food frequently. Adult learners often lack practice in sitting for long periods. A stretch break will pay for itself. A snack provides calories for learning. A full bladder prevents learning.

Selecting the Right Teacher

One person may carry the full teaching load, or two teachers may teach it as a team. Using more than one instructor reduces the burden by dividing up the tasks of teaching. Students' attention tends to drift if they listen to one person too long. Teams break this up. One teacher may prefer certain teaching techniques such as leading discussions, and another may have special professional skills. However, team teachers must plan materials together, work well together, and discuss each class immediately after the class to avoid repetition or discontinuity.

A good teacher doesn't need to be an expert in dementia; nor does she need prior teaching skills—liking or wanting to teach helps. Attributes of a good teacher include the following:

1. Has time to prepare for classes and can teach without being interrupted.
2. Likes the people she teaches. Showing respect and courtesy toward your students models the respect and courtesy you expect them to show to their clients.
3. Is trusted by the students. Ideally, learning is an open environment, but in reality it rarely is. You may supervise the people you are teaching or be in a position to report or discipline them. Students may fear that what they say or do in the classroom will affect performance reviews or workplace attitudes.
4. Has experience doing direct care. To teach others practical problem solving, you must have experienced the demands of caring for angry, distressed, and confused people, and you must have actually done activities of daily living (ADLs: eating, dressing, bathing, toileting, and walking) you now will teach. In addition, direct care providers are much more willing to learn from people who have worked "in the trenches."
5. Likes to care for people with dementia. Your enthusiasm is critical to successful learning.
6. Is willing to look at things in a new way and to reexamine past learning in light of new information.
7. Is often flexible and organized and has minimal tendency to be controlling.

Time Involved in Preparation

You can teach this material with very little preparation time. It was designed so that novice teachers who know little about dementia care may use it. However, learning will be greater if you invest time in making this course your own. Many experienced teachers estimate preparation time to be equal to classroom time. Preparation includes the following tasks:

Necessary:

- Reading through the entire course
- Using Chapter I to plan the course; selecting the units you will teach
- Selecting the materials within the units
- Reviewing the training materials, goals, and the course plan with management
- Familiarizing yourself with your teaching materials
- Selecting your students; arranging coverage
- Selecting your teaching methods
- Final review with management
- Photocopying materials; making overheads from provided materials

- Setting up the classroom; gathering equipment
- Arranging for the certificates
- Planning and posting a class schedule
- Letting all supervisors know about the course and who will be taking it

Optional:
- Modifying teaching materials to suit your needs
- Rehearsing teaching techniques
- Providing time for clinical hands-on teaching
- Providing one-to-one teaching if a student has a special need
- Purchasing student notebooks (a loose-leaf binder in which each student will keep materials)
- Making posters announcing the course

Teaching Methods

This section lists many different teaching methods. Some are the traditional: didactic lecture, video, and written materials; others are active learning techniques such as discussion and role play. Use a variety of teaching methods: some people will learn by listening, others by seeing, still others by doing. Try to balance both didactic and experiential methods in each class. The individual lessons do not specify which of the experiential techniques should be used. Select those you are comfortable with and you think your class will respond to.

Even shy students and adults who have never done experiential learning before will participate. The secret is that everyone must trust that *nobody can make a fool of herself in the classroom.* You may all laugh together, but nobody will ever be laughed at, no matter how big a mistake she makes. Let people become comfortable with the discussion format and then lead them gently into other methods.

Some of these techniques may be new to you. Practice in front of a mirror or with the video camera if you need to. Students rarely notice when their teachers flub.

Sometimes you may try an approach and have the class not respond. Sometimes even the best teaching approaches will flop, even in the hands of the best teachers. Have something (a lecture, video?) in mind for a backup.

The Student Must Know What Is Expected

The first step in successful teaching is to let the students know what they will learn, why they are learning it, and what the learning ground rules are. Post this information, and go over it in class.

In Chapter I you identified the program goals for the course, and in Lesson 1 you will identify, with your students, the goals for their course.

Because each lesson builds on what is learned in the previous lesson and because the course is designed to teach people to learn and think as a team, you must enforce a few rules. The rules apply to management and supervisors as well as nonprofessionals. (When supervisors "drop in when they can" or rush out when their beeper sounds, they disrupt discussions and distract from the learning process. They also convey the message that they do not think the course is all that important, and this discourages the students who may find themselves having to make major adjustments to find time for the course.)

1. Everyone who commits to the course should be present in the classroom at all times and attend every session. You must clearly define an attendance policy and state it at the first class. Post it or hand it out as well so there are no misunderstandings, for example:
   a. legitimate absences may be made up in another section of the same course, although this disrupts the teamwork method; or
   b. the student may be permitted to read the teaching materials you use, plus do extra credit if he or she is able to learn this way; or
   c. you may hold a one-to-one makeup session with the student.
2. People in the classroom must participate. There are no audits, drop-ins, or watchers. Of course, you will not pressure shy students to speak up, but this is different from people who drop in to observe.
3. Students in the classroom may not be doing something else (charting, talking to each other). Friends, children, and other nonstudents should be banned from the classroom. Decide in advance what to do when someone calls and says her sitter is sick and can she

bring her three-year-old. Provide frequent breaks to avoid bathroom trippers.

4. Clearly define and discuss the issue of freedom of speech in the classroom. If a student makes negative statements about management or a person with dementia, to what extent will this affect performance evaluations or job security? Be sure that the position you adopt will be supported by management and all supervisors. For example, what happens if the students come to class with information about a serious breach of regulations?
5. Define what the program will do for the student: for instance, certificates, extra credit rewards, paid time in the classroom, or free lunch. Be as generous as possible. These things are cheap in comparison with the improved learning they buy.

Privacy Issues

This course asks the members of the class to discuss ways to help clients known to them. Discussing real clients is important for many reasons; most important, it enables the students to test ideas and learn from experience. It also raises issues of client privacy. No matter how impaired clients are, they and their families are entitled to privacy. The Health Insurance Portability and Accountability Act of 1996 (HIPAA) establishes privacy standards. There are several ways to ensure appropriate client privacy:

1. You may choose to inform family members and clients that a course is being taught that will benefit the clients. Ask them to sign a limited release that grants permission to discuss individuals in the classroom. Family members are usually eager to support training. However, occasionally a legal representative or a client is not comfortable with this. Assure them that this person will not be discussed.
2. When all members of the class and the teacher work in the same facility, discussion of clients is acceptable.
3. If the teacher does not work in the facility in which she is training, she must have a *business agreement* with the facility.
4. When the teacher or class members do not all work in the same facility, refer to a real client by a pseudonym or as "this client," and do not reveal characteristics that would identify the person to others if you have not received a release from the responsible person.

Staff members are also entitled to privacy. Their behavior or ideas should not be discussed outside the classroom or with supervisors without their permission.

If you choose to videotape staff or clients for training purposes, you will need to obtain releases from both.

Lessons from George

George is a resident in a residential care home whose care taught many things about being a teacher.

George had apparently been a somewhat difficult person all his life. He was grumpy and not very social and sometimes drank heavily. When he developed a dementia, he presented serious problems for the staff members caring for him. He refused to bathe, became combative, insulted the other residents (particularly the women), and sneaked out twice and got drunk.

Almost as soon as the class began, the staff members raised their concerns about George. The teacher offered various suggestions, but none was helpful. A session or two later, George came up again, and the teacher asked the other students (from other facilities) what they would do. Next time George came up, the teacher asked the class members to use their newly learned care skills to solve the problem. But nothing worked, and she began devoutly to wish George would vanish.

Like most teachers, this one liked to appear to know what she was doing, and George was showing her up badly. She spent the rest of the class reexamining her teaching skills, and George continued to be a problem no one could solve.

Eight weeks after the course ended, the teacher visited this facility to evaluate the success of the training. "Remember George?" the staff members asked.

She groaned inwardly.

"He's the nicest man. And he doesn't do any of those things!" The teacher asked what they had done. The answer was *many small things*, some of which had been suggested in class, some of which the staff members had worked out for themselves.

The first thing George teaches is that this training system works. Instead of teaching staff members many different interventions to try, the staff members learned to change themselves, to observe George closely as an individual, and to select among a repertoire of interventions. The specific interventions used with George may not be replicated, but the process used to achieve results can be.

The second lesson George taught is that it is all right for the teacher to not have the answers. (This is a good thing because, in a discipline as challenging as dementia care, no teacher ever will have all the answers.) The learning process is a joint effort between the students and the teacher. Students are adults with a wealth of experience and ideas.

The class spent a lot of time on trial and error with this case. Let students know that trial and error is necessary. It is unlikely that anyone will hit on the right interventions the first time with a difficult person. Because the teacher didn't know what to do about George, she talked through her thoughts in the classroom. Sharing one's thinking, even when it is not going anywhere, helps the student learn to do the same.

This course empowered the staff who cared for George. When they returned to their facility, they felt they could find some solutions, and they knew they would be permitted to do so. They had been given, and they accepted, ownership of behavior management and life quality for George. This was a big change from their attitude when they came in.

Getting the Most out of Three Old Work Horses

Lecture and visual aids are didactic: the student learns passively. The teacher pours information into the student's eyes and ears and hopes that it sticks. Discussion is active: the student is required to do something.

Lecture

Lecture is the most familiar teaching method. Use it to introduce factual material, which you will reinforce with discussion or other techniques. Avoid depending heavily on lectures, and keep them short.

Lecturing effectively delivers a large quantity of information quickly and is necessary with large groups where discussion is not practical. People not accustomed to listening to lectures may not retain what they hear.

Strengthen lectures by meeting people's eyes, limiting lectures to 20 minutes or less, and using overheads, slides, flip charts, or chalkboards. Make your lecture animated; do not drone on. Be sure your spoken language is simple and well organized. Do not read your lecture. Break the lecture frequently for questions and discussion. Organize your lecture around three steps: (1) tell your groups what you are going to say, (2) make three points, and then (3) tell them what you told them. Move around, use props, tell stories, get close to your students.

This course includes material you will use in lecture form identified as lecture notes and as outlines with key facts.

Overheads/Handouts

Overheads/handouts or slides allow students to follow along as you talk. This provides both verbal and visual information, which reinforces learning. Each lesson contains materials that can be used for overheads, handouts, or slides or any combination of these. Because it is the same material, it is referred to as overhead/handout. Select overheads or slides depending on your equipment. It is easier, faster, and less expensive to make overheads, and you can write directly on them. Use the material identified for overheads/handouts.

Overheads are helpful when the members of your group have so few reading skills that they will not use handouts. Whenever you use an overhead, read it and talk about each point.

You may copy and distribute handouts for any of these materials. Handouts allow the student to take notes on them and to keep the pages for future reference. You may use handouts and overheads of the same material to double the message. Do not give students handouts you will not discuss in class, and avoid overwhelming the student with more handouts than she can digest.

All overheads/handouts are provided in the

lessons, and their use in the class is indicated. If you use handouts, give the students a loose-leaf binder or folder to keep their materials in. Do not expect them to keep track of their materials otherwise.

People do not learn well in a dark room. If they manage to stay awake, they do not concentrate. If you must darken the room, do so briefly and never after lunch.

When you will use the same overhead more than once, make duplicate copies so you do not have to shuffle around looking for the right one.

Discussion

Discussion is an excellent learning tool. However, you may have had experience with rambling, disjointed discussion groups that you felt were a waste of learning time. Leading a discussion successfully is a skill that you can learn.

You must walk a line between discussions that wander out of control and discussions that are so rigid that individuals' ideas are not expressed. You must listen to a discussion you are leading with a third ear, constantly checking: Are we on topic? If not, is what is going on important? Are we on time? If not, is what is being said important? Is everyone participating? What is the tone of this discussion? Is this discussion in line with the goals of this exercise?

Personalizing the material (students' own experiences or things they have observed in the people we care for) helps hold the students' attention.

Stop frequently, not just at the end, for questions. Questions and discussion allow people to fix the material in their minds.

Write down the topic you want to discuss, and list each of the points that you wish to make. These materials will help you do this. Write on your notes the amount of time you plan to spend on the discussion, and make a habit of starting to summarize things about five minutes before that time is up because it's easy to lose track of these things as one focuses on the flow of conversation. Review Chapter III for problems that arise in groups.

Try to avoid multiple conversations going on at once. People can attend to only one of them, and you have lost control of the group. It is best to lay down this ground rule before the first discussion and to remind people when it happens. If this happens often, ask yourself what is happening in the group to cause it. For example, is the group avoiding talking about the real issues, or is everybody this excited about the concepts?

When a discussion drifts, ask yourself whether it has become a bitch session or gossip or is addressing something else that is important. If possible, offer some positive intervention for the topic of bitch sessions: "That is a problem, and we are going to meet with the administrator about it, but right now, we must focus on . . ." Sometimes a topic comes up that is important to the staff and that you know will be addressed in a later session. If you think staff members will be distracted by their concerns and not focus on the current topic, you may choose to address the issue now.

Pay close attention to group interaction and tone. If you hear unspoken frustration, ask if this is the case.

At the end of the discussion, summarize the points that were made on the flip chart. If issues were not covered, tell the group what will be done: you will discuss this again, or you will talk about these issues privately.

Never ignore someone's input. This discourages the person from speaking up next time. Interject, "Louise has a good idea." Or tell the person that you will bring up her idea at the next discussion or will talk to her privately later. Be alert to "Why don't you . . . ?" discussion. Let the group offer a few ideas for someone's problem and then move them on. The answer to "Why don't you . . . ?" is "Because . . ."—and leads to a rehashing of what has already been tried or what won't work. This type of discussion does not force the student to work toward a new solution.

Active Learning Techniques

Active learning techniques make the student work things out for himself. They are highly effective in accomplishing the behavior change you want to achieve, but they are possible only in small groups, and they are more demanding of the teacher than passive approaches.

Role Play

Role play means different things in different contexts. Some people feel uncomfortable doing what they think "role play" is. This course uses a specific and narrowly defined process that helps staff members in training test interventions. In this book role play means walking through situations in a group setting where both the role players and the rest of the group can make constructive observations. The role players and the observers can often think of a different way to accomplish the same thing. By playing the role of people with dementia in a situation, the staff members may also gain a sense of what the person with dementia might feel.

Using these strategies will make role play work in your classroom.

1. Begin by doing much of this yourself.
2. Reassure people who have an embarrassed giggle, but do not allow staff members to use acting as a way to poke fun.
3. Spell out the reasons this tool is important.
4. Make role play a frequent and spontaneous part of your class.
5. Thank people and praise them every time they participate.
6. Always check for feelings.
7. Be calm and matter-of-fact.

The following three examples illustrate some of the many roles for which this versatile tool can be used:

- Ask a student to stand up. Take her by the hand and, walking quickly, tow her around the classroom. Ask her how that treatment made her feel. Ask the group to describe a better way to get a person somewhere. Ask the student to demonstrate a better way to walk with you. Ask how she felt leading you this way. Say how you felt.
- A student describes a person with dementia who clenches his jaws and cannot be fed. Ask another student who knows the same person with dementia to act as the person with dementia, and ask the first student to do what he usually does to feed the person. (Caution them against chipping a tooth.) Stop this after a minute and ask *both* students how they felt or would feel if the situation were real. Ask for group input. Ask two people to role-model the group's suggestions. Ask the group to analyze the situation. Who is standing where? How are they holding the person? Where are they looking? Things they were not aware they were doing may be evident.
- A home care worker reports that she is having trouble getting her confused, apraxic patient into the tiny, old shower. Using a corner and a few notebooks, she creates the "shower." With her role-playing the patient (because she knows this patient's behavior) and another student as nurse and the class as analysts, the group tries different strategies until someone hits on one that will probably work.

Role play may not seem very different from a discussion in which the students ask "Why don't you . . . ?" but it works much better. People don't notice many of the small but important body movements and facial expressions they make until their attention is drawn to them, as in this type of exercise.

Role play is far from a perfect tool. Students will giggle and do things differently than they would in "real life." It is also a time-consuming technique and can be done only with a small group (to avoid embarrassing the student). Still, it is one of the best tools for problem solving and teaching empathy and insight into one's own behavior. Students who become confident of this skill in the shelter of the classroom will continue to use it in clinical care with great benefit to their clients.

Clinical Experience

A primary objective of this course is to show the students that it is possible to implement change in the workplace and to teach them how to do this. Many students feel overwhelmed by the limitations of care, not the least of which is their clients' impairment. Clinical experience is intended to begin to counter this. You may have experienced clinical rotations or practicums in your training and know their value.

Most of the lessons in this text recommend a clinical experience for students. These experiences are simpler and much briefer than clinical experience in professional training. However, they facilitate the transfer of new information to the workplace. They correct the common problem whereby students hear what they were taught but fail to understand how it applies to their tasks. Planning clinical experiences allows the student to try out ideas in a safe environment. Trying out new learning in the clinical setting reinforces learning and determines whether, in fact, what students were taught will work with the people they care for. It also highlights problems in the workplace that will resist transfer of learning. When students are to test new roles with increased flexibility or new responsibilities, a clinical experience provides a low-risk setting. This method of teaching is time consuming and requires the commitment of workplace staff but is the most effective way to ensure that the course pays off in improved skills. Use these guidelines:

- Plans are made by individual students or small groups of students who work in the same setting.
- Planning is closely supervised. When a plan is not realistic, use constructive methods to encourage the student to modify it. Ask for suggestions from others in the group.
- The plan must be one that can be done in the setting, despite existing limitations. Do not let students drift into blaming the doctor, the physical plant, and so on.
- Plans must be simple, require limited time, and involve only one or a few clients. The student should not have to consume extensive outside time or learn independently. Plans should be something the student can easily implement into daily routine care.
- The student should identify the goal of the plan.
- Plans should address quality of life as well as more tangible care.
- Plans should be within the student's skills (for example, an aide may plan to visit with a client as she provides ADL care, but an aide would not plan to make medical diagnoses).
- Plans should have a realistic chance of success. Do not let the students select the most difficult problems or clients; they are not ready for these. Failures in clinical experience will teach the students that nothing can be done. However, when things do not work out as planned, work with the group to identify partial success and to modify the plan.
- Implementation of plans is optional but desirable.
- If the students implement their plans, they must obtain permission from supervisors. Either the teacher or the supervisor must be responsible for oversight. If required by regulators, chart these interventions based on the need of an individual client as a short-term intervention to test its efficacy.
- Implementation should be limited to one or two weeks.
- Students will make errors. Errors are part of the learning process, and students should not experience negative consequences. The client is protected by designing a plan that is within the student's skill level and is supervised.
- Outcomes should be discussed in the classroom and modified and tried again if they do not work at first. The goal is to help the student gain confidence in his ability to solve problems. Spend the first part of each lesson reviewing clinical experiences. Praise people for whatever they accomplished. You want the experience to excite people and encourage them to buy into change because the new techniques work.
- Students may not notice slight changes in clients: point these out. Your goal is to demonstrate that a change, even small things or slight gains, is possible. By the end of the course, students should realize that a sum of small changes benefits both the client and the care provider.
- Allow students to plan and report orally.
- Never use clinical experience to get more work out of an employee. This builds resentment, and little learning will occur. Seek plans that do not add significantly to the student's workload.
- If your students are not working in a clinical setting, try to find some opportunity for them to see a person with dementia, such as visiting a neighbor's grandmother or spending a few hours in a formal clinical setting. If no resource is available, substitute role play and discussion.

Here are some examples of simple student ideas for clinical experience:

a. Ann says there are men outside her window at night. We think she has vision problems and is seeing the bushes moving. We plan to close the curtains before dusk to see if that helps. We'll note whether she complains less about these "men."

b. George pushes us away and becomes agitated when we try to feed him, but he appears to be hungry. We can see broken teeth and sore-looking gums. We told the charge nurse that we thought George's teeth hurt him, but it will be a while before a dentist can see him. We decided to chop his food and have him eat in the little dining room, where it is quieter. We asked the kitchen to prepare some softer foods for him. He doesn't get so angry now during meals, but we can't tell whether he is eating more.
c. One aide was concerned about a man who seemed withdrawn and would not participate in planned activities. Her first plan was to discuss with the unit director whether the man might have an excess disability that affected his involvement. The unit director explained that the man was almost totally blind and therefore doubly disabled. When the class reached Lesson 5, this aide planned to try making dressing a social time, telling him what she was doing as she cared for him. Part of the group objected that this would take too much time, but the plan was tried for a week. It did not take noticeably longer to dress him. He did not respond at first, but by the end of the week he appeared pleased to be with her and tried to join in the conversation.
d. A student nurse working for a one-month rotation on a subacute care unit noticed problems with pain management in people with dementia. For two patients, she developed a more effective plan and taught the aides that by the time people with dementia begin to scream or act out, their pain is often out of control. Medication needs to be given before behavioral symptoms occur.

Using Carrots: Feedback, Rewards, and Extra Credit

Feedback

Feedback is a constant process in education. Students get feedback from your facial expression, their experience in the clinical setting, and other students, as well as more formal feedback such as test results, your comments on their performance, or video. This course asks students to change attitudes and behaviors: clear and frequent feedback is necessary for students to know they are on the right track. Positive feedback is one of the most powerful tools you have to urge students to make change.

Adult students respond much better to positive feedback than to negative feedback. Positive reinforcement (feedback) is stronger in almost all applications. Adults in the workforce often receive only negative feedback or none at all. They learn to tune out negative feedback or deny its validity. Consistent positive feedback works well with such people.

Do everything possible to focus on positive feedback. This does not mean offering effusive praise for shoddy work. Often it means noticing the small ways in which the student is moving in the right direction and saying little about the rest. Suggestions can be phrased constructively, such as "I'm glad you mentioned that. Also there's another approach . . ." or "That was a good idea to try, but because it doesn't seem to be helping, could you try . . . ?"

Occasionally you will be at a loss to find anything good to say about someone's work or comments. If all else fails, ask the class's opinion and let the student learn from her peers.

Instead of praising students effusively, teach yourself to make comments such as "right" or "good thought" often.

Encourage feedback from classmates and teammates. Ask, "What do you think about that?"

This course asks people to speak up in discussion, try new techniques, and explore new ways of thinking. Criticism at this point will be misunderstood as "Open your mouth and you get shot down."

Teach students to obtain feedback from the person with dementia. People with dementia often show flattened affect or apathetic responses. Remind students to notice faint smiles and muttered appreciation. Point out times when problems occur less often after an intervention.

Rewards

Rewards are an important part of learning. Some rewards are intangible: help your students see the small ways in which they are helping the people they care for. The administrator's pride in the course should be evident to the class: this is one exception to interruptions in the classroom—if someone important is getting the tour, point out the industrious students. Posting students' names and having a luncheon for them halfway through the course are other ways to reward them. Plan certificates of completion. Make them nice: many people frame these in their home as a mark of a major achievement. Nice snacks are a good reward—they give people the energy to keep listening.

Paying salary while a person attends the class or increasing salary a certain number of months after the person completes the course is an important reward and a clear statement of the value placed on what the person is doing. The latter helps retain people in whom you have invested training.

Extra Credit

Offering extra credit is a nice way to motivate people to do some independent thinking. Researching information that comes up in class, solving patient care problems, and doing work that is included in the lesson but will not be covered in the classroom are a few examples of activities for extra credit.

Be sure everybody knows what the reward is for extra credit and be generous. This is one way you emphasize the value you place on independent learning. A much loved reward is paid time off (usually by the hour).

At the class's option the entire class can pool extra credits for a group reward: a barbecue, desired improvements in the staff lounge. This teaches teamwork and helps the staff build a bridge with management.

Making It Stick in Their Minds

Case Examples

Case examples are used to translate general information into specific, individual information and to provide an environment that does not involve clients in which to test new skills.

Use case examples that illustrate the current topic to stimulate discussion and encourage students to find their own way to solutions. There may be no easy right or wrong answers to the case given.

Use real cases from the clinical experience of the group in place of the written examples whenever possible. The following guidelines are important when using real cases:

1. Know the full content of these teaching materials well.
2. Use your professional background. Omit concepts that you have been taught that are not congruent with these materials.
3. Know the people under discussion (if possible).
4. Be prepared to admit that you don't have an answer. Many teachers have a deep need to have answers, but there aren't many answers in this field.
5. Encourage the students by explaining that, even if there is no evident solution to the problem they present, care skills do help.
6. Be careful that cases presented by the staff do not become unproductive gripe sessions.
7. Try breaking up your class into small groups to discuss case examples.

When the group is having difficulty with a case example, lead the class step by step back through each lesson, reviewing principles and key points as they apply to the case at hand. Your goal is to teach students to use this orderly review on their own.

The problem with case examples is that when we present one, we single out the clues that are most important. But in clinical care, the student faces a patient with dozens of extraneous "clues." One of the most important skills in problem solving is to sort out the meaningful information from the rest. This is why it is important to use real cases known to you and the students as much as possible.

When students discuss a person with dementia, have them do so with respect. Avoid starting with the most difficult patient, as this can teach defeat.

Humor

Humor is a wonderful teaching tool. Students never forget a point linked to a joke or a vivid image. It breaks tension and builds teamwork. Humor will sustain direct care providers when caring is onerous. It is important to teach caregivers to laugh to release stress and to share the burden dementia creates.

Humor is also an excellent way to communicate with the person with dementia. When they are relaxed and trust the staff, people with dementia often reveal delightful humor. A laugh with the person with dementia may help a staff person accomplish a task as well. A staff person said, "I thought this job would be so sad, but we laugh a lot around here."

However, because of its great power, humor can also be one of the cruelest and most destructive weapons. What you teach and how you model humor is very important. Use humor to reinforce learning, to teach staff members to release their frustrations, but teach the difference between humor that is belittling and humor that is healing.

Try these suggestions:

- Laugh at situations, not people.
- Laugh at the here-and-now situation.
- Laugh at cartoons, published jokes.
- Laugh at yourself and teach your students to laugh at themselves.
- Never laugh at someone else, whether that be a person with dementia, a student, or a colleague.
- Avoid laughing at aging, race, ethnic groups, disability, or dementia.
- Make a point of reading cartoons and save a file of them. Save lots of them. There are books of cartoons in the library. Select your favorite cartoonists.

Role Modeling

Role modeling is not the same as role play. In role modeling, you use yourself as a living example of the tenets you teach. You do this all the time, whether you wish to or not. You role-model in three ways:

1. The way you approach your students. Staff members treat people with dementia in much the same way they are treated. If staff members are treated with respect, they will learn respect; if staff members are valued, they will value others; if staff members are treated with patience and acceptance, they will treat others with acceptance and patience. This principle underlies much of what this book says about management and about teaching methods.
2. Your behavior toward people with dementia. This is probably a more powerful tool than most provided in this book. Take time to listen, meet people's eyes, smile. Review your own behavior. Do you share the lack of grace most of us do: appearing rushed, not wanting to run into certain people, becoming bored with the same old problems? Are you patronizing toward the person with dementia or the staff person?
3. Deliberate modeling of positive interventions. You can better teach many things by doing them yourself. Staff members will not forget how you did something, and you will not need to say more. This allows everybody to "save face."

The instructor observed a nurse trying to give a woman with dementia a glass of orange juice. The woman had a grip on the nurse's arm that held the orange juice and was trying to get a grip on her other arm. Not wanting to make anyone feel bad, the instructor offered to try. The instructor offered the woman an empty mug to hold with her free hand and then gently slipped her finger between the nurse's wrist and the woman's palm. As the woman's grip transferred to the instructor's finger, the nurse gave the juice and the medication that accompanied it. No "how to" discussion was offered, but the staff had learned this trick.

Show and Tell

Tell people and show them how to accomplish what you are asking. Concepts such as dignity, choice, and not rushing people are difficult to implement when staff members are rushed, people with dementia are upset, or rules and family expectations get in the way. Tell staff in training how to implement these ideas, talk about how they might be carried out, and show people how to do things, either with a volunteer student or with a person with dementia.

Try to tell students what *to do* and not what *not to do*. (You will use this same technique with people with dementia.) If you tell a staff member not to put so much food on the spoon, you leave that person to figure out how much is the right amount. If you demonstrate by putting the right amount of food on the spoon, it is easier for the trainee to succeed. And, of course, it does not make the person defensive. (In the classroom it may be all right to ask the group, "How much food do you think should be on the spoon?" but in direct care avoid asking staff members to take a guess and risk being wrong.)

Repetition and Review

People learn best when they are given the same material several times in slightly different ways. Sometimes we are tempted to skip this process to save time, but without repetition people will miss key material.

At the beginning of each lesson, review the previous lesson. Mention any specific issues that came up in the previous class.

If questions were put aside until later, keep a list of them and recall them when you reach the right time to address them.

As the students discuss the issues of each lesson, ask them to review the concepts they learned in earlier classes.

Clearly state the connections between each lesson and those that preceded it.

Use several ways to communicate at once—for example, discussion, handouts, notes on the flip chart. Remind students to look back at handouts from earlier lessons.

Being Available

Good teachers are available to their students. Students may not want to ask a certain question in class; they may be having trouble understanding something and need extra help; they may have wonderful ideas they are too shy to share; there may be no time to discuss certain issues; or the group may be talking about something without bringing it to your attention. Commit yourself to a set period of time when you are available to your students. University students are accustomed to seeking out their professor, but people who are not used to being students may need a more informal way to reach you.

Mingle during the break. Consider this your working time and do not try to do other things.

Stay after class.

Be available, not rushed with something else, for a regular time on the unit.

Invite people into your office to discuss something that concerns them. They may be more comfortable in small groups than individually.

Spend time in the work setting.

Team Learning and Small-Group Work

Change in the clinical setting is best achieved through groups of people learning together. Many successful programs strive to create staff teams that work together, support each other, and solve problems as a group. This course asks students to learn together and to solve problems, work on case examples, and so on as a team. However, not all providers will be ready to relax the hierarchical managerial system or to empower low-level employees to this extent. You must be clear about the environment people will be working in and temper your teaching accordingly. Staff members trained to work as a team will be angered and frustrated by unilateral orders and hierarchical management. If you train only a small proportion of your staff, the rest of the staff may strongly resist the team approach that your students take back with them.

Team Learning

In discussions, homework, and addressing specific problems, ask people who know the same clients to work together. This strong emphasis on teamwork will help even people who have worked together for a long time to build new bonds. It also helps the group members support each other when they return to clinical care.

There are many ways to encourage teamwork:

1. Talk about the team concept. Staff members may not like the idea. Let them air their concerns.
2. Be sure that everybody has an opportunity to share ideas and input.
3. Make teamwork democratic. Discourage higher-ranking individuals from controlling input or decisions; learning to listen is part of everyone's training.

4. Identify individual strengths (e.g., "I am better with men," "I like problem solving").
5. Teach students to approach clients as a team (e.g., "You try, and if that doesn't work, I'll come along and distract him").
6. Teach staff members to share information. They may not do this automatically. For example, if the aide who works every other Sunday knows how to bathe Mary, have her tell, in her own words, what she does.
7. Have everybody learn what everybody else's job is and how others feel about it. This is particularly important for people of different ranks (e.g., "I never knew how hard it is to do this part of direct care" or "I never thought about it, but she is responsible if we make mistakes").
8. Often strong bonds will form among team members. Notice and support these. Find ways to reward them in the workplace.
9. If you train people from different settings, ask them to learn in groups of three or four and work together in small groups. If students do not work in a setting, consider forming stable small groups that will always work together through the course.

Sometimes a facility with a limited budget will want to send one person to a course with the hope that she will videotape or record the class and return to "share" her new knowledge. Probably the worst way to transfer learning is through hours of unedited tapes or the words of one returned staff person. One person in a class has almost no chance of effecting change in her program. Sharing this way may transfer some factual material, but it will not transfer the material needed to change behaviors.

Small-Group Work

Small groups are an excellent tool for team building and teaching people to solve problems. Students may resist teams and small groups because these are unfamiliar. Discuss this if necessary. Small groups without an instructor for each group will not compensate for an overlarge class. People taught this way may just spin their wheels.

If you use small groups, watch your groups closely: never leave the room. Are they staying on topic? Are they coming up with good ideas? Or do they tend to drift, giggle, or gossip? Is not much getting accomplished in the small-group time? To help them stay on track, give small groups clear, fairly narrow discussion tasks. If you have team teachers, each may teach a group, doubling the amount learned.

When groups come back together, list their ideas or decisions. Be sure to keep moving along, so that the last to report are not dumped for lack of time. This sends the message "work hard and you are ignored." Speak positively about contributions and observe and comment on group process.

Your use of small groups will depend, in part, on the size of the class and the ability of your students to work fairly independently. Students can improve this skill in the classroom.

Paper and Pencil

Reading Material

You may ask people to read handouts, texts they take home, quizzes, slides, overheads, and flip charts. Do not expect people who are out of practice with academic learning to learn from independent reading. Read handouts, overheads, and flip charts aloud as you introduce them. Pause in your reading to comment on the text.

This course uses written overheads/handouts to reinforce other teaching methods and to provide a written record the student can refer to.

The References and Resources section at the end of the text lists a number of recommended outside references. The richer your body of knowledge, the more your students will learn. Most libraries can obtain books for you through the interlibrary loan system, or you can access university libraries through the Internet.

Note Taking

Some students learn well by taking notes. Others, often those who are out of practice in the classroom, do not. People can learn very well by listening. Suggest that people write on their handouts, and give them notebooks to keep their handouts in. Remind them that they will be asked to refer to earlier classes as they go along. Do not be offended if nobody writes anything down.

Tests

Tests are important if a student must meet certain licensure or certification requirements. Some instructors think that students pay better attention if they know they will be tested. "Pop" tests are the ultimate example of this. However, it is the teacher's responsibility to keep the student's interest without relying on tests.

Though important, testing has disadvantages. For instance, tests measure factual knowledge, not attitude or behavior change. Because the goal of this training is to change attitude and behavior, tests have limited use. Another consideration is that alternative testing methods must be provided for students who have difficulty reading or for whom English is a second language.

Adult students, in particular, may be so intimidated by the prospect of a test that they do not pay attention to important detail. In addition, teachers or organizations sometimes use tests in a punitive way, or staff members fear that they will—this also limits behavior and attitude change.

An alternative to testing is goal setting. The materials in this book identify goals, ask students to set goals, and use the final unit to design clinical goals. The advantages of goal setting are that it matches performance (accomplishment of a goal) with the current resource levels (student ability, facility resources) and allows evaluation of all areas of interest. The student can evaluate her own improvement; the instructor can evaluate whether the goals of the course were met; and the provider can evaluate the extent to which goals were met.

Helping People Think for Themselves

Positive Reinforcement

A director of nursing observed that her staff did not use effective interventions in coping with aggressive behavior. However, there were occasional successes. When an aide did cope well, the director of nursing made a poster for the bulletin board, naming the aide as the staffer of the week and spelling out what she had done. (Another approach is to have the administrator mention the aide and the incident at a staff meeting.)

Select a method that does not embarrass the staff member. It is not necessary to point out why the intervention worked or to say much about interventions that don't work. Reward alone has a powerful impact. Other staffers will quickly try similar interventions on their own.

Asking Leading Questions

Often students think of an idea that you do not think will work. Avoid telling them that it is a poor idea, but do lead them to think through a better approach. Guide people's thinking rather than telling them what to do. Ask the question in a way that encourages them to think rather than to defend what they did: Say, "I see that you are having trouble with . . . " or "What do you want to accomplish with her?" or "Is there a better (or other) way to do that?"

The Aha! Experience

It is not uncommon for teachers planning this course and their students to work steadily through much of the material and then, quite suddenly, to think, "Oh! Now I get the picture." Look for this and celebrate it in yourself and others. Learning is much more than facts and more than the sum of facts. This aha! experience is the process of internalizing and internally ordering knowledge.

Don't Tell Them the Answer

Telling people the answer is what teachers do. We have handouts and overheads with the right way to do things, the correct answers. But students learn best when they are forced to figure out the answers for themselves. Try giving people all the information they need to solve a problem but let them figure out the answers. For math teachers this is easy: they teach the student how to add and subtract, but the student has to solve the exercise problems for herself. For the person teaching patient care, this technique requires some thought but is worth the effort. Here are some examples of staff members using their new knowledge to find answers:

On one occasion during a power outage, a quick-thinking aide handed the most restless man a flashlight and asked him to help her. He remained calm throughout the crisis. A week later another aide found a way to get the same man through his shower with less distress. The same "staffer of the week" approach was used for these aides who found their own solutions to problems.

The Bugaboo: Documentation

"Document what you did!" "Document why you did it!" "Complete these forms!" "Cover yourself."

In general, care providers would rather provide care than fill out endless forms, but documentation is essential for good communication. See Chapter V for guidelines in helping staff members accept the value of documenting what they do. Forms must be completed, and when staff members try something new, they must justify their actions. When students complain about time spent on documentation, don't lecture them on its necessity. Help them analyze why it is useful. Of course, much paperwork may not be necessary but is required. Talk openly about this. If you ignore the issue, staff frustration can affect care.

Advanced Teaching Tools

This section includes teaching tools beyond those provided earlier. These tools help you teach issues that are emotionally loaded.

- Consider whether your group is ready for these tools. Are they still experiencing the issues discussed above? Are they settled into learning? Do they trust you?
- Consider whether you are ready to deal with these emotionally laden issues. Will you be defensive? uncomfortable?
- Consider enriching the discussions with a co-leader.
- Ensure that you can carry the lesson to closure without interruption.
- Leave enough time to help the group wind down after the exercise.

Videotape: Seeing Is Believing

The exciting thing about video is that it teaches in a new way, but select your videotape carefully: a good video can teach bad things. For example, it can show a nurse gently giving medication while in the background two aides drag away a half-dressed resident. Your staff will learn both concepts. That's not what we want, but that is what we just taught, and that message, not the words spoken, will be the stronger message.

Use videos of staff members at work. Let the students view the raw videotape and comment on what they are doing right and what needs improvement. Replay sections so that the group can analyze closely what went on. Look for body language, patronizing behavior, and the creation of positive experiences for people. *Erase the videotape in the classroom. Never let anyone who is not a full participant in the course see any portion of the video. Never keep a video, no matter what was on it.*

This is by far the best tool for teaching about staff behavior that conveys respect (or a lack of it) or for evaluating how successful staff members are restoring positive feelings in patients. It also allows staff members to pick apart what happened (went wrong) by looking at the film several times. In the rush of the moment, it's hard to pinpoint what we did right or wrong. Let the students do this analysis: this way they are teaching themselves, and you will not fall into the role of critic.

Videotape daily care routines; don't try to film "good" or "bad" staff behavior. Try to film all staff members. Keep the video short, and do not edit it. Three or four minutes of one situation is more than sufficient. Have someone video you interacting with clients. Try a handheld camera and wander around randomly filming interactions between staff and clients. It is not necessary to tape care of people with dementia who are not fully dressed.

Show the film in the classroom. The usual first reaction is horror and giggling about personal appearance, so allow time for that. Reassure your students that video tends to widen images, so those horrible views of staff people bending over are not that bad.

You must obtain written consent from clients or their representatives and from staff. Give family members and staff members a letter stating that the video is to be used for the sole purpose of teaching the staff to treat people with dementia with care and respect. State that the video will be destroyed immediately after use.

Have someone videotape you in a typical activity. The more egalitarian this activity, the more successful it will be.

Never break the agreement of trust: show the video to no one who is not a participant in the class (this includes families and management); never keep the video.

Experiential Exercises

Experiential exercises offer the student the opportunity to imagine how the person with dementia feels. In this regard, they are similar to role play. Such exercises are valuable in helping the student become more sensitive to the realities of life for a person with dementia. However, be cautious when using this tool: students can occasionally turn such exercises into an opportunity to mock the impaired person. Assess your group's readiness before using such exercises, and stop the exercise if it drifts into misuse.

Two exercises are provided below. You may choose to design others to meet the learning needs of your group. Exercise 1 is less demanding of the student and takes less time.

Exercise 1. Experiencing Losses

Teacher: Make three columns on a flip chart, heading them: How would you feel? What would you do? What have you lost? Instruct the group members to close their eyes and imagine themselves in the following situation.

> You wake in a strange room. Some other person is sleeping in here, too. You start to hop out of bed, but your feet don't work right. The bed is wet. You know you didn't wet it, but it does make you wonder. You cannot find the bathroom. You walk up and down, becoming more and more frustrated; there is no bathroom around here anyplace. You decide to get dressed, but your arms and hands won't unfasten snaps, and you can't figure out how to get your clothes over your head. You try it every which way. Eventually a nurse aide comes along and does it for you. She seats you in front of your breakfast, but there is nothing there you want. You tell her so, but you can't make her understand you. Then you sit in the hallway for a long time. They told you what you were waiting for, but you forgot. You'd like to get up, but somehow you don't. Eventually someone comes and gets you. She is kind and gentle, but she is taking your clothes off.

Tell the group that the staff members providing care in this visualization are kind, gentle, and cheerful, and they help you pleasantly.

Ask the group members to open their eyes and think about how being in this situation would make them feel. List all responses in the first column. Responses include anger, frustration, grief, feeling lost. Then ask, "If you felt that way, what would you do?" Answers in the second column may include fight back, try harder to do things myself, and so on. Finally, ask, "If you were in this situation, what qualities would you have lost?" Answers in the third column will address the losses caused by the disease. The disease takes away independence, dignity, mastery, self-esteem, success. Loss of these qualities causes much of the frustration, anger, withdrawal, apathy, and fear exhibited by people with cognitive impairment.

Exercise 2. Experiencing Disability

The object of this exercise is to enable students to experience life as a person with dementia.

Use this as part of most longer courses. It will have a profound effect and is well worth the effort. Allow two hours. Work with no more than 15 students at a time. Prepare carefully in advance.

You will need to know your group well so that you can recognize whether they will be able to respond to the simulations. Some groups are not ready for this exercise.

You will need to have two teachers in the room, and one should have some training in group leadership or mental health. This helps in drawing out students' feelings. Should a student become upset by the exercise, the second leader can take him from the room and debrief him.

Experiential exercises have a potential (but highly unlikely) risk of injuring or emotionally upsetting someone. Explain this to students and obtain releases. Students using devices that restrict freedom of movement must exercise caution. A key role for the two leaders is to steer participants away from risk just as one does with a person with dementia.

Advance Preparation

Create an environment similar to the environment your clients experience. For example, if you use reclining chairs, use one or two in the exercise. If you use restraints, you will restrain one or two students. Arrange for students to sit in chairs at a table or tables.

Ensure that there are no interruptions: these would end the exercise. Make sure that there are no observers who do not participate, and never videotape this exercise. People cannot "get into" the task if they are being observed.

Arrange a group task. The most successful is to have a snack served that will require manipulating a cup and spoon. Custard, ice cream, or Jell-o with coffee or soft drinks works well.

Obtain adult incontinence wear of the type your program uses (or select a mixture of full absorbent types if students come from different settings). Have enough for all students. Encourage everyone to volunteer to wear the incontinence wear and to keep it on, against the skin, for two hours. Most of the people your students will care for will eventually have to use these products. They are uncomfortable, bulky, and itchy. Thus, wearing them is important for empathy. Plan advance time and more than one changing room for students to put on the incontinence wear.

Use eyeglasses, including some sunglasses. Coat them with Vaseline or hand lotion to simulate visual impairment. Ask most students to volunteer for some simulated visual impairment.

Use a sleep mask or opaque scarf to simulate blindness. Ask for no more than two volunteers.

Use earplugs (available from drug stores) to simulate deafness. Have no more than half the class volunteer.

Use Popsicle sticks and nonallergenic tape or similar device to splint second joints on fingers to simulate joint rigidity. Have most but not all of the group volunteer.

Plastic dry cleaner bags cut crosswise in strips about 10 inches wide can be used as ankle restraints to simulate a shuffling gait. Leave feet at least 14 inches apart. Use with only a few volunteers.

Include physical restraints if you normally use them. Restrain only a few volunteers.

Copy the roles in Exhibit II.1 and cut them into

Exhibit II.1. Possible Roles for Experiencing the Feeling of Dementia

- You feel restless and cannot sit still. Even if you become tired, you still feel too restless to stop moving.
- Drift around the room. Try rummaging in other people's handbags, making irritating noises, or trying bits of food from other people's plates. Imagine how it might feel to be looking for something but you do not know what. You do not understand why people become upset with you.
- Put your head down on the table. Think of a time when you felt very sad, alone, or sick. Do not respond when people approach you. Your sadness makes you feel very alone.
- You cannot understand what anyone else says, and you cannot make them understand you.
- You need help to use the bathroom, but everything you say comes out unclear, and you cannot get anyone to help you.
- Do a repetitive task from your chair like tapping or rocking. Do not stop for more than a minute at a time. This activity will keep you from eating.
- You have a role, but you do not know what it is. (To staff members: Completely ignore this person. Discuss the person in front of her in the third person.)
- You need to leave here right now and go home. You don't want to do this activity; you just want to get home. Focus your mind on a situation that might happen at home that would worry you.

individual slips of paper. You must match roles with the disabilities chosen (for example, do not give a wandering role to a "restrained" student).

Do not overload students. Two devices per student will allow each student some function and a strong sense of disability. Use no more than one role per student. Some students with multiple disabilities will not need a role. Too many handicaps reduce empathy.

The Leader's Role

The two leaders' tasks are to maintain an atmosphere of empathy, ensure safety, and withdraw any student who becomes upset. The co-teachers will act as direct care staff members. There is no need to play the role of the mean nurse; being kind and helpful will still give your students the feeling of disability. You may, however, use routine responses to behaviors (such as saying "Your mother died long ago. You have to stay in the nursing home now" to the person who wants to leave, or saying "Wait until I am finished with this" or ignoring the person who is acting the quiet role of the depressed person). You will need to hand-feed a few people, redirect others, and so on. Two staff members will be very busy.

The Exercise

Once everyone is ready, give instructions.

Tell the group that the exercise is voluntary. However, if a person does not participate, she may not stay in the room.

Explain to the students that the purpose of this exercise is to help them understand how people with dementia may feel. Focus on how being disabled would make the student feel. Explain what each item of the disability equipment simulates. Ask students to really get into this experience. The impact of the experience will be much greater if they use their imagination to enrich the experience.

Remind the students that the two group leaders will play the roles of caregiving staff members. Remind them that items such as restraints and those simulating vision and hearing impairments and arthritis can lead to accidents for them, as for people with dementia. The students must move carefully and do nothing that could cause injury to themselves or someone else.

Everyone should stay in the room. If at any time someone begins to feel anxious or wishes to stop the exercise, tell him to let one of the two leaders know and she will help.

Ask for volunteers for all physical simulations. Have the students assist each other in putting on their devices. Distribute slips of paper with each role. It is not necessary to assign all the roles. Select those most appropriate to the group, and do not overload the students.

Once everyone is ready, tell the students to begin to play their roles. At this point, you will no longer give any instructions or comments but will play your role as the "staff member" guiding and assisting the "clients."

Ending the Exercise

For each group there is a point at which the students begin to tire of their roles. You should be able to sense this change in the group and stop the exercise. Twenty minutes is a long time to carry out a role or to experience "disabilities." Announce that the role play has ended. Have the group members help each other out of their simulations at this point. Do this quickly so that the momentum of discussion is not lost. Have people remain in the room and continue to wear their incontinent garments until the end of the class.

Discussing the Experience

Students usually begin spontaneously to talk about how it felt to be disabled in these ways (often before they have completed removing simulations). Guide them to fully describe their feelings and to relate these to the experience of people with dementia. Encourage insights (for example, "I did not like it when you told me to wait" or "You served me black coffee, which I hate"). One man pointed out that one-size-fits-all incontinence wear is not comfortable for a man. Ask how the group felt about the behaviors of others. (For example, one woman, instructed to be bored, began banging and made others angry.)

Before dismissing the group, directly ask if everyone feels debriefed and comfortable.

CHAPTER III

TEACHING ADULT STUDENTS

Teaching adult students successfully requires a different approach than that used for teaching high school or college students. This chapter looks at both the students themselves and the ways in which we teach.

False Assumptions That Can Get in the Way

Training programs often make some false assumptions about training and about students learning long-term-care skills.

The first false assumption is that if we teach the right information, the quality of care will change. In fact, knowledge of good care does not ensure that good care will be provided. The teaching techniques, the students themselves, and the workplace environment all present obstacles to implementing new learning. To encourage the transfer of new learning into the workplace, this course asks students to identify new practices that they can reasonably implement and to try them in the workplace.

Students must practice good care. Without practice, students will revert to their "old" interventions when the demands on the student are greatest—the very time when new behaviors will be most successful with fragile people with dementia. Clinical practice and review of this experience in the classroom help students find ways to integrate new learning into their current care strategies.

Most students and their supervisors and teachers have never seen the best models of care for people with dementia. They do not know what they are striving for. Students and staff in training may not know which changes in caregiving or in patients' responses are realistic and which are impossible. For example, staff members are often confused about the realistic need for drugs that affect agitated behavior. They have probably heard that such medications should not be used, but their experience is that they cannot manage people without them. The lessons help answer this confusion. It is also important to point out subtle changes in clients as caregivers gradually modify their own behaviors.

The second false assumption is that training is independent of the workplace. The workplace in which the student is trying to implement new learning shapes what is possible and provides feedback about the success or failure of students' efforts. Regulations, client factors, available funding, the physical plant, the attitude of staff members who do not receive the training, the cooperation of noncaregiving support staff, and goals of management all determine how much new learning can be used in the workplace. To address this, exercises must focus on ways to adapt training at the same time that efforts are made to modify the workplace.

A third false assumption is that the students are a blank slate ready to be imprinted with skills and values. In fact, adult students come to the classroom with an established set of values and opinions regarding their work and the care of elderly persons. These values arise out of their culture, their views of themselves, and their experience. Few people give up strongly held beliefs on the basis of a short course. The majority of staff members take pride in their work, and they like the people they care for. From their point of view they are already doing a good job. Teaching in a way that asks students to adopt others' ideas without considering theirs negates their pride in their work and discourages their efforts. Training must begin by recognizing these opinions. The adult learner is often correct, at least in part.

Often she does not have all the facts. For example:

> Staff members were frustrated with the administrator for failing to correct a simple problem. The toilet adjacent to the activity room was out of order. This meant more work for the staff, and some clients could not attend activities. The administrator said that it was too expensive to fix, but the staff knew that one person's husband could fix it cheaply and quickly. What they did not understand were constraints on whom the administrator could hire and which complicated codes had to be met. An open discussion with the administrator helped.

Who Are Long-Term-Care Staff Members?

A growing literature about long-term-care staff members tells how direct care providers view their work, how they go about it, and what they believe about their clients.

Long-term care is physically exhausting and emotionally draining. The pressure to complete nursing and personal care has an effect on the behavior and attitude of all staff members. Staff members spend the day on their feet, on hard floors. Even in well-staffed facilities, they often feel overworked. High on their list of goals are making a living and using time- and energy-saving routines such as limiting long trips down the hall or cleaning up messes. Depending on their personality and their personal goals, people adopt strategies for managing their jobs. For example, some staff members keep their sights set on getting ahead, no matter how difficult this is; others endure and make no waves. Idealistic students may leave the system in frustration. Demoralized and defeated staff members, and those who have learned negative coping styles in destructive work settings, will also emerge in the classroom. While it is unlikely that you will change people's coping styles, it is helpful to recognize them. Target your teaching to use the strengths of each.

Adult students bring with them job-related problems. Long-term-care staff members, most of whom are women, often have experienced toxic management and manipulative, abusive, and unpredictable treatment from supervisors. Many staff members working with people with dementia have been injured by someone with dementia. These injuries are often assumed to be "part of the job," and staff members may be expected to continue working without even a short break to help them to recover emotionally.

It seems reasonable that the people we ask to care for our ill, difficult, and frail elders would receive strong support from management and protection from violence, but this is often not the case. When people become used to violence in the workplace and to toxic management, everyone loses compassion, dignity, humor, and affection. Such workplace situations teach burnout, learned helplessness, resentment, and an unwillingness to take responsibility for improving care.

Adult students bring with them the demands of their home life. Many staff members are responsible for children, dependent siblings, and parents. Many are caregivers themselves. They face the problems of limited funds and low-income neighborhoods. They may be up all night with a sick child, work a full shift, and then come to class. Professional staff members, although somewhat more affluent, still cope with the multiple demands of adulthood. Despite this, some care providers value their job because it takes them away from the problems at home. Unlike their personal situation, they are valued and respected on the job.

Whether or not any of these factors are raised in the classroom, they powerfully affect the learning process. They cannot be ignored or wished away. People cannot learn when they are exhausted, stressed, or angry. What they do take away from the learning situation they will interpret and implement in the light of their life experience.

Adult learners are sensitive to patronizing behavior from management and teachers. They may lack self-esteem or be defensive about "having to go back to school." Patronizing behavior, even when subtle and not intended, is inconsistent with teaching people to observe and to problem-solve. The recognition that one can cope with problematic situations improves self-esteem. You reach these students through the difficult task of devising a classroom experience that challenges them but enables success.

Far from being a disadvantage, the skills learned

in adulthood translate directly into good care, although bringing these out is a challenge to the teacher. Teaching staff members how to cope with a difficult job and outside personal demands allows the educator to role-model both problem solving and compassion. Recognizing and drawing on strengths instead of weaknesses helps better use staff resources. Teaching staff members to work as teams allows them to support each other.

Not all the factors that motivate students are altruistic goals for improved care. Money, getting ahead, getting out, gaining control over one's life, and gaining influence over others are important motivators. So is getting off one's feet and through another day. Training that pretends these goals do not exist can sabotage learning.

One of the most powerful motivators for adult students is the teacher who treats her students as adults and encourages them to find their strengths. Students learn *for* a good teacher.

Students with Diverse Backgrounds and Values

Often direct care staff members come from diverse cultural backgrounds and have different values and ideas. They may disagree with each other or not agree with the approach of Western medicine. View this cultural mix as a strength rather than a problem.

Identify and discuss these differences openly. Do not try to change the student's beliefs. Discuss the ways in which the student's values can help in caregiving. Explain that because (usually) the residents are from a Western culture, we have an obligation to care for them according to their values.

When two or more persons of ethnic minority background are together, they may form cliques or dump extra work on the other group. Usually this needs to be addressed by management. Use a cultural-sensitivity exercise. Ensure that supervisors are not unwittingly expressing biases.

Process or Content

Teaching consists of both process (how you teach, what happens in the classroom, students' input, and the like) and content (what you teach). In this training, process is as important as content. Students will be unable to transfer what they learn into the workplace unless process is effective. Because this is not the way most educators learned in school and because teachers usually are under pressure to deliver a planned amount of factual knowledge in a limited time, teachers may find focusing on process challenging.

Problems in the group are almost certain to emerge at some point. There may be anger and frustration at being taught things the students do not think they can implement; resentment toward supervisors, other departments, or each other; boredom; fatigue—the list is endless. There will also be times when your students simply do not understand what you are trying to teach. A good teacher knows when to abandon the teaching outline, despite time pressures. It is time to listen, to talk openly about the classroom problem you observe. If you do not address these problems, student learning will slow, or the group will stop hearing you. It may be most effective to plan the beginning of the next class as a time for the students to discuss their concerns with the appropriate supervisory person. This may mean that you will have to drop something from the teaching outline. Process means teaching well what you can rather than loading the students with content they will not apply.

When staff members of different ranks and assignments take the course together, natural discussion (process) will resolve many of these issues as each learns the other's viewpoint and problems.

In these situations, the authors' personal technique is to declare a coffee break and circulate among the group to try to gain a better feel for what is going on. It also allows time to regroup and plan what to do next.

Who Is Responsible for Learning?

When you went through college, you may have encountered the assumption that the student is responsible for learning and that if the student did not learn, it was the student's "fault." Even when faculty members were deadly dull or hopelessly disorganized, they droned on, and the students struggled to pass. At least some of the students who failed assumed that they were stupid or inherently unable to understand the subject. Many of the people who will take your course are lifetime academic failures. They have repeatedly had trouble with academic settings and believe that they are stupid or can't learn in the classroom. Some of them have given up, and some are angry with the educational system.

You will be more effective if you assume that it is the teacher's responsibility to make material accessible to the student. Skilled teachers work hard to help their students learn, and their students enjoy learning and gain self-confidence. Assure your students that this course does not require academic skills such as math or memorization—it is a course in learning to do.

Disruptions in the Classroom

Murphy's law guarantees that a disruption will occur just when you have gotten your group's attention or a good discussion has begun. Do your best to prevent students' just dropping in or bringing pagers. Do not videotape the lessons. Students will not participate openly if they are being videotaped, and a tape of a discussion is more than useless: it can be very confusing for people who did not participate.

Students occasionally bring their children to class (or their cognitively impaired grandmother whom they have to care for). The presence of children can be disruptive, but sometimes the adult student has no alternative.

Students may carry on personal conversations in class, do their charting, arrive late, or leave early. Address these problems individually if possible. When several people are talking, charting, or chronically late, try to find out why. Reasons range from anger ("When do you expect us to chart?"), to lack of commitment ("In-services come and go, but the work never changes"), to habit.

Routines

In most programs, because there is more work in the day than the staff can complete (work expands to exceed the staff ratio), organizing the work in a way that staff members can manage and cutting corners where they will not be noticed are job requirements. Successful aides are able to organize their work into routines that ensure that most of it gets done. The staff members are proud of the way they have organized things and believe that this is the best—and only—way to do things. Routines bolster the staff's sense of competence and control over the confusion of multiple demands. However, inflexible routines lead to problems. Staff members resist trying new care approaches because doing so would disrupt their routines. They respond by saying that "we can't do it that way" or "we would never finish."

Routines lead to other problems as well: staff members may fail to respond to a person who calls out because if they break their routine the day will fall apart. People may sit and wait for meals or other care while staff members finish their routines. No one listens to the halting voice of a distressed person. Families and advocates protest that care is inflexible and not patient-centered. Staff members may come to view clients as obstacles to their routines rather as individuals with needs.

This text will encourage staff members to stop and listen to clients, to bathe someone later if it works better. Many of these recommendations are time-neutral but require flexibility. Change in this area is difficult. The emphasis on task-oriented care complicates change. Staff members will be afraid of leaving someone uncared for, that an accident will happen, or that important tasks will simply not be done. Use the classroom as a place free of pressure to assist the staff to consider that their feeling that "we can't do it that way" can in fact become more flexible. Take very small steps to change. Teach the staff to prioritize tasks and to organize their day.

People Will Be People

Classes inevitably include students who are shy, deaf, or not too bright; know it all; talk too much; gloss over serious issues; are exhausted, distracted; have different social values; or do not speak English well. Consider them the challenges of teaching. Figuring out how to reach them requires budgeting for out-of-classroom time. They keep teaching from becoming dull.

Transferring Responsibility

Transferring responsibility from traditional roles will be difficult. For example:

> On one unit, supervisors post the bathing schedule, in order, with an assigned staff member and an allotted amount of time for each person. In contrast, on another unit, staff members accept that they have a re-

sponsibility to get everyone clean. In informal discussion with a supervisor, a staff member may decide who needs more time or a different approach. If one staff member has her clients clean and settled, she may spontaneously help another whose client load is difficult that day.

It may be difficult for a supervisor to give staff members more responsibility when they seem uncooperative, resistant, or poorly trained. It may be equally difficult for some staff members to accept even basic responsibility. Direct care providers have learned not to take risks or rock the boat. Their position is, "If bathing does not get done, let the supervisor take the blame." Others will be eager to undertake inappropriate responsibilities.

Changing who makes what decisions is a gradual learning process. When direct care staff members and supervisors participate together in the classroom, encourage them to make plans for small changes. Use the classroom as a risk-free setting in which to negotiate safe increases in flexibility and to review successes. For example:

In the classroom, care provider and supervisor agree that one person's behavioral symptoms require more time during bathing. Together they make a plan to carry this out and get other clients' needs met as well.

Do not leap into major changes: if they fail, both care providers and supervisors will be unwilling to try again.

"Stupid" Questions and Students Who Make Mistakes

There are no stupid questions. Remind your group that if a person has what she thinks is a "stupid" question, probably others have the same question but are afraid to ask. Dedicate yourself to finding a positive response. There are many variations on the phrase "that's a good point." Once in a while a student will ask a question that you cannot answer without putting the student down. The secret here is to ask the other students how they would address this question. This provides review and gets the teacher off the hot seat.

Students will make clinical mistakes and ineffective care plans. Avoid pointing this out. Look for ways to build on the experience. Make suggestions that will protect the client and keep the student from looking foolish. The process of learning requires trial and error. Students' clinical experience is reviewed by both the teacher and the supervisor to protect the client. Management must be prepared for mistakes.

Mistakes are an important part of learning. Most people remember making a mistake and never forget that issue again. People at all levels make mistakes, occasionally serious. Students must learn that it is okay make mistakes if they are to take the risk of giving good care. They must also learn that management can accept mistakes without punitive action. The individual's level of responsibility and the expertise of the team set limits on the nature of decisions and therefore the mistakes a person can make. Respond positively to mistakes, and help the group explore the consequences of an idea before it is initiated.

Students Who Blame Others for Problems

Many of the students you teach (whether professionals or not) do not see themselves as the problem although you may perceive them as needing to change. People blame administration or the demands of the job for difficulties in care. Commonly staff members see the person with dementia as the problem. You cannot shift this attitude by teaching. It is futile to try to argue students out of this position. When staff members blame management, involve supervisors and administrators in classroom discussions. Look for compromise. Always focus on answering the question, "Because we cannot change that, what can we do for the person with dementia?" Look for small modifications in the system.

No amount of information alone will stop people from placing blame on people with dementia, although information helps. Use empathy exercises and discussions of neuropathology in lay terms.

You may hear comments such as: "People with dementia are like children. They respond to being treated like children." This strategy protects staff feelings when clients treat them badly, but it fails because the person with dementia is not in on the secret. The person with dementia thinks she is an adult. Another comment you may hear is: "We'll take charge." This assumes that people with dementia are either bad or childish. It allows the staff to get the work done quickly and efficiently. It allows schedules and tasks to take precedence over individual goals or needs. Most people hate to be treated this way, and people with dementia will either withdraw or resist. Some will become overly dependent.

Anger and Frustration

You may hear negative remarks from students such as: "You choose: shall we chart or listen to you?"; "We already know all that"; "They won't let us do that"; or "We don't have time for that." Many staff members have seen courses and teachers come and go, but nothing much changes in the work setting—sometimes the workload gets worse. They are angry, frustrated, or demoralized. Learned helplessness—"there is nothing we can do"—is common among care providers. They perceive that the system will not change and that the expectation of training is that they do something without support. This course asks students to believe in themselves, to buy into change, and to invest themselves in the work. To accomplish this, we repeat what has been said throughout the text:

- Management must be prepared to support the transfer of learning to the workplace.
- Staff concerns must be discussed in the classroom. Denying or ignoring them or trying to talk students out of their attitudes will block learning.
- An understanding must be reached between management and students about what can realistically be expected of the course.
- Teachers must adjust the training to match this agreement.
- Guide the students to identify what they can realistically do, and use the classroom as a safe place to test ideas.

Students Who Are Forced to Take the Course

This is getting off on the wrong foot, but it often happens. Listen to the student's side and then ask the group members what they can gain from the course as long as they are stuck in it. Be honest and strike a reasonable compromise. Usually they will become excited as the course progresses.

PART TWO

LESSONS

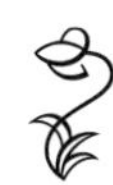

LESSON 1

HELPING THE PERSON BY UNDERSTANDING THE PROBLEM

Summary. This lesson lays the foundations for the course. It provides a basic understanding of dementia and an empathetic understanding of the experience of the person with dementia. Empathy is a powerful tool for problem solving. The factual base establishes that the manifestations of the disease are symptoms of an organic condition.

Section 1.1. The Voice of the Person with Dementia. Introduces students to the course by encouraging them to empathize with the person with dementia.

Section 1.2. Establishing Student Goals. Establishes student learning goals and links them to management goals for the training.

Section 1.3. Recognizing Terms and Differences. Explains the terms used in dementia care.

Section 1.4. Information about Diagnosis and Evaluation. Provides more detailed clinical characteristics for the assessment of people with dementia.

Using the Sections

- Introductory course:
  - Section 1.1 required
  - Section 1.2 optional
  - Section 1.3 select appropriate information
- Core course:
  - Section 1.1 required
  - Section 1.2 optional
  - Section 1.3 required
- Special audiences:
  - Staff members responsible for diagnosis, assessment, referral, and treatment: all sections, including section 1.4

Problems You May Have in Implementing This Lesson

Section 1.3, Recognizing Terms and Differences, is a lecture. Because lectures can seem boring, this may turn off students at the beginning of the course. Instead of starting this way, begin with Section 1.1 and with suggested Section 1.2.

Section 1.1. The Voice of the Person with Dementia

Objective

The student will learn to feel empathy with the person with dementia. Throughout the course, students will be asked to consider issues from the perspective of the person with dementia. This section initiates the process and is upbeat and moving.

Information and Instructions for the Teacher

Although this section may seem like "fun," it is vital to the success of the course. For any course to result in changes in caregiver behavior, caregivers must see value in learning and understanding the perspective of those they care for. This section is the first step in this process. The rest of the course builds on it.

Discuss briefly what this course is about. Hand out copies of the course outline you have selected, identify the major topics, and say how they will help the participants.

At the end of the class, give a brief, upbeat summary of what was covered and remind the group of the time, place, and topic of the next meeting.

Lecture/Discussion Notes to Be Presented to the Class

Overhead/Handout 1.1.
People with Dementia Still Communicate
and/or
Overhead/Handout 1.2. Alzheimer Patient Quotes

Point out that people who have dementia are real people with real feelings. Sometimes they can still express themselves, and we need to pay attention to what they are trying to say.

Hand out the list of quotations. Ask the students to read through them and select the two that move them the most. Allow time: you can see when the group is about finished.

Ask each person to read the quotation that he or she liked best. (If a quotation has already been read, ask the person to read a second choice.)

Start an open discussion by asking: "Why did you choose this quotation?" "Does it remind you of someone you care for or someone in your family?" "Do these words express your values about people?" You may ask if anyone has heard a person with dementia say something that he or she would like to share now. Ask if people have observed facial expressions or gestures that are meaningful. Occasionally, a student will report a statement that seems "funny" or cute but makes fun of the person with dementia. Explain that staff members should avoid doing this and should listen for the real feelings of the person with dementia.

You may not need to say much after this exercise. Let the impact of the exercise make the point.

Section 1.2. Establishing Student Goals

Objective

The student will be encouraged to "buy into" the course. This section creates a tool (list of goals) that you will use throughout the course to reinforce learning and creates a measurement (number of goals met) so that you and the student can evaluate the success of the course. It lets students know what they can expect and what can and cannot be accomplished in the course. (For example, we can expect to improve overall levels of problem behavior, but we will never eliminate all problem behavior.)

Information and Instructions for the Teacher

It is important for the student to identify goals in order to learn effectively. Follow the steps in the Lecture/Discussion Notes.

Lecture/Discussion Notes to Be Presented to the Class

Say what you will cover in this exercise. Talk briefly about goals and their importance. State that goals help us decide what is most important to do so that we can see whether we are making gains to give purpose to our work.

When we seek to improve care for people with dementia, we must keep in mind that many groups will have goals. The facility or provider has identified its goals in Chapter I. In this exercise the staff members in training will identify theirs. You may want to talk about the goals others have for improved care for people with dementia: What goals do people with cognitive impairment have? What goals do their families have? What goals do cognitively well people who live in the same facility have?

Ask the group members what they would like to learn from this course. (Your review of the course outline in Section 1.1 should have given them some ideas.) Try to obtain a response from everyone without forcing anyone to speak. Avoid overloading the list with any one person's ideas but do so without putting that person down.

Write all ideas on a flip chart, or ask small teams to list their goals; then write the goals from each team on the flip chart.

Even if students' ideas are naive, avoid discouraging them. You will help your students explore and test ideas as the course goes on. When goals are suggested that cannot be accomplished, emphasize that this course will work toward doing the best we can with what we have. When ideas are beyond the scope of the class, try to offer some resolution: "The administration is aware of that problem and is working on it" or "Perhaps we can find a way to compromise on that."

Tactfully suggest important goals that the group may have missed. This list must be the group's, not yours.

Go through the list and identify which class or classes will address this issue.

Optional: Share with the group the management's goals for this course. In discussion format, identify the points of agreement.

Keep the flip chart sheets. Once the group's goals have been defined, use this regularly with the class. Taking just five minutes at the beginning of some classes, put the sheets up and check off those goals that have been met. At the end of the course, you will incorporate these goals into the final workshop.

In a few sentences, state what was covered in this exercise. This is a good opportunity to reaffirm the tone of the course and compliment the group members on their goals and their participation.

Section 1.3. Recognizing Terms and Differences

Objective

The student will learn why care is done the way it is. This section is the basis for the remaining lessons. The student will learn that the dementias are diseases, that they are caused by organic changes in the brain, and that delirium resembles dementia but is different and must be noted and reported.

Background

The diagnostic criteria for dementia and related issues have been accepted for less than two decades. Many people learned earlier terminology. It is essential that students learn and use the accepted diagnostic criteria because these will influence decisions about care. A common language is necessary, and professionals must be able to communicate about their patients. Discuss any conflicts with what students have previously learned. These definitions continue to change. Stay current through the Alzheimer's Association.

Widely held myths still survive and must be dispelled in this lesson. Each is addressed in later lessons. Among them:

- "Everybody is going to become like this eventually." This belief causes staff members to distance themselves from those for whom they care.
- "There is nothing to be done." Hopelessness and powerlessness devastate good care.
- "She could do better if she tried" or "She is being manipulative." It is easy to form these misunderstandings of dementia, which result in applying the wrong strategies for intervention.
- "It doesn't really matter what we call it" or "It isn't worth the investment in a full-scale workup" or "There isn't any consensus about these things yet" or "All decline is just part of the dementia." These are all false. These ideas prevent people from helping those with dementia live as well as they can with their illness. Simply telling students that these concepts are wrong does not change the way they care. Use the text and discussion here and in later lessons to help students work through these biases.

Information and Instructions for the Teacher

This material can be presented as a lecture or as discussion. Alternatively, academically prepared students can read it at home and discuss it at the next session. Lecture or discussion, however, is usually more effective.

The complexity of your presentation should depend on your group. Nonprofessional direct care providers who have time for only a short course will require less of this information. Weigh what your group members need to know to do their job. For example, a nursing assistant should know that when people are sick they may become more confused or irritable and that this should be reported. The assistant may not need to know the definition of delirium. It is more important that lay staff members learn that there are differences in dementias than that they learn what those differences are; likewise, it is more important that the students know that the changes in people with dementia are caused by organic change than that they know what those changes are. Use enough of the information about how the disease affects the brain to lay a foundation for the understanding that these illnesses are organic in nature. This is the basis for many interventions. Many behavioral symptoms seem deliberate or manipulative until one recognizes the incredible complexity of the failing brain. Most students find this material fascinating.

This course presents a schematic, oversimplified explanation of brain function. The purpose of this material is to communicate that brain function is related to disease and to behavior. The course does not teach neuroanatomy.

Stop frequently for discussion and questions. Even the simplest presentation can confuse people when the concepts are new. If people are confused, try to find an alternative way of explaining things. It is much better to cover only part of the material and have students understand it well.

Focus on concepts rather than on memorized definitions. Only people responsible for diagnosis, assessment, referral, and treatment need memorize the distinguishing characteristics of dementia, delirium, depression, vascular disease, and Alzheimer disease.

When you stop for discussion, ask students to consider people with dementia they have seen who are typical and atypical of the syndrome you are describing (they will see both). If you are not sure that you can recognize these syndromes easily or don't know the people your students care for, don't guess. You will not be making diagnoses; you will be thinking about differences. The objective is to teach students to use their powers of observation and orderly thinking. Do not rely on chart diagnoses for the "answers" as these are often wrong.

Students may ask questions such as the following:

- "What does a person have who doesn't make sense when he talks?" Because this is only one area of mental function, help the students paint a broader picture of the person's other disabilities.
- "What about a person who just lies in her room and won't come out?" Students tend to think in general terms. Help the student find which set of characteristics best describes the patient (perhaps depression).
- "I know she has Alzheimer disease because she has a bad attitude" or "I know she had a terrible childhood, which explains why she is so nasty." Students tend to mix conclusions and extraneous information into definitions. Help the students learn to set aside such information and determine whether the patient fits the description of dementia. Jumping to these conclusions leads to faulty interventions. The things we would do to help a person's "bad attitude" would be different if the person had delirium rather than dementia.

You may be asked questions about topics such as drug treatments or specific people that you do not have time to answer or don't know the answer to. Respond to these in a way that does not discourage your audience: "That is an interesting question" or "I don't know, but . . ."

Lecture/Discussion Notes to Be Presented to the Class

What Dementia Is Like: Overhead/Handout 1.3. The Experience of the Person with Dementia *and* Overhead/Handout 1.4. The Progression of Dementia

Teacher: These two overheads are optional. Use them with students who have had little experience with dementia or whose understanding of dementia is inaccurate. As an alternative, guide a discussion of what dementia is like.

The Human Brain

The human brain is said to be the most complex thing on earth and perhaps in the universe. Galaxies, mathematics and physics, the rest of the human body—all pale in comparison with the human brain—like the one you have on your shoulders. It contains about 100 billion cells—an unimaginable number—visible only through a microscope. These cells are linked by long, threadlike axons. The brain works because these cells communicate with one another through faint electrical pulses and through chemicals called *neurotransmitters,* which the cells manufacture within themselves.

Nerve cells look somewhat like a many-branched tree with branching roots. Each cell may have several thousand branches (axions). In the center of the cell, the "trunk of the tree," is the heart of the cell, which keeps the cell working and contains the DNA (the operating instructions for life). When you think, move a muscle, or feel an emotion, a weak electrical message passes through the cell, out the "branches," and on to the next nerve cell. When you learn something new, a new, permanent connection is made along this pathway from one group of nerve cells to another, and the next time you recall that information, the pathway will be retraced.

The brain divides up the work of mental processes. For example, bundles of thousands of cells in the back of the brain analyze the signals from the eyes; another area on the left side contains bundles of cells that handle language. Muscle movements, reason, and judgment have their own areas. Farther inside the brain are areas that coordinate memories and other areas that process emotions. There are millions of individual groups of cells that handle different mental tasks.

If you imagine billions of cells doing all this work, it is easy to see why no two people are alike. Throughout adulthood, some brain cells and their branches die, but there are so many billions of cells that normal cell loss has no effect. If a few cells die, the rest of the cell bundle can operate perfectly normally. But if just one part of this process is damaged, the person's conscious awareness of the world will be damaged.

Damage to the Brain

If a person sustains a serious head injury, a large area of cells may be destroyed, and the person's abilities or moods will be changed.

The Definition of Dementia

Diseases such as Alzheimer's and cognitive loss from vascular disease are called *dementias*. These diseases affect several areas of brain function. There are about 60 dementias, of which Alzheimer disease and vascular dementia are the most common. Most of the others are quite rare. *Dementia* is an umbrella term that refers to diseases that cause memory problems and problems in other areas of mental function.

The Impact of Dementia

Four million people in the United States have a disabling cognitive impairment. They exhaust their families who care for them. Their care in nursing homes, in day care, at home, and in residential facilities costs millions of dollars each year. Most important, the nation has lost their talents and their contributions.

Whatever the cause of the dementia, the brain just cannot work: the person is trying as hard as she can, but nerve cells, cell branches, or necessary chemicals have been lost, including

- cells with memories in them;
- cells that make new memories;
- cells that make sense out of what other people are saying;
- cells that figure out how to behave;
- cells that express affection or anger; and
- cells that give instructions to move parts of the body.

Cells are destroyed unevenly, so the person's behavior may be hard to understand. Injured nerve tissue may work one time and not another, frustrating families when the person can do something one day and not another.

That not all cells are damaged evenly can be frustrating, but it gives us a great advantage in care: we can help the person by helping him use the brain cells he has left and by not asking him to use brain cells he has lost. This is what this course is about.

Vascular, or Multi-infarct, Dementia and Stroke

Later in life a person may have a stroke that destroys a large number of cells. A stroke occurs when a blood vessel leaks like a worn-out garden hose or when a small blood vessel is blocked by a blood clot. If a vessel bursts, blood flows into the brain cells, causing them to die. If a clot blocks a vessel, no blood, with its valuable load of oxygen and nutrients, will reach the surrounding cells, which then die. What is damaged depends on where the stroke occurred. You may have seen people who have had strokes in the language area of the brain and as a result can no longer talk. If a person has a stroke in the motor area of the brain, she will no longer be able to move parts of her body. Her bones and muscles still work, but the brain is unable to give instructions.

You may know people who have *vascular (or multi-infarct) dementia,* which is caused by one or more strokes. Sometimes a person has *transient ischemic attacks,* or TIAs, which resolve. These should be considered warnings of a stroke. Strokes can be so small that almost no damage is evident. However, if many such tiny strokes occur in the same area, they will damage enough of the brain that the person will be impaired. People with vascular dementia often seem similar to people with Alzheimer disease, but you may notice differences. These differences occur because with vascular dementia the damage is spotty: most of it is in the areas in which the strokes happened to occur. Undamaged areas will function normally. People with this kind of dementia may decline and then stabilize, then decline again as another stroke occurs.

Researchers are learning many ways to treat or prevent stroke and vascular disease. People who have high blood pressure or diabetes, who are overweight or have cardiovascular disease, or who have a history of heavy drinking are more likely to have large or small strokes. Taking high blood pressure medication and following the diet recommended by your doctor are important. If a person has a stroke, reaching an emergency room quickly is important. If the person is treated early, the damage caused by the stroke can often be reduced. (Your students may not know what high blood pressure means—that it puts more pressure on the blood vessels, making it more likely that one will burst under too much pressure.) Ask for discussion of lifestyles. Take this opportunity to do some teaching about the risk factors for strokes.

Optional: If people do not know what their blood pressure is, arrange for them to have it checked. Have a referral source ready for those who need it.

Alzheimer Disease

Alzheimer disease damages the long branches of cells and the chemistry within the brain cells. When this happens, old message traces we have had all our life just disappear, or new information may never be stored. Pieces of the brain's data bank are being erased, and other pieces are never stored. This is why people forget: the memory has been lost inside the brain. When you tell someone something and she forgets it a minute later, it is because her brain has stopped storing information. Scientists are now learning how these changes take place.

Alzheimer disease damages cells involved in memory and language. The disease may trigger a depression. As the disease progresses, the motor areas, judgment, and many other areas fail. Because the many areas of the brain work together, failures in one area have a domino effect, resulting in failures in many areas. Because not all areas fail, however, the caregiver sees strange patterns such as people who are able to recognize one person but not another or people who are able to curse but unable to use any other verbal skills. Most people are able to walk long after they have good judgment about where to walk; they can argue long after they understand another person's point; and they can strike out long after they have lost the self-control they might wish to have. Alzheimer disease shows itself slowly: the affected person gradually develops problems in memory and other areas. Mental functions usually decline over 5 to 20 years and end in total disability.

How Are the Dementias Transmitted?

There are as many causes of these diseases as there are diseases. Neither Alzheimer disease nor vascular disease is contagious.

Alzheimer disease runs in families. That is, some people will inherit the disease, some people will inherit the *risk* of the disease, and some people will not inherit it at all. In some of the people who inherit the risk of the disease, other factors, such as health, the environment, or lifestyle, probably determine whether they will *develop* the disease. Because Alzheimer disease usually begins late in life, some people who have inherited it will die of some other illness (cancer, heart disease) before the Alzheimer disease begins.

People may also inherit the risk of vascular disease, but probably other factors affect whether they will actually develop it (such as high blood pressure).

Treatment

At present, we cannot prevent or cure Alzheimer disease, and we cannot reverse the impact of vascular dementia. However, scientists are finding some medications that may help the person with Alzheimer disease function better. The care you give offers a lot of hope. Knowing how the disease affects the brain, staff members can adjust their care to help the person cope. They can help people use what brain tissue is still working and can find ways to keep them from being frustrated and upset by things they cannot understand. This is a powerful tool. There is a lot staff members can do so that people can live comfortably, laugh a little, or make friends, even though they do have a terrible disease. *Ask the group for examples.*

Normal Forgetfulness

Do you ever have the experience of forgetting what you were doing? going into the kitchen and forgetting why you went there? misplacing your keys? Ask the group if this means that a person is developing a dementia. Do all people develop a dementia when they grow old? What would mean that you are developing a dementia? (*Answers: Normal forgetfulness is com-*

mon. It is more common when we are tired, stressed, or depressed. When a person has other losses such as language or judgment as well as memory, or when mental problems interfere with daily life, the person should see a physician.)

Does Everyone Become "Senile"?

Until recently, it was assumed that serious memory problems were inevitable in old age. In fact, most people live to very old age without developing cognitive impairment; they remain just as alert and intelligent as the rest of us, even if they become a little absent minded. Dementia is caused by a *disease;* it is not something that is normal in old age.

A few people who are middle aged develop dementias, but this is rare. Of all people who are 65 years old, most will have no trouble thinking. Cognitive problems increase with age, yet of all 85-year-olds, many will be thinking well. This is important. As staff members and family members observe the tragedy of dementia day in and day out, they need to know that they do not have to look forward to the same fate.

To people caring for cognitively impaired elderly persons and people with Alzheimer disease, it can seem as though everybody has problems. It seems this way because these are the people we see all the time. Most elderly people don't need us, so we don't notice them. Think of the spouses of your clients: most of them are elderly and have no serious problems in thinking.

What's Good for the Heart Is Good for the Brain

Teacher: This research is still developing, so keep your information current through the Alzheimer's Association newsletters.

Researchers are finding that diet can postpone the onset of dementia or stroke. This information is especially important because the same changes in diet can reduce the risk of several chronic diseases, including Alzheimer disease, heart disease, and stroke.

Changes in diet are effective only over the long term. The effects of poor diet build up slowly and are not obvious for years. Changes in diet that last for only a month or two will have little effect on long-term health in late life, and crash diets may make things worse. A person planning major changes in diet should consult a physician before beginning.

Experts recommend the following for people who are developing symptoms of a dementia or are at risk of developing a dementia:

- A diet recommended by the individual's physician for a healthy heart
- Reduced levels of saturated fats and trans fatty acids
- A diet low in cholesterol and the treatment of high cholesterol
- Increased amounts of omega-3
- No iron supplements after age 50 unless there is a medical reason for them. (Many foods and vitamin supplements include iron, so it is necessary to read labels.)
- Increased folate supplementation to 400 mcg or more
- Increased thiamine supplementation
- For people who know that they are at risk of developing dementia or stroke, an antiplatelet agent such as coated aspirin if recommended by a physician
- Supplemental vitamin E if recommended by a physician

Understandings and Misunderstandings about the Cause of Behavioral Symptoms

If you look at the human brain, it appears to be a very wrinkled object about the size of a coconut. If you cut into it, it turns out to be like jelly. The neurotransmitters that bring the brain to life disappear quickly after death. Until recently, scientists have not been able to look at a brain and see how it works. They were limited to looking at the postmortem tissue under a microscope. This tells the scientist nothing about how thoughts and feelings work. Therefore, physicians made a best guess about mental function. Recent research makes it possible to update our knowledge extensively.

Every culture has developed a theory to explain human behavior. Some cultures believe we act as we do because of fate or karma, others because we have a succession of lives. The Western world developed the familiar theories of psychology. These theories have been popularized through magazines, books, and television. Everyone knows much of this pop psychology and assumes it to be true: behavior is thought to be caused by early childhood experiences and ways learned in infancy to cope with anxiety. It assumes things such as this: people who are depressed need to express their anger; seriously disturbed people had cold, remote parents; fears can be overcome through various learning processes; and so forth. These theories may make sense in the daily lives of people who are basically mentally well, but it is now clear that they fail to explain or help those with serious mental illnesses such as bipolar disease, schizophrenia, or Alzheimer disease. New discoveries tell us that these diseases involve the cells of the brain and changes in the chemistry that these cells generate. When we use the old pop psychology ideas to help people with serious brain diseases, we can do them more harm than good.

A better understanding of the major mental illnesses and dementia came with the recent discovery of the chemicals in the brain called neurotransmitters and the development of equipment that allows scientists to observe the living brain in action. With this new information, scientists can see that the problems that arise for people with dementia are caused by failures in the structure or chemistry of the brain.

The first neurotransmitters were discovered in the 1970s. In the 1970s and 1980s, drugs were developed that affect the neurotransmitters and bring relief to people with depression and schizophrenia. More recently, drugs have been developed that help those with anorexia, obsessive-compulsive disorder, and panic attacks. Imaging tools and studies of brain chemistry indicate that these illnesses are biochemical.

These research developments have come so fast and so recently that most students who care for people with dementia may hold inadequate or outdated explanations for human behavior. The new understanding of brain development and brain chemistry, the new miracle drugs, and the new imaging equipment expand our vision. Perhaps the most challenging thing the student will learn in this course is to revise old concepts and grow with new developments in order to provide the best care. (These changes will be discussed throughout the text.)

Section 1.4. Information about Diagnosis and Evaluation

Objective

The student will learn the clinical characteristics for the assessment of people with dementia.

Lecture/Discussion Notes to Be Presented to the Class

Dementia versus Delirium

This section describes the characteristics of two conditions: dementia and delirium. Either of these can be present with cognitive impairment, and they may be confused. It is important that the clinician recognize the differences and know when each is responsive to treatment.

There has been considerable confusion over terminology for cognitive problems. In the past 20 years an internationally accepted set of definitions has been developed. These definitions are simple, but people sometimes try to add to them and make them complicated. The reason for learning these terms is to be able to recognize possible syndromes and make appropriate referrals. It is not a substitute for clinical training.

Diagnosis of these conditions is made by a physician. The following information should trigger medical evaluation.

The definitions may differ from what you have been taught or what physicians in your area are using. This is usually because people learned earlier definitions years ago. The newer definitions are designed to eliminate confusion and ensure that patients receive the care they need. Using them protects the patient who may have a treatable condition or a partially treatable condition from being overlooked.

Dementia

Dementia is a syndrome (a group of symptoms) characterized as a decline in more than one area of mental function in a person who is awake and alert. Dementias are caused by many diseases, including Alzheimer disease and vascular disease. (See Exhibit 1.1.)

The Definition of Dementia

1. A Decline in Mental Function

   Has your client's mental function declined from what it used to be? Usually you must have a history from the family or someone else, or know the person for a while, to determine that he has declined.

   A decline in mental function discriminates between dementia and a lifelong disability such as mental retardation. The person who has always been impaired does not have a dementia unless that person has declined from his lifelong level of disability. Thus, a person with Down syndrome whose cognitive function becomes worse does have a dementia.
2. A Decline in More Than One Area of Mental Function, Including Memory
   a. Has your patient shown problems with memory (long term or short term) that she did not previously have?
   b. Memory loss alone is not sufficient to define dementia. Has your patient shown problems in any other areas, such as
      - short-term recall for five minutes;
      - impairment of long-term recall;
      - memory/recall ability (season, where she is, location of her own room, staff names/faces);
      - cognitive skills for daily decision making (needs help in new situations, needs cues or supervision, or rarely makes decisions); or
      - impaired ability to understand others?

   Several things have been left out of this definition:

   a. Severity: a dementia can be mild or severe.
   b. Potential for treatment: a dementia may be treatable or untreatable. Some dementias, such as those caused by thyroid disease and vitamin B_{12} deficiency, are potentially treatable.
   c. Chronicity: a dementia may be chronic or short term.

If memory or language is the only impairment, the patient should be evaluated for the cause of the disability, which technically is an amnestic syndrome or an aphasia, not a dementia, and could be treatable.

3. A Decline in a Person Who Is Awake and Alert

Is your patient awake and alert or drowsy and "out of it"? This is a judgment call. Practice and clinical training are needed to strengthen your skills. Be alert to the possibility that the person's cognition is clouded when the person is taking any medications or has even a mild illness.

There is an important distinction between cognition deficits in a person who is stuporous, comatose, unconscious, drugged, drowsy or asleep, or unable to focus even briefly and a cognitive impairment in a person who seems awake, alert, and able to pay attention at least briefly. The person who is drowsy or stuporous may fit the definition of delirium. (See the subsection "Delirium" later in this section.)

When a person is drowsy or stuporous, we cannot make a diagnosis of dementia. It is necessary to wait until the clouded consciousness clears before deciding that the person has a dementia (or Alzheimer disease). Elderly people in hospitals are often delirious as a result of their medical illness or the drugs used to treat it. When such people are given a diagnosis of dementia or Alzheimer disease for the first time, they must be reevaluated once the delirium has cleared.

This distinction is important to care. Delirium can often be reduced or eliminated by the treatment of underlying conditions. When delirium is mistaken for a dementia or Alzheimer disease, important medical care is overlooked, and the patient ultimately may not recover lost cognition.

If your patient has a decline in mental function in more than one area, including memory, and is awake and alert, suspect a dementia.

Old Terms

What happened to the term *hardening of the arteries?* As we developed better ways to study the brain, we learned that rigidity and narrowing of the arteries are not causing cognitive impairment. The term *senility* has been dropped because it carried connotations of hopelessness and of every old person becoming "senile." The term *chronic organic brain syndrome* was dropped because of the implication that all problems are chronic, which they are not. *Confusion* merely means that the person is confused. Occasionally this text uses the term *confusion* as a change of pace, but it can also mean that a person is confused about the instructions that came with his VCR!

Causes of Dementia

Dementia is caused by about 60 different diseases. Each has different symptoms. Diagnosis is important for several reasons:

- A few people have memory problems that we can treat, such as vitamin B_{12} deficiency and thyroid disease. Some conditions respond well if treated early enough but become chronic if neglected.
- Some people have conditions that we can partly help so that their thinking improves but is not cured (often including normal pressure hydrocephalus, brain tumors).
- Because some dementias, including Alzheimer disease, run in families, it is very important to other family members to know which disease the person has: the family may be worrying unnecessarily.
- Sometimes a person acts differently than people with Alzheimer disease do. Staff members can provide better care when they understand the disease.

Wally Brennon can still express himself very clearly—he has the "gift of gab"—and his friends and neighbors are convinced that nothing is wrong with him, but he cannot remember anything for even a few minutes. He thinks that his wife and son are stealing from him, and he hits his wife. His wife has read about Alzheimer disease and does not believe Wally has it. She thinks her husband, a former alcoholic, has just gotten meaner. When Wally was diagnosed as having an alcohol-related dementia instead of Alzheimer disease, she was able to accept his disease and change the way she responded to him.

- People with different diseases respond differently to medications, and staff members need to recognize this.
- Often the person also has other problems (e.g., Alzheimer disease and stomach ulcers; Alzheimer disease and depression). The brain is affected by everything that happens to the body. The combination of illnesses can make the person's thinking worse than the Alzheimer disease alone. If we can diagnose and treat these other problems or relieve the person's pain, the person will do better.

Albert DeNiro had done well in day care for several months, but recently he had become agitated and had hit staff members and other participants. The staff were not sure they could continue to keep him but knew that his wife could not manage without the respite that day care gave her. When Albert's physician discovered that Albert was having pain and chronic infections due to an enlarged prostate and treated this problem, Albert's agitation disappeared.

To group everyone together as having Alzheimer disease causes us to overlook ways to help people, just as the old term *senility* did.

Some of the dementias are listed in Exhibit 1.1. A diagnosis of Alzheimer disease—or any dementia—must be made by a physician using a history, laboratory tests, brain imaging, and often neuropsychological tests.

There are two ways to make a diagnosis:

1. Examination of brain tissue, now done only on autopsy
2. Clinical diagnosis. A clinical evaluation is an excellent method of diagnosis. To ensure the best care for your patient, review what was done at the time of diagnosis. A careful work-up by an experienced clinician will be accurate about 90 percent of the time. Diagnostic tests are being developed; however, no test, when it is developed, will be 100 percent accurate, and tests will not be a substitute for a clinical diagnosis.

Alzheimer Disease

At present, Alzheimer disease is irreversible, ending in death, but often the quality of life can be enhanced by reducing excess disability.

Alzheimer disease is characterized by insidious (gradual) onset, usually over months or years, and specific changes in the structure and neurochemistry of the brain.

You may have observed symptoms that seem characteristic of Alzheimer disease, but be cautious in assuming they apply to all clients.

Vascular Dementia

Vascular disease accounts for about 10–20 percent of all cases of dementia.

Vascular dementia is characterized by

- often abrupt onset;
- a stepwise decline, which may fluctuate;
- "patchy" intellectual loss; and
- evidence of cerebrovascular disease, hypertension, or diabetes.

This type of dementia often accompanies cerebrovascular disease, hypertension, or diabetes. Lesions will frequently be visible on brain imaging. Recognizing the different symptom patterns will make care easier. Although there is a potential for slowing or preventing this disease, clinical experience has so far had limited success. New research is expected to benefit this group of patients.

Vascular disease and Alzheimer disease often occur together in people with dementia.

Other Dementias

Among the other dementias is Lewy body dementia. People with this disease often have some stiffness, slowness, and balance problems and are at risk of falling early in the dementia. They frequently have hallucinations and paranoid ideas but often have side effects when given neuroleptics.

People with the frontotemporal dementias (or lobar dementias), including Pick disease, may make rude remarks or do things that are dangerous. Language skills may be lost early.

All the remaining diseases together account for about 10 percent of cases of dementia. A good evaluation can usually determine which disease the person has because there are differences in symptoms. People who have abused alcohol are more likely than others to develop a dementia. Because their language skills remain good while memory, judgment, and inhibition are lost, staff members and others may not recognize the extent of their difficulties. These people may become agitated or do things that are inappropriate or dangerous.

When the dementia is not currently treatable, as in Alzheimer disease, we can treat symptoms to improve the quality of life. In diabetes we manage the person's kidney disease: in many dementias we manage the feelings—like being lost and afraid—that make people act out.

Delirium

Delirium is different from dementia.

Even though delirium is very common, it is frequently overlooked. Recognition of delirium is important because people who are delirious are at greater risk of dying; in addition, if the underlying problem can be treated, the potential for helping the person is great. Hands-on staff members and supervisors are often in the best position to recognize delirium early.

Delirium is sometimes mistaken for dementia. People with dementia are vulnerable to delirium, often from minor causes. Delirium worsens function, can increase agitation, and can lead to combativeness. Delirium overlaid on dementia is sometimes mistaken for a worsening of the dementia and left untreated. When delirium is treated, the person's cognitive function usually improves, although the underlying dementia may not.

Because delirium affects cognition, a diagnosis of dementia cannot be made if a delirium is present or suspected.

Delirium is characterized by

- a clouding of consciousness;
- development over hours or days;
- fluctuation during the day;
- may include perceptual disturbances, incoherent speech, disturbed sleep cycle, drowsiness, disorientation.

Delirium is present if the following symptoms are different from the resident's usual function (a worsening of symptoms or a new onset) over the past seven days:

- The person is easily distracted (e.g., has difficulty paying attention; gets sidetracked).
- The person has periods of altered perception or awareness of surroundings (e.g., moves lips or talks to someone not present; believes he is somewhere else; confuses night and day).
- The person has episodes of disorganized speech (e.g., speech is incoherent, nonsensical, irrelevant, or rambling from subject to subject; person loses train of thought).
- The person has periods of restlessness (e.g., fidgeting or picking at skin, clothing, napkins, and so on; frequent position changes; repetitive physical movements or calling out).
- The person has periods of lethargy (e.g., is sluggish; stares into space; is difficult to arouse; has little body movement).
- Mental function varies over the course of the day (e.g., sometimes better, sometimes worse; behaviors sometimes present, sometimes not).

Usually a specific organic factor (illness or medication) causes the delirium, and it often resolves when this factor is treated. (See also Lesson 3 and Section 11.5.) When delirium is suspected in anyone, search for an organic cause. In people who already have a dementia, even slight problems such as a urinary tract infection or constipation may trigger a delirium. Even low doses of medication may be responsible. Not all elderly people fully recover from a delirium: prompt treatment is thought to increase recovery rates. A change in behavior may be the first sign of a delirium.

> Mrs. Wong entered the hospital for treatment of pneumonia. The pneumonia resolved uneventfully, but Mrs. Wong remained confused and combative. The staff concluded that she had Alzheimer disease. In fact, Mrs. Wong's cognition had been clear until the pneumonia made her delirious. The sedatives she was given to treat her restlessness in the hospital continued the delirium. She was intermittently agitated, was unable to focus on her meals, dozed much of the day, and scored poorly on a test of cognition. Her physician prescribed Atavan to calm her so that a nursing home admission could be arranged. Instead, Mr. Wong took her home and decreased all medications. Very slowly Mrs. Wong returned to her prior clear mental status.

There is no level of severity in the definition of delirium. In elderly persons and in people with dementia, the onset of delirium may be subtle: observant staff members report "seems more irritable," "seems listless," "didn't want her breakfast." When several such minor changes occur, suspect the beginning of a delirium.

Although the definition of delirium describes an acute onset, delirium in frail elderly people may be longstanding if the underlying condition cannot be or has not been resolved.

Exhibit 1.1. Some of the Dementing Diseases

Metabolic disorders
- Thyroid, parathyroid, or adrenal gland dysfunction
- Liver or kidney dysfunction
- Certain vitamin deficiencies, such as vitamin B_{12} deficiency

Structural problems of the brain
- Normal pressure hydrocephalus (abnormal flow of spinal fluid)
- Brain tumors
- Subdural hematoma (bleeding beneath the skull, which results in collections of blood that press on the brain)
- Trauma (injuries to the brain)
- Hypoxia and anoxia (insufficient oxygen)

Infection
- Tuberculosis
- Syphilis
- Fungal, bacterial, and viral infections of the brain, such as meningitis or encephalitis
- Acquired immune deficiency syndrome (AIDS)

Toxicants (poisons)
- Carbon monoxide
- Drugs
- Metal poisoning
- Alcohol (Scientists disagree about whether alcohol can cause cognitive impairment.)

Degenerative disease (causes generally unknown)
- Alzheimer disease
- Lewy body dementia
- Huntington disease
- Parkinson disease
- Frontotemporal dementia, including Pick disease
- Progressive supranuclear palsy
- Wilson disease

Vascular (blood vessel) disease
- Stroke or multi-infarct disease
- Binswanger disease

Autoimmune disease
- Temporal arthritis
- Lupus erythematosus

Psychiatric disorders
- Depression
- Schizophrenia

Multiple sclerosis

Overhead/Handout 1.1. People with Dementia Still Communicate

"I'm still me, but not sort of." It is not true that "everything" is lost in people who have a dementia. Some aspects of memory and language may be lost, while feelings and aspects of personality remain. As we go through these lessons, we will talk about what is lost and what is retained and how to help the person make the best of "still being me." People with dementia are still the people they have always been, only disabled now. Even very impaired people often still sense the feelings of others.

A retired nurse who had had Alzheimer disease for several years found an elderly woman crying out in pain. She did her best to put a pillow under the person's head and then walked back and forth between the nursing station and the person, trying to get help. She had a dementia herself now, but she had spent a lifetime as a caring nurse and in her heart remembered her skills and obligations.

A young nursing aide, obviously pregnant, seemed tired and discouraged as she cared for her client. The woman, who was quite confused, gently patted the aide. "I know you feel . . . I can see you do . . . Let me be your—your friend."

One woman never forgot how to play the piano. She could remember only one song, but she always smiled with delight when the staff commented on her skill.

When the doctor asked a person with dementia to remember three words as part of a memory test, she responded, "Young man, how dare you ask me such a thing."

An impaired man clearly enjoyed rocking a baby who was visiting the unit. But when the infant began to cry, he remembered just what to do: he quickly handed the child back to the mother.

A woman had had a major stroke and could no longer speak. She sat in a wheelchair while her family visited. When a staff member noticed that her robe was wet and urine was pooling under the chair, the staff member quietly put a lap robe over her to conceal her incontinence from her family. The woman smiled as best as she could and took the staff member's hand and kissed it.

Overhead/Handout 1.2. Alzheimer Patient Quotes

Alice, who has Alzheimer disease, said to her daughter, "I don't remember when I was born, but I'll be OK if you don't lose me."

A confused patient to her aide: "You're not so much as the other one. I like you more."

The doctor was interviewing a man with dementia. When the doctor asked how things were going for the man, the man replied: "Life's not so bad. After all, I'm only as old as seventy miles."

Hannah Wilson said: "It feels so good when people listen to you sometimes instead of telling you to do so much, so much, so much."

A woman was searching through her dresser drawer, saying to herself, "I've lost all thought. I don't know who I belong to."

Sarah, who often wept, said, "I've lost them. I've lost them. I've lost all anything of my life."

A person with dementia said to her nurse, "It all seems so gone. I don't say so much so I won't cry."

A woman with dementia said to her son, "I don't know what you all are so upset about. I'm the one who doesn't know who I am."

A man with dementia said, "Well, I'm not so bad. You know, sometimes I can do it. Some things go. If I can stop and try it out, I like to do that and I do that. You can't make yourself own up. Well, I couldn't do that. Like all I had to do was that. So I'm not so bad."

When a staff member began to undress a man before his bath, the man said, "Why do you make us guys look so dumb?"

Overhead/Handout 1.3. The Experience of the Person with Dementia

Dementing illnesses do not abruptly or uniformly disrupt a person's thinking: they gradually and selectively impair intellectual functions. In addition, other illnesses, a nonsupportive environment, fatigue, or stress can make persons with dementia even more impaired in function and intellect than they need be. The seemingly strange contradictions of impaired and spared areas of intellect are probably as frightening to persons with a dementia as they are to those who care for them.

At first, individuals may be aware of their failures and become deeply discouraged and frightened. They may fear that they are going insane. As the disease progresses, however, they will forget their forgetfulness and be unaware that they are ill. They will try to continue to do what they have always done—go to the office, prepare meals, or drive—unaware that they are getting lost or making dangerous mistakes.

People with dementia may be frustrated to the point of rage when they can no longer do simple tasks, such as button a dress or jacket or tie their shoes. Their environment becomes filled with inexplicable obstacles—once familiar tasks now lead to failure and embarrassment. Unable to understand why they fail, they may struggle to cover up their failures, or they may not understand what is wrong. Their clumsiness can be humiliating. As the disease progresses, they may not know who they are and may experience extreme and ongoing terror. They may cling tenaciously to the one person who seems familiar. When individuals with dementia are no longer able to convey pain or fear, no one may respond to them, although they will be unaware that no one can understand them. Yet their ability to enjoy human companionship—and to give and receive love—appears to continue some time after they have lost the ability to talk clearly or to care for themselves.

Source: U.S. Congress, Office of Technology Assessment, *Losing a Million Minds: Confronting the Tragedy of Alzheimer's Disease and Other Dementias,* OTA-BA-323 (Washington, D.C.: U.S. Government Printing Office, 1987), p. 59.

Overhead/Handout 1.4. The Progression of Dementia

At the beginning of the disease, people experience memory loss and a lack of spontaneity. They may have a change in language or handwriting or trouble doing mathematics. They lose the ability to make rapid hand and fine motor movements. They may cover up these difficulties, although many become depressed. Individuals may be uncharacteristically moody or exhibit sudden outbursts over trivial issues. They will be able to care for themselves and may be driving a car, cooking meals, or even living alone. The disease may go unrecognized until some event calls attention to the problem: they may get lost coming home from work, be asked to resign from a job, or have a car accident. Some minor additional stressor often precipitates a temporary decline in abilities, so that the individual's difficulty comes to the attention of others.

As the disease progresses, apraxia (problems carrying out purposeful movement) and aphasia (problems with language) appear and worsen steadily. People will be unable to remember new information for even two or three minutes, but their memory of the past will deteriorate more slowly. These individuals will no longer be able to work or to care for their personal needs independently. Such people cannot be left alone: they do not comprehend their limitations and therefore are at serious risk of accidents. At this point, most are still physically vigorous, and some cause significant problems by trying to walk away from their home or care setting.

During this period, people with dementia may show angry outbursts, sudden shifts of mood, suspicion, fearfulness, or violence. They need help in dressing, in eating, and eventually with using the toilet. Many of these individuals are awake and active at night. They do not recognize their need for care and often vigorously resist help.

The late stages of the disease often begin with the onset of incontinence. Gradually the apraxia progresses until these people are unable to walk without help. Many are bedfast. They will need to be bathed, fed, dressed, and taken to the toilet. They will be essentially mute; language will consist of only one or two words or cries. Behavior problems disappear due to the severity of the overall impairment.

Seizures are common. These people become feeble and emaciated. They may refuse to eat or be unable to swallow without choking, so that artificial feeding may be required. They are at risk of developing bedsores, infections, and pneumonia. Pneumonia is a common cause of death. There is significant variability in the symptoms from person to person, and some symptoms never appear in some individuals.

Source: U.S. Congress, Office of Technology Assessment, *Losing a Million Minds: Confronting the Tragedy of Alzheimer's Disease and Other Dementias,* OTA-BA-323 (Washington, D.C.: U.S. Government Printing Office, 1987), p. 67.

LESSON 2

HELPING THE PERSON BY UNDERSTANDING HOW THE BRAIN AFFECTS BEHAVIOR

Summary. This lesson links the brain damage due to dementia with function and behavior. This understanding is basic to all successful interventions. This lesson describes behavioral symptoms in which the brain damage is a primary cause. Each symptom is defined. The student is not expected to learn terminology or be able to make neuropsychological diagnoses.

Section 2.1. Understanding the Role of Brain Damage. Introduces the concept of the brain damage as the origin of behavioral symptoms in people with dementia and explains the impact of specific cognitive losses, such as loss of memory, language skills, and motor skills.

Section 2.2. Recognizing the Capacities That People with Dementia Commonly Retain. Teaches the student to recognize spared abilities. This understanding makes possible supporting self-esteem, dignity, and independence, which in turn are the essential tools for addressing dysfunctional behavioral symptoms.

Section 2.3. The Interplay of Personality, Life Experience, and Cognitive Losses. Describes the interplay of cognition and personality. The student learns to use personality to support the person's identity but never to explain behavioral symptoms.

Section 2.4. Abilities Commonly Impaired in Dementia. Teaches the student to recognize behavioral symptoms that may be caused by damage to the brain and to develop interventions that will help to improve quality of life for the impaired person.

Using the Sections

- Introductory course:
  - Section 2.1 required
  - Section 2.2 required
  - Section 2.3 use a few examples
- Core course:
  - Section 2.1 required
  - Section 2.2 required
  - Section 2.3 use a few examples
  - Section 2.4 required, but use only some items as relevant to the course

Problems You May Have in Implementing This Lesson

Many students are not aware of the range of cognitive functions that may be impaired in people with dementia. Take as much time as needed to help them understand the concept. To correctly identify which areas of mental function are impaired in an individual requires the skills of a neuropsychologist. Do not encourage students to "diagnose" deficits. Instead, focus on the concept that behavioral symptoms—which they can identify—are the result of neurological damage in the brain. With this knowledge, the student can separate behavioral symptoms from personhood, that is, "I like you, but your behavioral symptoms cause problems."

You may encounter the idea that this is "too medical," but the beginning of understanding a person includes understanding her strengths and weaknesses and that her behaviors are rooted in her illness.

Many programs will not have the skills of a neuropsychologist available. In the absence of specific information about spared and impaired functions, ask the students to define functions as clearly as possible without using diagnostic terms. For example, instead of saying a person has an apraxia, state that she can no longer button buttons but can still put her arms in her sleeves; or instead of saying a person has an agnosia, state that he seems not to recognize familiar people.

You may be concerned that otherwise unprepared lay staff members will have difficulty with these concepts. However, we have taught this material to many such groups and found that they not only enjoy it but also are quite adept at applying this knowledge to care. This knowledge of the underlying problems is essential to successful care.

Section 2.1. Understanding the Role of Brain Damage

Objective

The student will recognize that behavioral symptoms in people with dementia are profoundly influenced by damage to the brain caused by the dementia. Mental skills are lost unevenly: some remain, while others are lost. We help the person by recognizing this and by placing no demands on lost skills while enabling the person to use retained skills.

Background

Hundreds of individual mental functions are required for the smooth functioning of the human mind. As these are damaged by dementia, some losses (such as language function) are obvious, whereas others are not obvious. Combined, they may cause a single behavioral symptom or may appear in multiple behavioral symptoms. Do not expect students to learn this terminology or to be able to state which deficits cause which symptoms. The goal is for the student to learn that cognitive deficits account for many behavioral symptoms. Staff members can care for people well without putting a name to the cause of symptoms.

This understanding is essential for successful care of people with dementia and is the underlying framework for this course. Many of these ideas may be unfamiliar or counterintuitive. You will review these concepts throughout the course. Take time in this lesson to allow the students to integrate these ideas into their thinking.

Students will accept that changes in the brain account for some behavioral symptoms: loss of memory, difficulty understanding others and being understood, and loss of motor skills. The challenge is in helping students realize that damage within the brain also accounts for many other behavioral symptoms, such as loss of judgment and insight, arguing unreasonably, or inability to control impulses. A complex mix of spared and impaired functions may look to the layperson like "manipulation," "denial," "personality," or "life experience." Students bring with them the point of view of their culture, religion, awareness of recent research, and pop psychology. This combination may not include the new understanding coming from neuropsychology and psychiatry. Our understanding of the human brain is expanding rapidly and contradicting old ideas. Not enough time has elapsed for this information to reach the lay public.

Pop psychology, which many of us accept (including many mental health workers), holds that personality and life history explain people's behavior and that people are in control of their behavior most of the time. These assumptions are clearly not valid when the brain itself is damaged.

People with dementia who have a lifelong history of annoying behaviors complicate our understanding when these behaviors continue through much of the dementia. They tempt staff members to attribute current behavior to the old patterns. However, because the person has lost insight and memory, he no longer has the potential to change. He is probably continuing habitual behaviors but no longer has the option for learning new ways to cope with anxiety. We must respond to him differently.

This approach is not a medical model. However, it is necessary to understand the physical underpinnings of the behavior of a person with dementia. Why teach the different functions within the brain? Because if the student does not internalize the organic basis of the behaviors she must cope with, she will continue to respond to people based on her old assumptions. Also, this course teaches students to solve problems, which requires a set of correct assumptions about their cause and the ability to identify the specific problem.

This text provides merely a starting point: it describes only a few of the many cognitive deficits and gives only a few examples. *It does not list all the possible causes of a behavior and all potential interventions. The same symptom may have different causes in different people; there is great variability among individuals; there will be multiple causes for many problems—and, of course, the picture changes as the individual's disease progresses.*

Information and Instructions for the Teacher

Make the following points throughout the lesson:

- The person with dementia is trying as hard as she can. She is no longer able to choose or change lifelong personality traits or habits.
- Life experience and personality play important roles in the life of the person with dementia, but their role is in sustaining personhood, not in explaining behavior.
- Common sense or pop psychology approaches do an injustice to the person who is struggling to function despite serious deficits. Expecting the person to cope otherwise is tantamount to expecting a person with no legs to "stop whining" and walk. Such explanations for behavioral symptoms short-circuit the problem-solving process by applying pejorative labels that do not correctly describe the problem. Labels prevent us from seeing the person behind the behavior.
- The goal of treatment is to recognize which abilities have been lost and which remain. The care provider can then place few demands on lost functions and support those that remain.

Everyone wants to know how the brain works, and this makes the material fascinating. This lesson is fun: keep it lively, not academic. Acquaint yourself with the lecture notes and then present the material in your own words. Take as much time as needed to allow students to explore these new ideas. Stop and do a reality check often. Is this making sense to the students? Ask for students' ideas and questions.

Encourage discussion of each point as you go along. Ask for and suggest ways in which the care provider can place fewer demands on lost functions and support remaining functions. Discuss clients known to your group. Focus discussion on the easier clients until the team develops some expertise.

Use your knowledge of Sections 2.2, 2.3, and 2.4 to help you. The exhibits are for your guidance; do not hand them out.

The Mini-Mental State Examination (MMSE) tests seven important areas of mental function: orientation, registration, attention, calculation, recall, language, and spatial perception. It is helpful to review a completed MMSE from someone known to your group and discuss how these impairments affect function in this person. Often students will be surprised by certain losses. (See p. 359.)

You may choose to use the terms *aphasia* and *apraxia* or the lay terms "problems in talking," "problems in understanding words," and "problems doing familiar motor tasks."

By the time you have completed the introductory lecture, you will have covered deficits in the following areas: aphasia, apraxia, affect, insight, judgment, impulse control, long- and short-term memory, interpreting vision, coordination of mental functions, agnosia, postponing impulse, choosing among items, perseveration (inability to stop an activity), sequencing, and distractibility. More examples and discussion of these deficits are included in Section 2.4.

Lecture/Discussion Notes to Be Presented to the Class

Our brains do countless tasks so smoothly that we hardly notice. The brain is responsible for everything the body does and everything we think and feel, from drawing breath to planning a vacation, falling in love, or adjusting heart rate when we exercise. The brain always does many tasks at once. Only when the brain fails—when a person has a stroke, Alzheimer disease, or a severe head injury—do we think about how the brain works.

The brain is unimaginably complex. Because it is so complex, scientists are only now beginning to understand how it works. In Lesson 1 we talked about the brain cells and the billions of connections they make to do the tasks of running the body, thinking, and loving.

Scientists know that the brain divides these tasks so that different activities are carried out in different parts of the brain. The nerve cells and the approximately 200 chemicals are specialized for each job. When a stroke, head injury, or dementia damages some of these cells, the jobs they are responsible for do not get done. Other brain cells, however, continue to work normally.

Overhead/Handout 2.1. Some Mental Losses

For example, talking and understanding are carried out by an area of the brain located here: *(Teacher: put your hand on the left side of your head in front of and above your ear.)* This area of the brain handles speaking and understanding words. When you want to say something, this area "looks up the words in its dictionary" and then it puts the words in order. This part of the brain understands what your ears hear in the same way. When a person has a stroke in this area, he can no longer talk, but the rest of his brain may be functioning. Difficulty making yourself understood or difficulty understanding others is called an *aphasia.* Suppose you had lost the part of your brain that controls your ability to make sense when you talk but no other part of your brain? What would you feel (frustration, isolation, grief)? How would you act?

(Teacher: put your hand slightly behind your ear on the left side, draw a line toward the top of your head.) This is the part of your brain that moves your arms, legs, hands, and fingers and the rest of your body. In Alzheimer disease, damage to this area progresses slowly, from the person's being unable to do small tasks such as buttoning buttons or picking up food with a fork to stumbling or being unable to walk. This is what has happened if a person doesn't respond when people try to get him to walk or stand. When the brain can't tell the body to move but the bones and muscles are not damaged, this is called an *apraxia,* or problems in doing familiar motor tasks.

Alzheimer disease does not just affect *memory:* it affects each of these other functions as well. Often these other mental losses can disable the person more than problems with memory.

When a person has had a stroke or head injury, some areas may be severely damaged, while others are able to function normally. When a person has Alzheimer disease or another dementia, the disease gradually cripples cells in many areas of the brain and changes the availability of chemicals that those cells use. Some areas of the brain, which do certain tasks (e.g., memory), are damaged earlier than other parts of the brain. What we observe is a person whose abilities gradually decline. At the beginning, the person may have a problem just with memory; later she may have difficulty making herself understood, then gradually may develop more problems with eating and walking, and finally be bedfast and unable to speak. In the end, the brain may be unable to tell the lungs to keep breathing.

But the brain does not just dim out. Some skills remain longer than others. This is why we see people who can walk well but don't know where they are going or people who can argue but don't understand what we say to them.

The brain cells that control our emotions are located in several parts of the brain. Stroke or Alzheimer disease may damage these brain cells, so that a person is tearful, depressed, or irritable. People may have strange emotions that are not logical—evidence of the damage to the brain. Well people can control the extent to which they express their feelings: if you are furious with the boss, you may choose not to show your anger; or if you don't want your lover to know he has hurt you, you may laugh it off. But the person with dementia may lose this ability and cry or explode over even minor things.

(Teacher, put your hand on your forehead.) This area is responsible for knowing what you are doing (insight), judgment, and controlling impulses. This area is often damaged, but not destroyed, in Alzheimer disease, so people do things that don't make sense to us. Suppose you lost the motor part that moves your legs and you lost insight (you did not know you were disabled). How would you act? (You might try to walk.) People who keep trying to get out of a chair even though they would undoubtedly fall have this problem.

> A man insisted that he could drive just fine, although his son kept telling him he had had several accidents. Even when the son pointed out the dents in the car, the man insisted he had not caused them.

This man had lost insight, or the part of the brain that gives feedback about actions. No matter how much the son argued, nothing changed. Logic, reason, and dents in the fenders have no impact on a brain that has lost its feedback system. Because other parts of his brain were still working, however, there were ways to solve this problem. This man's doctor told him he could not drive. He had always done what his doctor told him, so he sadly stopped driving. This does not make much sense unless we understand that processing feedback (knowing what he had done) and obeying the doctor are different mental tasks.

By taking some cognitive skills and leaving others, the disease makes it harder to understand that the person is impaired, and this can make his caregivers frustrated and angry.

Alzheimer disease devastates the areas of the brain in which memories are stored. This devastation begins with the parts of the brain that store new memories—what happened this morning or yesterday. Memories of events in past years are usually remembered longer. Therefore, people lose short-term memory (memory for recent events) before they forget events long past. A person may remember her children when they were little and think that she lives in California although she now lives in a nursing home in Georgia.

Can you forget that you don't remember? (Yes.) If you don't remember, how would you know what you forgot? Cognitively well people often do remember that they have forgotten something; they just can't remember what. That is, the memory is in their mental files somewhere, but they can't find it. People with dementia never file the new information; they often don't know that they were told the information.

In the back of your head is the area of the brain that receives the messages from the nerves of the eye. If you damaged this area, your eyes would see things, but you would not know you saw them. So if the doctor said, "I know your eyes can see," and you said, "I don't see anything," who would be right? (Both.)

Deep inside the brain are important areas that coordinate the tasks of various brain areas. When these areas are damaged, complex mental functions are impaired. Also deep in the brain are some of the areas that affect feelings and that may be affected differently than memory.

People with dementia cannot help the damage to their brain—they are often not even aware of it, or they may sense that something is wrong but not know what. But that damage affects how they behave: whether they become angry, deny things that are obvious, or forget what you said. *They are trying as hard as they can to function with the brain cells and chemical messengers called neurotransmitters (see p. 51) they have left.*

In this lesson we will talk about some of the brain skills that people with dementia often lose. We can help the person by recognizing what is lost and doing those things for the person. But because many skills remain, we also help by knowing what brain skills remain and helping the person use those.

Because the brain is so complicated, understanding what is happening to a person gets very complicated. Let's review a few important points.

Overhead/Handout 2.2. Key Points to Remember about Brain Damage

Teacher: The notes below are to guide you in your discussion. Ask your group for examples of each point.

The disease causes most of the behavioral symptoms we see. The person is trying as hard as she can. It's the brain that is letting her—and us—down. If the person were herself, she might be difficult or sweet, smart or dull, but she would not be like this.

Some abilities are lost, while others are retained. Each person is different. What seems to be happening and what works in caring for one person will not help with another. The changes in the brain make caregiving individual. For example, some people quit driving on their own; others don't understand what the doctor said. Some will do what a son asks; others won't. If a family member fixes the car so it won't run, some people with dementia will give up; some will fix the car. (How can a person who does not know he had an accident fix the car? This is a classic example of the uneven nature of brain damage early in the dementia.) All these responses are powerfully influenced by changes in the brain that the person cannot help.

The person cannot help her behaviors, and explaining them to her may not help. When you try to care for someone, remind yourself that her behavior is caused by the disease, not by the person, and your goal is to help the person cope with the disease.

Because the brain is so complex, a person's abilities may come and go. The mind does not just fade away. It works like a flickering light bulb: sometimes it connects and sometimes it does not. This makes care providers and families think that the person can still do things if she wants to. A person may recognize her daughter sometimes and sometimes not or may recognize one daughter and not another. Sometimes a person who has not spoken for weeks suddenly speaks. Or a person can feed herself some days and not others. Although this might seem like evidence that the person can choose to talk or eat, it is really evidence of the brain damage. Doing something occasionally does not mean the person is getting better; it means the ability is gradually being lost. Accepting that the person is doing the best she can with what she has left and that these weird things have to do with brain cells is the best way to help the person.

The same behavior may have many causes. Solving problems would be easy if the same behavior always had the same cause. It doesn't. The same behavior will have different causes in different people and even in the same people at different times. Often you will not know why a person is doing what he is doing. Fatigue, stress, health problems, or multiple cognitive difficulties change the picture dramatically. There are many things you can do to help, and the remainder of this course will teach you how to help, even when the wondrous brain remains a mystery.

Making a Sandwich

To illustrate some of the brain skills we take for granted but that people with dementia often lose, I am going to tell a story about making a sandwich. Sit back and imagine you are this person.

> You are sitting at home watching television. To watch TV, you must be able to *understand what is being said* and you must be able to *remember* from moment to moment what is going on. People with dementia often lose both these skills.
>
> You decide that you want a sandwich but that you will wait until the commercial comes on. You are able to *postpone*. The ability to postpone is often lost in dementia.
>
> When the commercial comes on, you go to the kitchen and open the refrigerator door. Inside is part of a moldy pizza, a piece of pie, a jar of jelly, part of a roast, some bread, and some mayonnaise. You pick out the roast, the bread, and the mayonnaise and leave the rest. You are *able to choose among items,* a skill people with dementia may lose.
>
> You slice the bread. Slicing is a *motor skill* that dementia may damage. You stop slicing when you have enough for your sandwich. *Stopping* is a behavior that is lost for many people. People with this loss would go on slicing until the whole loaf was sliced.
>
> Next you lay out the bread, spread the mayonnaise on the bread, and put the roast beef on that. You are doing things in the right *sequence.* You can imagine what happens when you can't sequence things.
>
> The dog is walking around at your feet begging for some of the roast, but you ignore him. You are able to *tune things out.*
>
> Now it is about time for your show to come back on, so you decide to clean up during the next commercial. But the person you live with comes into the kitchen and says, "Look at the big mess you made." This irritates you but you don't want to get into a fight, so you clean it up quickly. You are able to *control your impulse* to argue, a mental skill often damaged in people with dementia.

The brain does these tasks and hundreds of others just to enable a person to get up from the TV and make a sandwich. Suppose you can do some of these things but not others. If you can't choose among items, you will get moldy pizza and jelly in your sandwich. If you can't sequence, you will spread mayonnaise on the table instead of the bread; if you can't tune things out, you might feed all the roast to the dog.

Overhead/Handout 2.3. How We Help

Teacher: Briefly discuss what each of these means.

- Once we recognize the problem, there is so much we can do to help.
- We help by enabling people to do what they still can.
- We help by not expecting people to do things they cannot.

These are the things that we can do to help. For example:

- Suppose a person with dementia is trying to make a sandwich but has difficulty choosing among items. If someone sets out just the things the person needs and takes away the moldy pizza and jelly, the person can still make his sandwich.
- Suppose a person can no longer control her impulse to get angry. If people avoid the things that upset her and take her to a quiet place to calm down when she does become upset, she'll still be able to manage in the day care group.
- Suppose a person feels sick today and can't make himself understood to tell anyone. Only if others recognize it from the way the person walks or the fact that he looks pale will he receive the care he needs.

Scientists have not found a way to cure these problems, but staff members can make a big difference by helping people do the best they can with their disease.

Exercise 1. Limiting Demands on Lost Functions

This exercise is a series of cases. Each case (1) defines the problem, (2) defines the cognitive deficit involved, and (3) suggests some interventions. The object is to help students reframe behavior in terms of the dementia. Use any or all of the cases. Encourage the group to discuss how the cognitive disability led to the problem and why the suggested interventions might work. Point out that the interventions are individual.

Case 1

Problem: Sally says she must go home for dinner. You tell her she does not live there now, but she says she has no money to pay for dinner.

Cognitive deficits involved: Memory, orientation.

Interventions: Furnish Sally's room with her own things and remind her that this must be her place, since her chair is here. Possessions say to the person, "This must be you because these are yours." Use a white lie: tell her that her daughter already paid for dinner. Tell her she can go home later, but invite her to eat with you. Make her feel like a welcome guest. White lies avoid confrontation and capitalize on appropriate social skills.

Case 2

Problem: Gene cannot make himself understood. Sometimes he becomes angry or cries because he tries so hard to make you understand.

Cognitive deficit involved: Expressive language.

Intervention: Listen closely to the first few words Gene says. Often these will give you a clue before he rambles off into confusion. Watch his body language closely. Don't say you understand when you don't. White lies here can get you into trouble because he may think you do understand. Ask him if he means. . . . Try interrupting if he seems to be rambling on and has forgotten the subject. Remind him of what he started out to say. See if this stops his building frustration. Pay attention to him.

Case 3

Problem: Tera comes out of her room with her bra and panties on over her running suit.

Cognitive deficit involved: Problems in sequencing.

Intervention: Save her pride: don't offer to help her put her clothes on right; instead, find an excuse to help her change into her favorite outfit (or a similar task that will allow you to get her underwear in the right place). If she objects, leave her alone. This is not a dangerous behavior. Document the reason for your decision, so that surveyors or family members understand.

Case 4

Problem: Vince pounds with his fists. He pounds on chair arms, walls, table tops. He does not appear to be upset, and he does not pound hard. He just pounds.

Cognitive deficit involved: Inability to stop a repetitive task.

Intervention: Check to see that he is not injuring his hands. Let him pound. Take advantage of his ability to do repetitive tasks, such as sanding, stacking silverware, carrying clean linen with you. Provide more one-on-one time—he may be seeking stimulation and attention in the only way he can.

Exercise 2. Cognitive Deficits and Empathy

The object of this exercise is to gain empathy for the person with dementia. Copy Exhibit 2.1. Cut these apart so that each item is on a separate slip of paper. Give one to each student. Ask each student in turn the question, "If you couldn't . . . , how would you act?" (Assume the person has lost insight, i.e., does not recognize her disability.) Encourage the group to think about how impairing these losses are. Student answers might be "I'd feel angry," "I'd cry," or "I'd say nothing was wrong."

Clinical Experience

Teacher: If you think that your group is not ready for the clinical experience, use the exercises instead. This lesson contains more exercises than you will need. This gives you the option of selecting exercises that will match the needs of your group.

Select a person with dementia known to you. Make a list of the specific ways in which problems in memory affect this person's daily life. List the ways in which the person reacts to this problem (for example, memory problems do not seem to bother her, or memory problems frustrate her, or she blames others for her memory problems).

For the same person, select one of the other mental losses the person experiences and do the same thing: list how this loss affects her daily life and list how she responds. Be specific.

In later lessons you will learn ways to help the person. In this lesson you are learning to observe and think about these losses.

Section 2.2. Recognizing the Capacities That People with Dementia Commonly Retain

Objective

The student will recognize abilities that remain in people with dementia. It is essential for successful care that the student see not just another patient with a failed brain but an individual with remaining abilities, no matter how limited.

Information and Instructions for the Teacher

This can be a fun and highly rewarding section. One of the most successful ways to reduce frustration and anger in people with dementia is to help them do for themselves the things that they can do. Recognizing spared functions makes it possible to support self-esteem, find a way to keep a person occupied, sustain independence, and plan activities. This is necessary if combativeness and agitation are to be reduced.

Sometimes the staff member's attention is understandably focused on the massive losses that interfere with care, and retained abilities are overlooked. The following exercise sensitizes the student to retained skills.

Retained skills change as the disease progresses. If you serve people at all stages, discuss the retained skills of each individual or divide the discussion into skills that are often retained in each stage. Refer to this material as you teach Lessons 5 and 6.

All care plans and evaluations should list the person's retained skills and strategies for encouraging them. Use staff meetings to identify an individual's retained skills, particularly for difficult people. A little humor is helpful; "He can hit people very hard" is a retained skill! It translates into "He has good upper body strength. Maybe we can find an activity for him."

Lecture/Discussion Notes to Be Presented to the Class

We have talked about the kinds of mental functions that are often lost when people develop a dementia. But the mental functions that people retain, at least for a while, are equally important.

The two main strategies we have for helping people are (1) not to expect people to do things they can no longer do—things that frustrate them and upset them—and (2) helping people to do the things that they still can do. That they still have some independence helps them feel good about themselves. This helps reduce angry outbursts.

At the beginning of the disease, people can still do many things. It's important not to take over more than necessary for the person. As the disease progresses, we can often help a person by finding out which parts of a task she can't do and which she can do. Maybe she can still dress herself if we hand her clothes one at a time, or maybe she can still water the garden if we don't care how much water is spilled. Late in the disease, only a few things will remain. We want to celebrate those: the ability to walk with help, to smile, to hold hands with a friend.

People who are depressed or who are upset and angry most of the time will be challenging, but we can usually find small things they can still do.

Exercise 3. Identifying Retained Skills

Emphasize the reasons why recognizing and respecting remaining strengths is important. These observations will be particularly valuable when the staff person is providing activities-of-daily-living (ADL) care. Then ask the class to form small groups. Each group will select a person known to them and make as complete a list as possible of that person's retained skills. Students often have difficulty thinking of any retained skills in difficult clients. Therefore, suggestions are provided in Exhibits 2.2, 2.3, and 2.4. Suggestions are listed by (1) stage of the illness, (2) skill category, and (3) a few real case examples. Use the examples in your presentation to help students get started. Do not hand out these long lists. Urge them to make their own lists. Regroup and discuss the remaining skills they have identified. Use this approach in later lessons whenever a difficult case is discussed in class.

Clinical Experience

For one of the people discussed in the exercise, develop a plan to encourage or support her remaining function or to provide more time for this person to function in a positive way.

Section 2.3. The Interplay of Personality, Life Experience, and Cognitive Losses

Objective

The student will learn about the relationship between life experience, personality, and dementia.

Information and Instructions for the Teacher

Present the brief lecture notes, emphasizing the idea that dementia distorts the personality we observe. Ask for examples from people the students know, and discuss how the dementia affects their behavior. These concepts will be new to many students.

Remind students that our goal is to improve the quality of life and find solutions to behavioral problems. Assuming that a behavior is manipulative or the outcome of past experience is a dead end: it places responsibility on a person who has no insight and cannot change and consigns that person's pain to the "nothing we can do for you" category. When we see a suffering person who cannot help himself, often the only one who can change is the care provider.

The second part of this section lists some common misunderstandings students may have. Use them only if they apply to your group, or come back to them in later lessons when the issues arise.

Lecture/Discussion Notes to Be Presented to the Class

In Section 2.1 we talked about ways in which brain damage influences behavior. But in practice, when we care for people, we often wonder whether what they are doing is the result of brain damage or their personality, or whether the way they were raised, their childhood, and life experience made them this way.

Perhaps as we talked about brain damage you wondered if we had forgotten that each person is a unique individual, with a personality, a particular style of coping, and a history that makes her special. In this section we will talk about these issues.

The dementia does not take away any of these things. The individual's unique personality, coping style, and history continue to be important to care providers and to the person with dementia. *However, we use our knowledge of these things to support the person's identity and self-esteem and never to explain behavioral symptoms.*

Imagine that you are looking through a lens that distorts things. The dementia distorts the way we see the individual's personality. For example:

> Mrs. Massenda was a gracious, charming woman who could become strong willed and irritable when pressured. As she developed a dementia, she felt pressured so much of the time that she seemed to her home care worker to be always nasty and never gracious.

> Mr. Luong's lifetime coping style was to boss people around when he felt stressed. His wife and employees knew and accepted this because he was usually a good employer and husband. As he developed Alzheimer disease, he felt lost and useless and shouted at his care providers much of the time. When the staff helped him feel comfortable and good about himself, he fell back on his bossy style less often.

In each of these individuals, staff members are seeing personality, history, and coping style through the distorting lens of the illness.

When a person has a dementia, we use personality to sustain identity and personhood but not to explain behaviors. We can easily see how the mental losses change how people behave. For example:

> Elisa's family said that in the past she was often critical of them, complaining and making them feel bad. Now Elisa's illness has taken away her ability to make sense when she talks. Because she can no longer criticize, Elisa seems to her family to have become much nicer.

> Mary has always had a sweet disposition. She was always pleasant and hardly ever appeared to be angry. But the disease has taken away her ability to control feelings of frustration. Now Mary blows up over minor things.

How personality changes (or appears to change) is different for each person.

> Ray had been a charming gentleman. His wife had always waited on him and looked after him, but he had a way of making her feel glad to help him. He did the

same thing at his job. He got others to do most of the work, but in such a nice way that everyone loved him. Ray settled into the residential care home easily. He was content to sit and let others do for him, but he was liked by everyone.

Mr. Winsted was a strongly independent man who preferred to do things himself or to closely control others. This independence did not fit in well in a group setting, where his disability meant that he should let others do for him.

The effect of personality seems different at different times in the illness. We see many old personality traits in the early stages of the illness, but later, personality can seem to change. How we see personality depends on our viewpoint. Sometimes families say, "He is not the same person he used to be." Other families, even late in the illness, say, "I can still see her old self, sick as she is."

A person's apparent personality will be influenced by what she thinks is going on.

Anna apparently thought she was in a hotel. Her behavior was that of a person who expected to be waited on, even though it was really her daughter, not a hotel maid, who was caring for her. Anna's daughter did not understand this misperception and thought Anna no longer loved her. When Anna moved to a residential care home, the staff allowed her to think she was on a cruise ship. So long as she could give orders, play bingo, and enjoy meal service, she was easy to get along with. (This was unique to Anna. It will not work with most people.)

Teacher: The following are questions that staff members may ask or assertions that may be reflected in staff attitudes. This material is intended to guide you in addressing these issues. Select only those issues that are relevant to your group, and discuss them in your own words.

- *"Doesn't he know how much trouble he's causing?"* To know how much trouble he is causing, the person must remember what he did to cause trouble and have insight into his behavior. Early in the illness, some people seem not to understand the impact of their illness on the caregivers. This can be difficult to accept because at this point the person seems to be only slightly impaired. If it happens, it is most likely linked to complex and subtle changes within the brain.

- *"She's in denial."*

Myrtle could not manage at home any more. It was time for her to move to a nursing home, but she insisted that she could function as well as ever. When her daughter pointed out the rotting food in the refrigerator and the burned saucepans, Myrtle insisted that they weren't there.

If we understand that Myrtle's loss of insight means that she does not connect the problem with her behavior, her answer makes sense. Instead of trying to argue with her, her family can help her cope with her feelings of loss. She may be able to help select things that are special to her or determine who is to get certain things "when she does have to move."

- *"She's trying to get attention."*

"Honey, I have to go to the bathroom," Zelda called out to every person who walked by her. When someone took her to the toilet, she passed only a few drops of urine. "You just went," staff members usually said. But this made Zelda cry.

Urinary frequency is often caused by medications or urinary retention. Zelda may feel an urge all the time. (These symptoms are frustrating to anyone.) Treating the medical problem may make her more comfortable.

But what about Walter? Walter does not have a urinary tract infection. He reaches out for a staff person and asks for something, but he forgets what he wants as soon as the person stops to listen. Is he just trying to get attention? Can Walter remember he has already asked? Are Walter's needs being met when he can't communicate them? Could he just need attention?

- *"She's being manipulative."*

Betsy doesn't like her dinner. Her caregiver brings her another one, but Betsy doesn't like it either. She says she wants eggs, so a special dish of eggs is made for her, but she doesn't want that either. The home makes every effort to serve what she likes, but she still complains.

Does Betsy remember that she has now asked for her third dinner? Did she remember that she ordered eggs by the time they got to her?

To be manipulative, the person must be able to remember how others responded the last time she tried the behavior. If a child has a temper tantrum and the mother gives in, the child remembers that temper tantrums work. But if the person can't remember your response to her behavior, she can't manipulate you. She probably will rely on old habits to get through. If temper tantrums were a lifelong habit, it may be the only behavior available to her. The difference is that now she has no option of changing.

- *"Isn't he just stubborn/willful/deliberate?"* Deliberate behavior requires that the person be able to plan and anticipate what the outcome will be. To be deliberate, the person must know the purpose of his act. Usually it is obvious that the person has lost these skills. But sometimes it is hard to understand.

  Mark urinated in the wastebaskets. The staff thought that he did this deliberately and pointed out that he did this only when no one was watching. But it is unlikely that Mark's dementia allowed him to think, "I'm going to get back at those nurses, so when no one is looking, I'll do it in the trash." It's much more likely that Mark was disoriented about the trash cans but still had a need for privacy.

  Stubbornness, willfulness, and deliberateness are behaviors that are useful and respected in successful people (think of football coaches). When a two-year-old is stubborn, we say he will have a strong personality. The trouble is, these same strategies don't work very well when you can't take care of yourself and others have to take care of you. By looking at these as effective strategies that just don't fit any more, we can find ways to care for a person and let him be himself.

- *"Does personality change when the person develops a dementia?"* When we speak of personality, we mean the sum of the mental and behavioral characteristics that make each person unique. Personality is made up of many cognitive qualities, and as the dementia progresses, personality seems to remain and yet be lost and to change. Often staff members will not know for sure whether personality or other factors are responsible for the behavior they see. But good staff members know how important it is to help sustain the person's sense of who he is and that he is special.

- *"Doesn't he act that way because that was the way he was brought up?"* Or "because of what happened when his brother died?" or "because of the way her husband treated her?" "Isn't she hoarding things because she went hungry as a child?" "Isn't she crying now for the sister who died twenty years ago?"

  Each person's life story is important. We use it to help the person maintain a sense of self. It is not as useful in explaining behavior for the same reason that personality is not: the relationship between behavior and life experience is very complicated, and it does not help us find a way to help. What is happening right now in a person's life often helps us understand and intervene. The person who is hoarding things may have always taken a snack to bed with her, but now she has lost track of how much spoiled food she has. The person who is crying is more likely to be crying because she is depressed, is frustrated, or feels ill.

  Liu cried easily and often. The staff did not know very much about this 83-year-old man with cancer and dementia. They did know that he had lost most of his family in a purge in China many years ago and that he had left a wife and five children behind when he escaped to the United States. They assumed that his tears expressed grief over these terrible losses. But Liu was old and ill. He physically felt sick. He was totally lost in the nursing home, where he was the only Chinese man. When the staff focused on dealing with his present predicament, Liu perked up and obviously enjoyed the elderly Chinese visitor they arranged for him.

- *"She's always been like that."* Many people use strategies such as manipulation, denial, dependency, and control throughout their lives. It is difficult for such people to change when they have no dementia—even psychiatric care often falls short. These people may continue to use the same ways of interacting after they have a dementia. But things have changed. The person can no longer remember what she just did and rarely has any insight into how her behavior affects others. It is too late for her to change. She is probably carrying on her annoying behavior out of habit.

All her life, Mavis complained of various ailments—some real, others more a symptom of her anxiety. Her children said she would "get sick" every time she wanted them to do something. Now Mavis says, "I'm sick, I'm sick. I'm dying," although she is in good health except for her Alzheimer disease. She has always talked about illness and that is what occupies her now.

It's unfair to blame a person for continuing a behavior past the point where the person has an option for change. Behavior modification rarely helps because the person does not remember what she did for more than a few seconds.

Perhaps the best solution for Mavis is to give her lots of attention and reassurance and to divide up the time spent with her among the entire staff so that she does not upset anyone.

When we label behaviors, we shortchange the person and stop the caring process.

People's life stories, our knowledge of their past personality, and their coping mechanisms help us sustain a sense of who they are. It helps us enormously to understand the person and to find and celebrate what is left. It is not useful as a tool to explain behavior.

Section 2.4. Abilities Commonly Impaired in Dementia

Objective

The student will learn to recognize behavioral symptoms that are influenced by damage to the brain and be able to suggest possible interventions for each symptom discussed.

Background

Rather than moving directly to teaching caregivers how to manage ADLs and behavioral symptoms, this course teaches three basic concepts: cognitive abilities, excess disabilities, and stress. Only after learning these concepts can the student effectively provide care (Lessons 5–11). The specific interventions in this lesson are examples of *concepts* rather than formulas for intervention.

This section is critical to the course. It discusses complex behaviors that are, to a great extent, caused by the brain damage, and it presents many strategies for care. The student's ability to select the right intervention for an individual is improved when the student learns to think of problems in terms of specific individual cognitive (or functional) deficits.

This approach enables the student to think in terms of reducing demands on specific lost functions and, equally important, planning ways to support retained functions. It reduces the distress and behavioral symptoms of the person with dementia.

Most behavioral symptoms are the result of a combination of the brain damage, excess disability, and stress (caused by environment, fatigue, and other factors). The balance between these factors varies. The behavioral symptoms listed in this lesson appear to be strongly influenced by the damage to the brain. Lessons 3 and 4 address excess disability and stress. When the students understand these three factors—brain damage, excess disability, and stress—they will have the basic tools for individualized care.

Knowledge of these underlying causes of disability in people with dementia greatly improves the student's ability to make changes within his existing setting. This information can easily be taught to unsophisticated students. Students with no background can understand and apply the concept that brain function underlies disability and that specific kinds of lost function result in specific disabilities. Use the MMSE (see Chapter VI) routinely with staff members to identify common deficits. Share information from neuropsychological testing, which is increasingly common and which provides a wealth of information about spared and lost functions. Professional staff members can translate technical terms into lay terms.

In the absence of specific neuropsychological information, students will always have to guess. This is done by defining the specific problem in terms of lost function in as much detail as possible. Even when no one is sure of the precise term for the deficit, defining the problem in this way will enable students to clearly see individual interventions.

This section expands on the concepts presented in Section 2.1 and provides suggestions for interventions. Successful interventions are individual: those suggested are to get the student started. The remaining lessons (beginning with Lesson 5) provide additional guidance in applying these concepts to such areas as ADL care, communication, and sustaining relationships.

Information and Instructions for the Teacher

There are several ways to use this material.

Use it as background for your own preparation as you teach the remaining lessons.

As problems arise in Lesson 5 and subsequent lessons, teach those behavioral symptoms that seem to apply to individual cases.

Teach as much of this material now as your students can internalize without becoming overwhelmed. Each impairment is described in the text. Keyed to the text are exhibits describing common symptoms of each impairment and suggested interventions. Select one impairment at a time. Hand out the exhibit or use it as an overhead. Use the accompanying text to describe it. Ask for similar examples. Discuss how this disability will impair function. Stop the presentation often and discuss clients known to the group or discuss the meaning of the material. Use functional rather than medical terms, and encourage your students to do so also. By using functional descriptions, you will avoid the pitfall of mislabeling impairments.

While you do not want to overload your students, the more of this material they understand, the easier it will be for them to plan interventions for people with dementia. Take as much time as needed, and teach the material in two class periods if necessary. If your students understand the first four lessons in this text, they will quickly grasp the subsequent lessons. By using basic language rather than technical terms, you ensure that even the least-prepared students will be able to understand this material. Look for ways to make your presentation relaxed and interesting.

Lecture/Discussion Notes to Be Presented to the Class

Briefly review Section 2.1. Make the following points. Use Section 2.1 to refresh your understanding of these points.

- Cognitive deficits are a factor in behavioral symptoms and disability.
- Close observation will help identify what the person can and cannot do, although you will often not be able to diagnose the specific neurological deficit.
- Three common behaviors indicate problems in mental function: refusal to do a task, failure in the performance of a task, and evidence of increased stress. These behaviors indicate problems in mental function and not stubbornness or personality.
- Usually a behavioral symptom is the result of multiple deficits.
- Some deficits (language problems, memory, motor skills) follow the course of the illness; others are much less predictable.
- Some disabilities occur in all people with the same disease; others are infrequent or may not occur at all.
- A behavioral symptom may be caused by different things in different people or even in the same person at different times. For example:

  Bob said, "No, thank you" because he did not know what he was being asked and used this to save face. Lewis said, "No, thank you" because he was depressed. Sarah said, "No, thank you" because her arthritis hurt her. Lucy said, "No, thank you" angrily because she was stressed.

- Different cognitive symptoms may cause the same behavioral symptom.
- When the underlying dementia is not treatable, the person cannot be retaught these cognitive skills.
- Psychoactive medication will not change the underlying difficulty.
- Despite these factors, there is almost always something the staff can do to alleviate the person's discomfort and reduce behavioral symptoms.

Present and discuss Overhead/Handout 2.1 if needed. For professional groups, consider using Exhibits 2.5 through 2.21 as overheads/handouts.

Some Cognitive Abilities Affected in Dementia

Agnosia. Agnosia is the failure to recognize a familiar object. A common and devastating agnosia is the failure to recognize familiar faces. These people have not forgotten the relationship with a spouse or child but are no longer able to recognize the face. They may say, "You look like my son, but you're not my son." They may fail to recognize themselves in the mirror and instead insist that some stranger (for example, the wife's putative lover) is in the bathroom. Reassure the family that this is a neurological failure and not a failure to be aware of the relationship or of intimacy. Agnosias resist intervention, and medication is often not helpful. Accept the phenomenon and adapt the environment. (See Exhibit 2.5.)

> Mrs. Barnes did not recognize her husband. She would ask him where she had met him and insist that he was not her husband. However, she would warmly greet all of her five grandchildren. She did not know their names, but she did understand that they were her grandchildren. The Barneses had had a difficult marriage. Mr. Barnes had been unfaithful, and in the years that followed, Mrs. Barnes had treated him coldly. The family felt that she deliberately denied knowing him to "get back at him."

It is more likely that Mrs. Barnes had a facial agnosia

and lacked the cognitive skills to plan and carry out this behavior as a way of punishing her husband. Agnosia can be eerily selective. It is not unusual for a person to have an agnosia for one person but not for others. When other children visited, the staff suspected that Mrs. Barnes thought all young children were her grandchildren.

Apathy. Apathy is not laziness. Damage to certain areas of the brain results in considerable apathy. Often nonparticipation is caused by many potentially treatable conditions. Apathy may indicate the presence of depression, pain, or illness. Do not assume it is primarily cognitive. If these other factors are ruled out and a cognitive cause for apathy is identified, a balance must be created between not letting a person become isolated and encouraging the person to be more involved than he can tolerate. People do not have to be involved at a predetermined level, but adequate social stimulation must be provided. The level of involvement must be based on the individual, the diagnosis, and the person's wishes. Restlessness or tearfulness may indicate overstimulation. (See Exhibit 2.6.)

Aphasia. Aphasia is loss of ability to express or understand language or problems in communication. Communication is one of the things that makes us human and makes relationships possible. As it is lost, both the person with dementia and the family suffer. Caregivers may overestimate or underestimate the extent of loss. There are many ways you can help. People may be able to use the first language they learned longer than languages they learned later; however, in progressive dementias, all languages will be lost. Lesson 6 focuses on language problems. There are many different types of language disorders.

Expressive language is the ability to speak and be understood. It is lost gradually: difficulty finding words may occur early, while later the person may ramble on but not be understood. The first three or four words may have the most meaning. Knowing the name of something is different from knowing what it is or what do with it.

When a nurse conducted an MMSE, she showed Bob her pen and asked, "What is this?" Bob took the pen and wrote with it but could not say what it was. Lucille also could not name the pen, but she could describe it as "a thing you write with."

Receptive language is the ability to understand others. It may not be lost in parallel with spoken language. It can come and go: never say things you do not want the person to understand. Do not assume that skill or loss in one skill means a similar skill or loss in the other.

A woman was able to talk quite coherently, although on close examination there was little substance to her conversation. She said things such as, "Thank you, honey. You are so pretty. You are so nice." The staff did not realize that she comprehended almost nothing of what they said to her.

In contrast, another man could not express himself but took everything in.

Apraxia. Apraxia is difficulty carrying out motor functions. As Alzheimer disease progresses, people lose the ability to do motor tasks even though their bones and muscles are still intact. The brain stops telling the muscles what to do. In general, fine motor skills such as buttoning buttons, picking up small items, and handwriting are lost first; then ADL skills such as using eating utensils are lost. Eating with the fingers usually remains after the person cannot use utensils. Later the person may shuffle and have difficulty stepping over ledges. Late in the illness the person may lose the ability to walk, sit down, and maintain balance. Old, overlearned motor skills such as dancing and playing the piano may be retained for a surprisingly long time. Rocking a baby is often retained until very late in the illness and makes a nice activity for severely impaired people. Problems in apraxia are discussed throughout the lessons. By assessing the motor tasks that each person can still do and those that are lost, staff members can facilitate a high level of independence. Because people with an apraxia also cannot learn, adaptive devices such as walkers and built-up handles will help some but confuse others. The MMSE assesses changes in handwriting and drawing that reveal a subtle apraxia.

If you ask a man to get up out of his chair and he cannot do it, try sitting down beside him and then get up. Often a man will rise too. (The old habit of rising when a woman does may cue him successfully.) Try similar cues for other problems. (See Exhibit 2.7.)

Changing Sets. Changing sets is the ability to change from one movement or task to another. (Perseveration and initiation are also involved.) The person lacking the ability to change will continue to repeat the same task.

A woman washed one arm over and over. No matter how much the home nurse encouraged her, she did not wash the other arm or her legs.

Sometimes touching the body part you want the person to start washing will trigger a change. Try gently touching the person's spoon to another food to prompt her to eat a different food item. (See the subsection "Perseveration" later in this lesson.)

Changing tasks (as from activities to mealtime) or changing spaces (as from bedroom to dining room) will upset people who have difficulty changing sets. Allow extra time, increase all sensory cues, use one-to-one assistance to bridge the change.

Choosing. Choosing among items is the ability to select from among several things those that one wants. Difficulty in choosing among items is only one of several deficits that may lead to these behaviors. (See Exhibit 2.8.) (The first two examples in Exhibit 2.8 may also be perseverative, and the person who cries may be overly stressed by the question. This is an example of the same behavior having different causes.)

Compensation. For part of the illness, people may retain the capacity to conceal or compensate for disability. This is a strength that should be encouraged; unfortunately, the compensations the impaired person finds often exasperate the caregiver. Tact is important in providing care while allowing a person to hang on to the compensatory strategies.

A woman had some stress incontinence but had lost the ability to organize washing out her panties, so she hid them in her closet. She denied her incontinence. Instead of indignantly hauling the panties out of the closet and confronting her, her niece discreetly washed them for her.

A man was unexpectedly incontinent of stool. When the staff found him, he had smeared stool on the bedding and the walls. At first the staff thought that this was a new bizarre behavior, but in fact the man had tried to clean up the accident, gotten stool all over his hands, and then tried to clean his hands. Because of his dementia, he had made a terrible mess, but his intent was to clean himself.

People sometimes lose the ability to compensate for deficits. This problem often occurs in combination with a failure to know that there is a need to compensate (insight). People with this problem will not compensate for sensory deficits: they will not turn on a light to improve vision or tell you they can't hear you. They will not walk carefully if they are unsteady. They may remove hearing aids because they are uncomfortable. Tasks of compensation must be done for them by staff members. (See Exhibit 2.9.)

Disorientation. Disorientation is failure to know where one is, who one is, and/or date or time of day. People may behave in public as if they were in private by disrobing or toileting; they may mistake staff members for intimates. Disoriented people may mistake daughters for wives. Inappropriate sexual behaviors are often simply disorientation. People may go to sleep in others' beds, walk into strangers' homes. These symptoms may have many causes. Determine individually whether reorienting helps reduce stress. There are many symptoms of disorientation: two that cause problems are listed. (See Exhibit 2.10.)

Distractibility. Distractibility is the inability to focus on one thing and ignore other things. If a person cannot focus his attention, he won't be able to register what you tell him. People who are easily distracted may reach for other objects as you dress them, wander away from activities or meals. These people are unable to tune out extraneous cues. Cognitively intact people routinely ignore noises, people, or multiple objects. People who have lost this skill will be distracted by many things around them. When there are several things for a person to focus on, she may feel increased stress. (See Exhibit 2.11.)

Impulse Control. Impulse control is the ability to control, divert, or postpone the expression of feelings such as anger, frustration, fear, and anxiety. The loss of this ability leads to striking out, shouting, and other explosive behaviors. This control varies with the individual, the occasion, and the situation. It is not necessarily logical: control may be lost over minor issues or over only some issues. For example, while some people cannot contain the impulse to strike out, few exhibit the impulse to run down the street naked. This behavioral symptom can be successfully managed by reducing the stress that leads to frustration. (See Lesson 4.)

Initiation. Inability to initiate is the inability to get started. The person with problems initiating behavior cannot start a movement, action, or task such as walking, feeding himself, getting out of a chair. Once started, these people can often successfully continue the task. Initiating motor tasks is difficult for people with Parkinson disease. You may need additional or different strategies to help them. Not participating may be due to problems in initiating, depression, motor skills, apathy, pain, illness, overmedication, or Parkinson disease. (See Exhibit 2.12.)

Insight. Insight is the ability of the brain to monitor what one is doing. People who lack insight have no way of knowing that they have a dementia or that they are making mistakes. This is not denial. Insight gives people feedback about how they are performing. Right now your insight is telling you that you have your clothes on, that you are acting all right, that your hands are not in someone else's lap. Without insight, you would not know whether you were acting right in the classroom—but you also would not know that you did not know.

Insight is lost early for some people and somewhat later for others. If a person has some insight in the beginning of the disease, she may have concerns about her illness, sometimes be depressed, and be able to participate in planning for her future. (Depression may be part of the disease process or part of the person's awareness of loss.) Other people lose insight early in their illness and vigorously deny any illness or deficit. Arguing is counterproductive.

While caregivers will discuss the illness and plans for change with the former group, there is little point in such discussions with people who have no insight into their illness. These people may be persuaded to stop driving, make a will, and so on through other reasons.

People often have partial insight—insight into some things or a vague awareness of failure or awareness that comes and goes. For example, one woman was able to tell her friends that she had a memory problem, but she insisted that she was handling her checkbook well, even when she was not. This infuriated and frustrated her family but was characteristic of the uneven nature of insight loss.

Loss of insight means profound change and creates behavior that can seem totally illogical. Because many people lose this ability early, while they can still argue, they are often seen as being difficult, stubborn, or nasty. What does it mean *not to know* that your memory is gone, that your feedback system is destroyed, that you don't have good judgment?

Care providers can turn loss of insight into an advantage. People with limited insight may enjoy interpersonal time or activities without being aware of their obvious limitations. For example, a woman who did poorly on her MMSE was not aware of her "wrong" answers and cheerfully enjoyed her visit with the therapist. (See Exhibit 2.13.)

Judgment. Judgment is the ability to make critical distinctions and to arrive at sensible decisions. It requires memory, insight, and other complex cognitive skills. Judgment is often lost early in the disease, at which time caregivers have difficulty determining whether the person's judgment is disabled or whether the person is being eccentric. Vestiges of judgment surrounding lifelong goals and values (such as a long-intended wish to make a person one's heir), a sense of propriety, morality, and social appropriateness often remain for much of the illness. People may also retain the ability to make immediate decisions about things they want or like, such as what to wear or which staff member they like.

A person may show good judgment in some things but not in others. For example, a staff member explained to a daughter that her mother's willingness to give money to dubious charities might well be evidence of a decline in judgment. But the daughter responded, "She shows very good judgment about when to call the doctor."

The capacity of a person to make responsible decisions is more complex than is often assumed. The advice of a neuropsychologist is helpful. Care providers should guard against taking too paternalistic a stand. Keep in mind that cognitively well people often disagree over what is good judgment.

If a person must make a will or assign durable power of attorney, the family should consult an attorney regarding the exact legal definition of competency. Judgment may vary from day to day. Helping with problems in judgment must be done on an individual and problem-by-problem basis.

Learning. Because they can't remember things, people with dementia have extremely limited ability to learn. Since learning comes so easily for us, we often assume the person can learn at least simple things, such as daily routines. This assumption frustrates both staff members and the person.

Once in a while, someone does learn something, but this is the exception rather than the rule. It does not prove that the person can learn anything else. Avoid tasks or behavioral interventions that depend on learning. Celebrate the occasional learning without expectation.

People with dementia do seem to "learn" general impressions, such as which people in the room are their caregivers—and therefore the ones they must depend on. People with dementia are often better able to retain information that is associated with emotions:

> A woman who had been bruised seemed afraid of one staff member. She could not name the person, but her memory of fear was probably accurate.
>
> A staff member gradually coaxed a shy woman into laughter. After that, each time she saw the staff member, this woman would smile and reach out.
>
> A man and woman who could not remember the way around the unit, and who were both almost mute, would smile and hold hands whenever they came across each other.

Use frequent reminders and orientation to place and person, and do not expect the person to learn these things.

Memory. Memory is the ability to recall past events. There are many terms for the different aspects of memory: short term, long term, emotional. Be cautious about making assumptions about the nature of memory: scientists are learning that many of our assumptions are wrong. Memory is an exciting area of research for neuropsychologists, who are discovering that it is much more complex—in all of us—than had been previously understood. We all probably remember some things and forget others. This is why so many husbands and wives disagree over the details of their wedding, although they agree that there was a wedding. Memory associated with feelings is probably stored and retrieved differently than memory for facts. Memory in any person is not a tape that plays back events accurately. It is rapidly, but unevenly, devastated in dementia. (See Exhibit 2.14.)

Registration is the ability to hold information in mind briefly. It is tested for in the MMSE. If a person cannot register information, she cannot remember things for even a minute or two. If you tell this person why you are taking her clothing off, she won't remember by the time you get to the next button.

Recall is the ability to remember something that happened or something the person was told a few minutes earlier. The person may recall some things but not others. What a person remembers can be unpredictable and may not be what you want him to recall. This is tested for in the MMSE.

Short-term memory is memory for events that happened not long ago. If a person is impaired in short-term memory and you tell her she needs to have a bath because her family is coming in the afternoon, she may have no idea why you want to bathe her by the time you get to the bathing area. People with short-term memory loss may not recall having visitors, what you just told them, why their leg is in a brace, or that lunch will soon be ready.

Most people lose the ability to register information or hold it in short-term memory fairly early in their illness. This is the hallmark of the dementia and is the most profound reason that compassionate care is essential. A person with problems in registration or short-term memory must absolutely trust those around her, yet most of us don't have a life experience of trusting strangers to undress us and toilet us. The care provider's understanding and approach largely determine the degree of anxiety the person experiences.

The anxiety over not knowing what is going on explains why a person will not let a spouse out of her sight (as soon as the spouse disappears, the person cannot remember where the spouse went) and contributes to the caregiver's frustration ("I just told her!").

Long-term memory is memory for things that happened weeks or years ago. It may be better preserved for a longer part of the illness. People may remember marriages, children, work, homes from long ago. Long-term memory is selective: people may not remember some significant events (such as weddings or traumatic events) but remember others. People may remember relationships but fail to recognize pictures of the people themselves. Sometimes people remember the long past and forget the present. Be aware that the "facts" a person tells you may be distorted by distance or flawed memory. The person may always relate the same bit of memory, unaware that she has told you many times.

This long-term memory is one of the greatest resources for sustaining the person's identity and for conversation topics. Do not try to correct accounts or "dig" for additional memory. Use the existing memory and the time together to support identity and a sense of self. Tap long-term memory of objects: even severely impaired people may recognize kitchen utensils or common tools.

Amnestic syndrome is a condition in which the cognitive deficit affects only memory. This is often observed in people with Korsakoff syndrome. People with amnestic syndrome characteristically remember the distant past clearly, the middle past spottily, and the recent years not at all. When their diagnosis is unrecognized, they can be frustrating for staff members. Their language and motor skills are essentially unimpaired.

> A 76-year-old man wrongly diagnosed as having Alzheimer disease was sure that he was 46 years old, that Nixon was president, and that he was a salesperson in another state. No evidence to the contrary, such as his aging body, persuaded him. He often eloped ("going to the office") and so eloquently charmed the police that they did not believe the nursing home director. He had married three different women in the past 30 years, forgotten each marriage, and failed to obtain divorces. He was not a fraud: he truly lived only in the world he remembered.

Mood (Affect). Irritability, depression, restlessness, and other moods are caused in part by the neurological changes in the brain. However, problems of mood are highly responsive to environmental change or medication (or both). Stress and difficulty comprehending the environment and other people are also major factors. For example, Mary did not realize that she needed a shower, so she became upset when her nurse suggested she bathe. Symptoms of problems in mood are discussed in Lessons 4 and 9.

Damage to specific areas of the brain can lead to odd symptoms of mood.

> Bob Hamilton cried easily and often. The staff knew that years earlier Bob's brother had committed suicide. The staff felt that Bob had never properly grieved, so the staff social worker spent time encouraging Bob to "get his feelings out." Bob cried copiously, but after many weeks nothing seemed to have changed.

A psychiatrist found that Bob had damage to the frontal lobe that may have caused him to mirror or to exaggerate the expression of emotions. We all tend to feel like weeping when others cry and tend to smile when others do, but Bob's emotions swung uncontrollably with those around him. He did not need help coming to terms with the past: he needed an upbeat environment to help him experience positive feelings. This syndrome is uncommon but reminds us that even mood is influenced by the illness.

Perceiving an Object as a Trigger. This is the tendency of a person to respond to everything she notices. It is related to distractibility. In this symptom, the object functions as an irresistible trigger for behavior. People with this deficit will grab at everything that catches their eye: bits of clothing, the caregiver's hair or wrist. If the person notices a door handle, he will open the door whether he wants to or not. Concealed latches and recessed door knobs are helpful. Giving the person a cloth, cup, spoon, or other object to hold helps prevent the person from grasping your hand. We can relate to this a little by imagining a box of chocolates lying on the table in front of us. It seems to say, "Eat me, hurry, eat me." (See Exhibit 2.15.)

Perception of an Object. Being unable to *perceive an object as a whole* is the inability to see things as an organized whole unit: if a person loses this skill, he may not be able to recognize things, take hold of things, or put things down in the right place. A person may lose the ability to see related things: the cutlery is related to the plate; all three items on the plate are food. He will have problems in eating. Perceiving a gestalt is necessary to complete the pentagons on the MMSE. (See Lesson 5 and Chapter VI.)

Perseveration. Perseveration is the tendency to "get stuck" doing the same activity or motion over and over. It is common and can occur at any point in the illness. It is the cause of many behaviors. If the behavior is not dangerous, allow it to continue. Being unable to let go of something may also be perseveration—getting stuck gripping. Perseveration is the opposite of initiating. Many of these behaviors have multiple causes of which perseveration is only one. Pacing is often an expression of stress; rocking and pacing are often an effort to provide oneself with stimulation. In the MMSE the person will get stuck drawing the same part of the pentagrams. (See Exhibit 2.16.)

Phantom Boarder Syndrome. Some people with dementia become convinced that an outsider is living in the house or that people are "working upstairs" in a one-level center. They may believe that there is an animal such as a snake in their room. It is an uncommon symptom but distressing to families. Arguing does not help; going along in a low-key way without outright agreeing usually helps. It is frustrating to both parties to try to argue someone out of something he absolutely believes. This is not always a hallucination and usually is not responsive to neuroleptics. (See Section 9.2.)

Planning. Planning is a complex skill that enables a person to carry out tasks of more than one step. It takes planning to get out of the chair, walk down the hall, and use the toilet. Task breakdown and reminders can replace planning and often enable people to function.

Postponing. The inability to postpone is the loss of the ability to wait to have needs met. For example, if you say, "Just a minute, Mary. I'll help you as soon as I finish with Ann," Mary may not have the capacity to wait. This problem is familiar to the parents of two-year-olds, who may not seem to understand the concept of "in a minute." Two-year-olds will grow out of this, but the staff must plan to help Mary. She may feel lost and forgotten. If she has a physical need (e.g., toileting), she may feel helpless. The person may become angry or accuse the caregiver, or she may forget what she is waiting for. (See Exhibit 2.17.)

Recognizing Boundaries. Recognizing boundaries is the ability to know where the edges of things are: corners of rooms, door frames, edges of plates, rims of glasses, seats of chairs. The person can see these things but not be able to adapt his motor behavior to compensate for them. (See Exhibit 2.18.)

Sense of Time. Loss of the sense of time is the loss of the awareness of the passage of time. Everyone has a clock inside her head that makes her aware of the passage of time. Some people can even wake up at exactly the time they plan to. People with dementia lose the sense of the amount of time that has passed. These symptoms may also be due to memory loss or the inability to postpone need. (See Exhibit 2.19.)

Sequencing. Sequencing is the ability to do things in the proper order. The inability to sequence is common at all stages of the illness and is very disabling. When sequencing is done for the person, she will be able to maintain a higher level of independence. These behavioral symptoms may be due to more than one disability. (See Exhibit 2.20.)

Spatial Perception. Spatial perception is the ability to perceive where things are in relation to oneself and other objects. People with difficulty in this area may not know where their body parts are in relation to others or may walk into walls. They may miss the chair as they try to sit (also characteristic of apraxia), may trip on stairs or ledges, will have trouble with crafts or tasks such as bingo, which require putting a marker in a certain square. Allow more space between people, use high-contrast boundaries, touch the person's body parts to cue him. (See Exhibit 2.21.)

Wayfinding. Wayfinding is having a mental map of an area. Even something as simple as a small apartment requires a map. Something can be in plain sight, but if one does not have a mental map, one can still not get to it. People with problems in this area may decline to go anywhere, or they may drive the car and become lost. People may lose some mental maps and retain others. People who can find their way at home may not be able to find the bathroom in another place. People may retain old maps but not be able to make new ones. Families planning a move may want to do so early enough in the illness that the person can learn her way around a new home. Environmental cues are more likely to help people in the early and middle stages of the illness.

Clinical Experience

Select a person known to you. Identify one disability and plan an appropriate intervention. Discuss your plan with the class.

Teacher: You must determine whether your students are ready to try a plan in the clinical setting. Some will be ready only to plan and discuss an intervention; others will be able to carry out a simple intervention with the person with dementia. Guide the student to select small, simple interventions that are likely to succeed. Point out small positive gains. Example: Mrs. Smith forgets within a minute, so we will remind her where she is going several times. Outcome: Mrs. Smith is somewhat less anxious.

Exhibit 2.1. Cognitive Deficits and Empathy

Initiate getting up out of your chair.
Understand the order of the steps in making tea.
Decide when things in your refrigerator have been there too long.
Remember what you are told for one minute.
Figure out who this person is who has come to visit you.
Understand why your husband wants to put diapers on you.
Put up with all these people milling around.
Get home to take care of your children.
Recognize that you have wet yourself.
Control your feelings of irritation or frustration.
Know that you have acted badly.
Find your way to a place that seems familiar.
Find anyone around who seems familiar.
Find anything that seems as though it is yours.
Figure out what your job is here.

Exhibit 2.2. Examples of Strengths We Might See (listed progressively from early in the illness to late in the illness)

As the disease progresses, the person's remaining skills change, but there are always some remaining abilities. For example, the person may be

- able to make decisions about daily routines and choices
- able to walk independently in a familiar area
- able to use prepared and labeled frozen meals
- able to do own personal care
- able to help with dressing if we tell her one step at a time what to do
- able to enjoy gardening
- able to enjoy family visits if only one person at a time visits
- able to chop vegetables and stir soup in activity program
- able to smile
- able to rock a visiting baby
- able to pet the unit's cat
- able to enjoy sitting in the sunshine
- alert, responsive

Exhibit 2.3. Examples of Strengths We Might See (listed by type of skill)

People retain skills in many areas of life. These are examples of skills a person might retain.
Activities of daily living:

- Can brush teeth if toothpaste is put on brush
- Puts on shirt if it is held in right position

Other activities:

- Can still play piano—needs help finding piano
- Remembers words to songs
- Can say rhyming words
- Likes spending time with animals
- Likes to "read" the newspaper

Social skills:

- Likes to dress well
- Rises when a woman comes into the room
- Comments on others
- Gives smiles

Communication:

- Can use and understand facial expressions and body language

Orientation skills:

- Knows she belongs here
- Knows which way to walk toward her room
- Recognizes people she dislikes

Handyman/homemaking/volunteer skills:

- Can roll a pie crust
- Can staple flyers

Humor:

- Laughs at a staff member who came in wearing a silly hat
- Will smile if coaxed
- Can make jokes

Overlearned motor skills and perseveration:

- Can wipe tables
- Can wash dishes
- Can sand wood
- Can rake lawn

Motor skills:

- Able to walk
- Able to swing in a glider

(continued)

Exhibit 2.3. *(continued)*

Music:

- Likes to sing
- Likes to tap out rhythm

Compensating for losses:

- Keeps lists
- Makes notes
- Is able to use signage
- Hides embarrassing accidents

Emotional capacity:

- Appears to retain a fully intact emotional capacity
- Experiences fear, excitement, pride, anxiety, sorrow, shame, sympathy, although their expression is not always understood

Awareness:

- Has an awareness of environment and a responsiveness to change occurring within it, even if events are not accurately or fully comprehended

Exhibit 2.4. A Few More Examples of Strengths We Might See

These real cases illustrate the feeling many staff members have that the person is still functioning.

- Although no one on the unit seemed able to find the bathroom, several different people led a visitor to see the baby birds in their nest.
- Annie and Joe found each other and made friends. They liked to sit together during activities and to hold hands.
- Katie was very impaired, and the staff members were beginning to worry because she was unsteady on her feet. However, she loved to dance. Whenever music was playing, Katie would begin to jive, twisting with perfect rhythm and beaming.
- Admiral Jones was a difficult man. However, he was unfailingly polite to women; he rose when they did and held the door for them.
- Mrs. Glick liked to sit in a chair opposite the elevator. She always had a big, indiscriminate "Hello" for everybody. And she would often say, "I didn't see you for such a long time. Come and sit with me."
- The staff members could not understand anything Harry said, but his smile told them he enjoyed telling jokes, so they laughed when he did. Both Harry and the staff member had a good moment together.
- If a woman wore a short skirt, Adelaide would say, "I see England, I see France, I see doctor's underpants," although she did not. Some staff members were offended by this; others saw this as one way Adelaide continued to interact and be herself—critical and opinionated.

Exhibit 2.5. Behavioral Symptoms of Agnosia

Symptom	How We Help
Fails to recognize familiar faces	Support the family; an agnosia does not mean the person has forgotten the relationship; use multiple sensory cues; accept.
Believes spouse is an imposter	Reassure the caregiver that the relationship is not lost; use different caregivers; sometimes hearing the caregiver's voice helps.
Fails to recognize own face	Soap, cover, or remove mirrors *for this individual only.*
Fails to recognize familiar objects: shower, eating utensils, food	Often overlooked. Be alert for. Provide multiple sensory cues. Avoid shower, use finger foods.
Believes the house is not one's home	Try cueing with familiar furniture, "This is your old chair." Don't argue; try light, smell as cues; move to a different setting if too upsetting.
Mistakes a daughter for the once young wife she now resembles	This is not incest. Do not shame the person. Reassure and support the family. Arrange the visit so the person has no opportunity to make overt gestures.
Fails to recognize familiar pictures	May be an agnosia, vision problem, memory problem.
Talks to pictures, mirrors	Don't use pictures. If person not disturbed by this, no intervention is needed.

Exhibit 2.6. Behavioral Symptoms of Apathy

Symptom	How We Help
Says he doesn't want to do anything; resists being involved; prefers just to sit	Search for noncognitive cause. Would this activity have interested the person in the past? Evaluate for depression. Simplify the challenge: "sit by me" instead of "join the activity group"; use one-on-one contact; shorten the time span for involvement but increase frequency—greet the person every time he goes by instead of stopping for long conversations. If diagnosis confirms a cognitive reason for the apathy, don't press the person to participate. Provide plenty of social contact, but do not force into activities.

Exhibit 2.7. Behavioral Symptoms of Apraxia

Symptom	How We Help
Becomes frustrated by her inability to do things	Observe what the person cannot do, and do it for her.
Does not want to do things	Do not expect people to do tasks such as crafts that require lost skills.
Can't do essential tasks	Simplify tasks, such as substituting Velcro for shoelaces. Encourage finger food. Use motor cues such as touching the back of the knees to trigger sitting down.
Can still play piano, slice bread, etc.	Do everything possible to support retained skills. Recognize that skills are not lost in a sequence that seems "sensible" to us. Watch for unexpected retained skills, and encourage the person to use them.
Has problems rising from chair	Ask the person to grasp arms of chair, lean forward, put feet underneath him, not out in front.
Changes in gait, odd apraxias, or slow shuffles	Changes in gait may indicate concurrent health problems. Uncharacteristic changes in gait may indicate a different dementia. As person begins to shuffle, secure throw rugs, make floor area safe, eliminate changes in level, objects person could trip over.

Exhibit 2.8. Behavioral Symptoms of Difficulty Choosing among Items

Symptom	How We Help
Gets out all clothing	Allow as many choices as the person can handle, but reduce the number of choices where needed (hold up two dresses).
Stirs food	Reduce the number of food items on a plate, but set the rest of the plate's contents nearby.
Fiddles with items instead of making a choice	Make choices for the person.
Cries when asked which item she wants	Present fewer choices. Reduce choice to one. ("Would you like this?")
Stops doing a multiple-choice task, such as grocery shopping	Give cues. ("I think we should buy Starkist tuna.")

Exhibit 2.9. Behavioral Symptoms of an Inability to Compensate for Deficits

Symptom	How We Help
Does not use glasses, hearing aids	Adapt the environment. In a group setting, label each person's hearing aids.
Does not use grab bars or compensate for unsteadiness	Use verbal reminders, make grab bars more visible. Have the person hold your arm.
Enters unsafe areas	Do not expect the person to avoid unsafe areas; prevent access or make them safe.

Exhibit 2.10. Behavioral Symptoms of Disorientation

Symptom	How We Help
Disorientation is the cause of many behaviors.	If not dangerous, allow or gently reorient some people if this reduces stress.
Masturbates in public; makes advances to a daughter; fondles staff members	Gently reorient the person. It is not necessary to scold, for the "mistake" is in orientation, not purposeful or sexual.
Yells at people; fights with other residents	Fighting with other residents may occur if the person thinks the other resident is someone else at some other time. Explaining does not often help. Separate the two.

Exhibit 2.11. Behavioral Symptoms of Distractibility

Symptom	How We Help
Becomes upset around multiple people, in noisy settings; wanders away from activity	Simplify the environment: reduce number of people, noises.
Does not pay attention to you	Work with the person when he is not tired.
Picks up objects on dresser or on wash basin, or picks up objects as you dress or care for him	Reduce objects around the person.

Exhibit 2.12. Behavioral Symptoms of an Inability to Initiate

Symptom	How We Help
Does not get up from a chair or bed when asked	"Start" the person: begin the arm movement for toothbrushing or start feeding the person; put an extra spoon at the table for the person to pick up; watch for signs that the person will carry on once the motion has been started for him.
Does not do a task when asked (The staff member puts a toothbrush in the person's hand and says, "Now brush your teeth," but nothing happens.)	Give verbal encouragement in addition to, not instead of, starting the motor movement.
Sits and looks at food or stops eating and does not start again	Help the person get out of a chair, etc.; but always give the person an opportunity to carry on.
Holds pencil or spoon but does nothing	
Says "yes" but does nothing	

Note: Each suggestion in the "How We Help" column can be used for all the symptoms listed.

Exhibit 2.13. Behavioral Symptoms of a Lack of Insight

Symptom	How We Help
Blames someone else or ignores wet clothing Does not associate own behavior with damage (messes, dented car, trouble given to caregivers) Insists his memory and cognition are fine, even in face of overwhelming evidence	Insight cannot be replaced, and no amount of explaining—or proof—will help. Accept the person's point of view. Caregivers must understand this loss. Don't argue; if someone says the man in the next bed struck him, express sympathy. Let people keep their self-esteem. Use other means—advice from a colleague to make a will, orders from the doctor to stop driving; suggest a change of clothing "because some water got spilled on yours."

Exhibit 2.14. Behavioral Symptoms of Memory Loss

Symptom	How We Help
Does not retain information for even a minute or two	Repeat important information every 2–3 minutes.
Asks the same question over and over	Accept repeated questions.
You are uncertain whether long-term memory is accurate.	Accept what the person says he remembers (don't put him down).
Cannot follow through on immediate instructions	Try writing a note the person can keep (e.g., "Your wife will come after lunch") or give frequent oral reminders.
Remembers one bit of information but not the rest	Give less information at one time.
Insists on looking for her small children, spouse	Encourage the person to talk about children, look at pictures, promise that she is cared for, do not contradict.

Exhibit 2.15. Behavioral Symptoms of Responding to Everything (Object as Trigger)

Symptom	How We Help
Grabs at clothing pulled over her head; grabs at everything in the shower; wanders away without completing toileting task; wanders around picking things up; carries things	Reduce the number of objects. Make the most important item very noticeable, right in front of the person, bright red. Accept behavior.
Pays attention to only one or two visitors and ignores the rest	Reduce the number of visitors, explain behavior to family.
In some cases, seeing the doorknob triggers going out	Make door and closet handles less conspicuous or conceal them; paint door frames and doors to match walls; reverse this for doors or handles you want the person to use.
Takes other people's things	Taking others' things is not theft; replace items discreetly, redirect.
Touches other people	Distract.
Grabs your hair, braids	Tie your hair out of the way when caring for the person.
Takes another person's food, especially if that person is served first	Serve the person first; arrange clearer boundaries.
Urinates in the wrong place	If the person is urinating in wastebasket or flower pot, move it, put a lid on it, change its appearance dramatically.

Exhibit 2.16. Behavioral Symptoms of Perseveration

Symptom	How We Help
Repeats words, parts of tasks Washes part of self, wipes table without stopping Stirs food without stopping Colors or draws same spot over and over	Take advantage of this to provide meaningful activities (especially for people who lack a sense of how long they have been doing something). Interrupt motor behaviors with a motor task, vocal behaviors with a vocal task.
Repeats a word over and over	Ask him to sing.
Rolls up skirt	Provide textured apron, lap robe.
Picks at clothing, rocks back and forth	Ignore if not harmful.
Grips your hair or wrist and does not let go when asked	To get a person who is gripping something to let go, ask the person to hold something else. Touch the person's hand with the object you want her to hold.
Puts on too many clothes	Accept the behavior. Lay out clothing. Secure closets so that the person can find only one outfit.

Exhibit 2.17. Behavioral Symptoms of an Inability to Postpone

Symptom	How We Help
Becomes impatient, cannot wait	Don't expect people to wait; take them to meals at the time the meal arrives, not earlier; to the doctor at a time when they won't have to wait. Give the person something to hold for you if the delay is very short. Take the person with you for what you must do first. Wait until the last minute to tell people about something.
Becomes restless or irritable waiting	Take people to meals when the meals arrive, not earlier.
Becomes upset at the doctor's office	Schedule appointments at a time when the person will not have to wait.
Gets angry when other clients go first—getting on bus, entering room, being served for meals	It may be more important to help this person immediately than to take people in "turns," which they won't remember anyway. Get someone to help you.

Exhibit 2.18. Behavioral Symptoms of an Inability to Recognize Boundaries

Symptom	How We Help
Misses seat of chair when sitting	May be an apraxia; move chair under person, gently touch backs of legs to chair.
Falls out of bed	Multiple causes; low bed may help.
Stumbles on stairs	Increase visibility of edges: Does color of risers and steps confuse or help?
Pushes food off plate	Use colored band on plate, plate guard.
Takes food from other people's plates	Multiple cognitive disabilities; position person opposite others, use place mats that delineate boundaries.
Unable to step over edge of rug, up onto scales	Multiple cognitive deficits; increase visibility of edges to help a person step up.
Tries to step over things that are flat	Decrease contrast when a person tries to step over nonexistent edges.
Confused by black-and-white tile floors, afraid to step on black bands	Give touch cues; eliminate rugs; cover tiles if possible.

Exhibit 2.19. Behavioral Symptoms of a Loss of Sense of Time

Symptom	How We Help
Asks the same question over and over Asks what time it is over and over	These behaviors are not dangerous, although they can drive the caregiver crazy. It is more successful to support the caregiver (give her frequent breaks) than to drug or frustrate the person. Ignoring repeated questions may precipitate an angry outburst. Try writing down the answer for the person and giving him the notes to keep.
In day care, becomes restless to go home or seeks the caregiver moments after she left	Try having the caregiver write and sign a note reassuring the person and saying when she will be back. Make many copies of this note in case it is lost.
Wakes at night	Diversionary activities like sing-alongs after the evening meal can reduce nighttime wandering and wakefulness.

Exhibit 2.20. Behavioral Symptoms of an Inability to Sequence

Symptom	How We Help
Puts clothing on in the wrong order	Sequencing is easily done for the person. For example, lay out clothes in the order in which they are to be put on.
Prepares familiar recipe in wrong order	Give step-by-step instructions.
Drinks water but does not take pills	Give the person her pills before you give her water, or give pills one at a time.
Becomes lost	Redirect.
Gets task steps out of order (puts toothpaste on toothbrush and lays toothbrush down upside down and says she is finished)	Use task breakdown. Use verbal cueing at each step.

Exhibit 2.21. Behavioral Symptoms of Problems in Spatial Perception

Symptom	How We Help
Misses chair when sitting	Position chair as the person is about to sit.
Eats off other people's plates	Use a square table (corners help define space). Use high-contrast place mat and plate.
Gets stuck in corners or alcoves	Design to avoid alcoves or block them off.
Bumps into corners or furniture	Use high-contrast tape to mark corners; in the home, remove low furniture such as coffee tables.
Has difficulty dressing	Guide one arm or leg into garment at a time.

Overhead/Handout 2.1. Some Mental Losses

Problems speaking or understanding

Problems doing familiar motor tasks

Problems with insight, judgment, impulse control

Problem with memory

Problems with postponing things

Problems choosing among items

Problems doing things in the right order

Problems tuning things out

Overhead/Handout 2.2. Key Points to Remember about Brain Damage

The disease causes most of the behavioral symptoms.

Some abilities are lost, while others are retained.

Each person is different.

The person is trying as hard as she can with what she has left.

A person's abilities may come and go.

The same behavior may have many causes.

Overhead/Handout 2.3. How We Help

Once we recognize the problem, there is so much we can do to help.

We help by enabling people to do what they still can.

We help by not expecting people to do things they cannot.

LESSON 3

FACILITATING FUNCTION BY TREATING EXCESS DISABILITY

Summary. People with dementia often have other health problems that exacerbate their disability; when these are treated, often there is improved function and behavior. Common excess disabilities include concurrent illness, pain, medication reactions and interactions, sensory deficits, dizziness, stress, and psychiatric and mood disturbances. This lesson discusses the effects of illness, pain, medication reactions, sensory deficits, and dizziness. Stress, mood disturbances, fatigue, and psychiatric disorders also cause disability and are discussed in later lessons.

Section 3.1. The Importance of Treating Excess Disability. Defines excess disability, its impact, and its common causes and teaches the student to recognize the characteristics of excess disability.

Section 3.2. Illness, Pain, Reactions to Medication, Sensory Deficits, and Dizziness. Discusses the impact of concurrent illness, pain, reactions to medication, sensory deficits, and dizziness as causes of excess disability in the care of people with dementia.

Section 3.3. Factors That Influence Excess Disability in People with Dementia. Describes the interaction between the concurrent condition and the dementia.

Section 3.4. Information about Excess Disability and Delirium. Discusses the success rate of interventions and the prevalence of excess disability. This section includes materials on identification and interventions.

Using the Sections

- Introductory course:
  - Section 3.1 required
  - Section 3.2 optional
- Core course:
  - Section 3.1 required
  - Section 3.2 required
  - Section 3.3 required
- Special audiences:
  - People responsible for diagnosis, assessment, referral, and treatment: entire lesson, including Section 3.4

Problems You May Have in Implementing This Lesson

The student should have few difficulties with this lesson. However, some programs will encounter serious limitations in the availability and response of medical professionals. Ideally, registered nurses, physicians, and mental health professionals need to be available and to respect the input of nursing assistants and family members. A prompt response is essential because people with dementia decline rapidly and behavioral symptoms worsen. Because people with dementia are fragile, the medical team will need to try again and again if the first intervention tried is not successful. Medical professionals need skills in geriatrics. Unfortunately, not enough such professionals are available, and funding policies often discourage their involvement. Compromises can work. For example, nurses often find ways to work with existing medical resources. When problems do exist, it is important to be open with the staff about these and encourage them to look for ways they can do as much as possible with what they do have.

Staff members must know their individual patients if they are to recognize the changes that signal health problems. The facility must have in place a system that allows a team of staff members to care for the same people with dementia. Home care, families, and researchers all emphasize the importance of consistent staffing. When substitute staff members are used in any setting, a system must be in place to provide basic information for them.

If you, the educator, are not a registered nurse (RN), ask one to co-teach this with you. Nursing skills are necessary to help the student recognize problems in excess disability.

Section 3.1. The Importance of Treating Excess Disability

Objective

The student will learn that health is essential to function and that direct care providers play a major role in maintaining health. The goal is to alert students to the effects of health problems on function and behavioral problems.

Background

The importance of excess disability in dementia care cannot be overstated. Illness, pain, and medication reactions and interactions exacerbate cognitive impairment. In addition, the person with dementia cannot correctly comprehend or communicate feelings associated with illness, pain, medication reactions, sensory deficits, and dizziness. This means that even mild problems can result in much more disability than necessary. Identifying these conditions and treating them to the extent possible will result in small gains for most people with dementia and dramatic gains for a few. This ongoing monitoring and intervention—judicious tinkering—over the course of the dementia is a hallmark of good care. Direct care staff members, who spend the most time with the person with dementia, are in the best position to observe subtle changes.

It can be difficult for young people to relate to the aches and pains of old age. Young people have more energy, have extensive reserves, and recover more quickly; they can cope with illness, a family, and a job without becoming confused or overwhelmed. As you teach, remind students to think about this difference. The older, damaged brain is like an old, slow computer: it takes longer to get the job done.

The question of a medical model versus social model may arise. Neither model is completely appropriate for people with dementia: health issues increase the cognitive deficit and the capacity to function, limiting the person's ability to enjoy social interchange and to experience success and autonomy. Thus, it is necessary to improve health to the extent possible to meet psychosocial needs.

The treatment of excess disability is not a magic bullet. The underlying dementia will continue. Some problems are treatable in theory but will not respond or cannot be treated in some people. The teacher must maintain an optimistic balance between improving treatment and the realities of clinical care.

Most commonly, multiple small interventions in areas such as a person's health status, staff behavior, or environment will result in change. This lesson provides a basis on which subsequent skills will be taught. Some, but not all, individual problems can be resolved through the skills learned in this lesson.

The changes that indicate excess disability in people with dementia are subtle and are often behavioral rather than medical. Physicians and nurses simply do not spend enough time with the person with dementia to notice these changes unassisted. To successfully address excess disability, staff members who spend the most time with the person with dementia and their immediate supervisors are in the best position to monitor clients. This may mean assigning more power and judgment to people with limited medical knowledge. For some care settings, this is a change. Staff members may be reluctant to accept this responsibility, and supervisors (and physicians) may be reluctant to give it. Errors in reporting symptoms result when staff members are inexperienced. However, with practice, aides, volunteers, and family members can become expert reporters. Teach them the importance of symptoms, the importance of their role, and which symptoms should be reported. Reassure them that they will not be asked to make diagnostic or treatment decisions but only to report observations. Ensure that they do not experience disapproval when they think there is a problem and none is found. A supervisory and medical system must be in place to respond promptly to staff reports. Strengthen this system as much as possible.

Information and Instructions for the Teacher

The overheads/handouts provide teaching points. Familiarize yourself with the text that supports each point, and present it in your own words.

Ask questions that give your students confidence

that they can recognize excess disability by helping them connect what they are already observing with the presence of excess disability. Ask questions that trigger observations the staff members already make: How do they know when someone has a urinary tract infection? is constipated? is tired? is hurting from arthritis?

Ask questions that help the staff members identify situations in which they have observed improvement when an illness or other problem has been treated or a medication stopped. When have they seen confusion, apathy, or irritability improve? When has calling out declined? When did people become more responsive? When they observed even slight improvement, ask them to think back and identify the clues that the person was having problems. Staff members providing subacute care will often see improvement as their patient's acute condition resolves.

Point out how similar these symptoms are to things we might think were just part of the dementia (dulled from medication; irritable from the flu) and ask them to think of examples they have seen in the people they care for.

Emphasize the positive side of excess disability: that this is one area in which we can make a difference.

Lecture/Discussion Notes to Be Presented to the Class

Overhead/Handout 3.1. The Definition of Excess Disability

What is excess disability? Excess disability is more disability than can be explained by the dementia alone. Imagine a person already physically disabled and needing crutches. Then imagine adding a ball and chain. This would be excess disability.

People with dementia often have excess disability as well as their dementia. If you can find the "ball and chain" that adds to the person's problems, you can make the person more comfortable and reduce behavioral symptoms. This lesson is particularly exciting because direct care staff members can often make real changes for the person with dementia.

The brain is affected by everything that happens to the body. The flu, an infected knee, medication, *everything* affects the cells of the brain. Can you think of a time when you had a bad case of flu or when you had taken a medication and felt that your thinking was not as sharp as usual? Medication or illness can affect people who do not have a dementia, but it does not affect them as seriously. When the brain cells are already damaged, the brain can't cope. The result is that you observe a person who seems drowsy, more irritable, or less able to do tasks.

What causes excess disability? Illnesses besides the dementia, pain, reactions to medications, sensory problems (e.g., poor vision, poor hearing), and dizziness are the most common problems that cause excess disability. The good news is that often these problems can be treated, and the person's overall function will improve. Excess disability from these causes is very common and will occur over and over again throughout the course of the person's dementia.

People with dementia often cannot say how they feel. They may also not show the same kinds of symptoms as others do. For example, a person who is developing pneumonia may not run a fever but may only become more irritable and resistant to care. For this reason, direct care staff members are in the best position to notice changes in function or behavior that may be signs of excess disability. Knowing the people you care for and observing them are essential skills you need to keep them as healthy as possible. Only the staff members who take care of people and their immediate supervisors are going to notice these things. Without direct care staff members watching over them, people with dementia will have unnecessary disability a lot of the time. Doctors and nurses do not provide the direct care you do and therefore will not notice things until the person is seriously ill.

Let's look at some examples of people with excess disability:

> You are trying to get Clara to eat. She usually watches you and opens her mouth for the spoon without clueing. Today every time you put food on the spoon and say, "Clara, open your mouth," Clara glances at you and returns to plucking at her skirt before you can even put the spoon to her mouth.
>
> The second shift noticed that Clara took a longer-than-usual afternoon nap and woke up tearful, which was unusual for her. The nurse checked her vitals and found nothing wrong, but the next morning Clara was

barely responsive. The doctor found that she had pneumonia.

Clara's first symptom was a change in behavior. The first symptoms were mild, but they signaled a serious illness.

Mrs. Benson lived at home with her husband. She had Alzheimer disease, some arthritis, and osteoporosis, but with the help of a visiting nurse and day care, they were managing well. She could become irritable and threaten her husband or the day care staff, but everyone had learned what things upset her and how to avoid pushing her. Then almost overnight she became combative. She hit her husband and one of the day care clients. She was particularly explosive when anyone tried to get her into or out of a chair or to help her with activities of daily living (ADLs). The physician started Mrs. Benson on a neuroleptic drug, but this made her so groggy that he discontinued it. After trying several things, the physician found a compression fracture of the spine. Pain medication and back support helped, and Mrs. Benson's combative behavior decreased as her pain was controlled.

Agitated or combative behavior is often the result of pain or illness that the person cannot tell you about. Because she could not describe it, it was difficult to find Mrs. Benson's problem. It could easily have been overlooked. A clue here was that sitting or rising from a chair or other movements that hurt her back made Mrs. Benson more combative. When people caused her pain, the only thing she knew to do was to strike out.

Mabel is mildly impaired. She cannot manage living alone. She needs help with dressing but can feed herself, is continent, enjoys the residential home's activity program, and is usually easy to get along with. But Mabel has recurrent urinary tract infections. When she has a urinary infection, she becomes severely confused, sometimes incontinent, unsteady, and cranky. For Mabel, the urinary tract infection creates excess disability—more disability than is caused by her Alzheimer disease.

Urinary tract infections are common and sometimes not considered serious. But staff members know that, when untreated, they contribute to behavioral symptoms. As with Clara, the first and primary sign that Mabel had another urinary tract infection was the change in her behavior.

George is severely confused and needs a lot of help. With reminders, he remains continent and can manage his meal if his food is cut up for him, but he is unable to participate in most craft activities, and he can be explosively irritable.

Because of his irritability, the doctor put George on a neuroleptic medication, but George got much worse. He became doubly incontinent, able to walk only with support, and apathetic. He did not recognize his caregiver and seemed to lose interest in everything.

The medications that we hope will help the person often create excess disability—more impairment.

The person with dementia may not recognize pain or illness, although he feels it as much as others do. He may not make the connection between walking on a sprained ankle and the pain he feels. Because he often cannot explain what his problem is, it is the direct care staff members who notice changes.

Overhead/Handout 3.2. Outcomes of Excess Disability

Excess disability has serious outcomes. People experiencing any illness, pain, medication reaction, or sensory deficit will be less able to function than they would be with the dementia alone. They will almost certainly show increased behavioral symptoms or need more care. (For example, the person who can usually feed herself may need to be fed, or the person who is usually continent may become incontinent.) Excess disability is a major cause of falls. The person who is experiencing stress due to illness or pain, who is more confused because of medications, or who has sensory deficits is more likely to shuffle, experience weakness, or move without thinking—any of which can lead to a serious fall. Studies have shown that excess disability is a predictor of death. Both illness and pain are predictors of death in these frail individuals, and falls can lead to terminal injuries. Thus, all staff members must take seriously any indication of excess disability, for the outcomes for the person with dementia as well as her quality of life are at stake.

Overhead/Handout 3.3. Things to Watch For

You may be thinking that all the people you care for are like this all the time. The key to identifying illness, pain, and medication reactions usually is to look for *change* in behavioral symptoms. Any behavior, mood, or level of function that is a change from what is usual for a specific individual is a warning sign for excess disability. If a person always is easily distracted and confused, this maybe usual for him. However, when something is not usual for this person, report it, even if the change is minor.

Often behavioral change is the only indicator that the person is ill, in pain, or reacting to a medication. Whenever behavioral symptoms or functional abilities decline over hours, days, or a few weeks, suspect that the cause may be excess disability. An increase in the person's level of irritability is a common symptom of excess disability.

Instead of becoming irritable, some people become quiet, passive, or lethargic. It's easy to ignore such people because we are so glad they are not causing us problems, but being more quiet than usual is likely to indicate problems for them.

Even mild symptoms may be evidence of excess disability. If they are observed and treated early, more serious symptoms may be prevented.

Listen to complaints. People with dementia do say things that help us know that they are having problems, but because they have difficulty expressing themselves and understanding you, their complaint may not be very clear. The person who repeats "help me, help me" may be in pain. The person who says her head aches may have a stomach ache but cannot find the right word for "stomach." Never assume that complaints are attempts to get attention or just part of a complaining personality. This is rarely the case. Even if the person has always complained, complaints indicate that the person needs something but cannot tell you what. When the person is "just complaining," remember that these people, too, are frail and can become sick.

To summarize, certain kinds of changes commonly indicate that a concurrent problem is likely to be present: the person is drowsy, unusually irritable, combative or angry, less able to focus on your or others; she dozes off, is less able to do ADLs or refuses to do ADLs, pays less attention to surroundings, seems more sluggish, is harder to understand, is less alert; her behavior or abilities vary from morning to evening. The person may seem bewildered by things that he can usually handle, such as needing assistance in the toilet or eating. He may fail to recognize people he usually can recognize. A high-functioning person may have trouble with tasks he usually manages.

When the person begins new drugs or has any new illness, new glasses, or a fall, watch for excess disability. *(Teacher: Take time to discuss these symptoms so that your class knows what to look for.)*

Overhead/Handout 3.4. How We Help

Direct care staff members help by *watching for even slight changes* in behavior or function. This means that you must know the people you care for.

Usually it is not the job of direct care staff members to diagnose or treat the underlying problem, although you may have a good idea what it is. (If you know that a person often has urinary tract infections, you will know that these changes look like the ones she has previously had. If you know that the person is in pain from her cancer, you can recognize when her pain is increasing and she will need more pain relief.)

Whatever changes you see, *report them promptly* —before your shift ends. A person who seems slightly more confused in the morning may be seriously ill by evening.

Continue to observe the person for changes. If the intervention helps, you will be the first one to observe the improvement. Watch for very slight improvements—the person eats a little better, seems to be calling out less. Report these: this is the only way that the doctor or nurse can know what treatment helps. Because problems often recur with people with dementia, the physician will know what to try next time.

People with dementia are difficult to treat. The first treatment the nurse or physician tries may not work. The medication to treat the problem may make the person more confused. Sometimes it is very difficult to ease the distress of someone with an incurable condition such as stroke or cancer or arthritis. Your close observation of slight changes—for better or worse—guides the medical professionals in what to do next.

Never assume that worsened behavior or a decline in skills is a natural decline due to the dementia. Of course, there is a natural decline, but if we mistake excess disability for the dementia, we overlook things that would help the person—and ourselves. Whenever a decline occurs, the physician and nurse first check to see if an illness or medication might be the cause. Only when we are sure there is no excess disability do we assume that the decline is part of the dementia.

What about the person with dementia who complains all the time? Don't assume that because you can't find anything wrong, there is nothing wrong. The person may not be able to tell you, and health problems are often difficult to find. The person probably can't remember that she has already complained, so each complaint is the first for her. She probably lacks the cognitive ability to deliberately complain just to get attention. If you cannot find a problem, reassure her frequently. Some illnesses show few clinical signs in any people with dementia.

Exercise 1. Recognizing Excess Disability

As a class or in small groups, discuss the following: When have you seen problems that you think may be excess disability? Use information from your teacher or supervisor to help you.

Section 3.2. Illness, Pain, Reactions to Medication, Sensory Deficits, and Dizziness

Objective

The student will learn to recognize and report possible excess disability and to understand why intervention is important in care.

Information and Instructions for the Teacher

This section focuses on each of five causes of excess disability. Use the overheads/handouts as talking points. The text presents some further information about each point. Present it in your own words. This section presumes that the teacher or a registered nurse is able help students learn to recognize subtle changes in health. Read Sections 3.3 and 3.4 to prepare yourself for this section. The points as presented are important but, of necessity, brief. Be prepared to discuss or expand the material from your own nursing knowledge. Exhibit 3.1 lists additional causes of excess disability. Do not hand out this exhibit; use it for your own information.

Lecture/Discussion Notes to Be Presented to the Class

In this section we will look at illness, pain, reactions to medication, sensory deficits, and dizziness individually. Each causes excess disability.

Illness

The cognitive impact of illness is real, biological. It acts on cells and tissues to lower functional and mental ability. People who are in acute or subacute care or who have just been transferred from acute care are likely to have some excess disability. As their acute illness improves, you can expect to see improvement in behavioral and functional symptoms. People with dementia who develop illnesses in any setting such as nursing home, residential care, day care, or home care may also have excess disability. The dementia and the concurrent illness usually interact and make care more difficult than the management of either condition alone.

Alice lived alone. She had diabetes, which she had managed successfully for years. She had been clear of mind and able to get out and be active. However, she gradually became incontinent of urine and stopped going out. Her niece, who helped her out, noticed this and told the doctor, but Alice denied the problem when asked about it. Then Alice fell and spent two days in the hospital. The hospital staff discovered that her sugar levels were too high and adjusted her insulin dose. She seemed quite competent and did not tell anyone about her incontinence. But at home she deteriorated rapidly: she was disheveled, and the house was unkempt. Her niece was concerned that she was not eating right, and her incontinence worsened. Now the niece thought that Alice had Alzheimer disease, as she was often confused and incoherent. One day the niece found her almost comatose.

Alice's beginning dementia interfered with her ability to manage her diabetes as she had done in the past. But whenever her sugar levels got too high or too low, this caused an excess disability, which showed up as incontinence, confusion, and an inability to care for herself or her home. Alice would need someone else to manage her diabetes.

Overhead/Handout 3.5. Some Common Illnesses That Cause Excess Disability

There are many illnesses that cause excess disability. These are just a few ideas. Often it is not major illnesses that cause problems but seemingly minor things such as constipation that can make a person with dementia much worse. What other illnesses have you observed that cause the person to have additional problems? *(Teacher: Review the indications of excess disability in Exhibit 3.1.)*

Don't expect illness symptoms to be the same as in other people. Symptoms of a particular illness may not be the same in people with dementia as in other patients. Symptoms may be subtle, almost unnoticeable. Older people may not run a high fever.

Ada was new to day care. Her husband did not give a very clear report, so the staff members were trying to assess her quickly. She seemed irritable and would curse and threaten other participants as they walked

> around. But when the director tried to do a mental status test, Ada dozed off between questions. Even when she was awake, Ada would seem puzzled, as if she didn't "get" the question. She would mumble and look away toward the arm of the chair and then doze off again. Ada's inability to focus or pay attention and her drowsiness are characteristic of the confused state that indicates illness or a reaction to medication.

We have talked about acute illnesses in which you will see a change as the illness develops. However, some people with dementia have chronic illnesses in addition to their dementia. These people will have the same symptoms of illness: excess confusion, restlessness, irritability, lethargy, difficulty paying attention, and fluctuating symptoms, but you may not see a change over hours or days. For these people, the excess disability has become a "normal" addition to the dementia. Suspect an additional excess disability in anyone who has another chronic condition. The medical team may be able to find ways to manage the person's chronic illness more effectively. In any event, these people will need extra understanding and support.

Sometimes no one knows that the person has another illness. You may suspect a problem and report your suspicions. Often only a complete medical evaluation will uncover excess disability that might respond to treatment.

Sometimes problems can be only partially treated, or the treatment adds to the person's confusion.

> No dental care was available to treat John's oral abscesses. The doctor gave John an antibiotic, which irritated his stomach. The stomach pains made him agitated. The kitchen prepared a soft diet, which John did not like. He threw his food at staff members. The problem was ongoing. The antibiotic worked for a while, and John calmed down, but the staff seemed to be constantly juggling diet, irritability, and medication. Had dental care been available, John would still have had to be heavily sedated for the procedure and would have had to adjust to using dentures afterward.

Overhead/Handout 3.6. How We Help

Check for other signs of illness (fear, unsteadiness, being slowed down, fever, pain, blood pressure); ask the person if she feels bad; ask other staff members (including the previous shift) if they have noticed any change; ask the family if they see a difference; check the chart to see if the person has a tendency to develop a particular illness; write down the change you noticed; see if it gets better or worse; watch for other changes.

Get medical care. Report the problem to your supervisor; get a nurse or physician to see the person. Act right away—these problems can't wait. Report the change, and then watch the person for further change. Tell your supervisor and the next shift. Recording symptoms in the log may not get treatment quickly enough.

Be supportive. Allow for a shorter attention span; allow for the person to be more tired, more irritable, worse in the evening; allow for less tolerance for stress; skip stressful or difficult tasks; make things quieter and calmer. Have the person lie down in her room if she will; skip activities; settle her beside the nursing station so she receives more reassurance and affection. Protect the person from falls and other risks.

Overhead/Handout 3.7. Pain

Teacher: Sometimes direct care providers trivialize complaints of pain. The object of this unit is to teach the staff to take pain seriously.

Pain often signals illness, injury, or problems such as decubitus ulcers and fractures. Even mild pain (arthritis, stiff muscles) can lead to considerable excess disability—a decline in ability to do ADLs or worsened behavior. In addition, pain can directly cause harm through muscle spasm or reduced mobility. People with dementia usually become more confused when they are in pain. Resistance to care, screaming, and asking repeatedly for help are common indicators that the person is in pain.

One researcher found that when combative behavior remained even in good care, pain was usually the culprit. Note when the person strikes out. If it occurs during ADLs, when staff members are moving the person's limbs, arthritic pain may be the problem.

It is easy to overlook pain—even serious pain—because of the person's inability to report it accurately. It is also easy to overlook pain in a person who complains a lot because we tend to take his complaints for granted. Always take any complaint of pain seriously.

Esther's husband asked for an emergency visit to the outpatient dementia clinic because Esther had recently started resisting everything and would try to hit him when he got her out of bed, led her to the table, or showered her. While the doctor talked to the husband, the nurse examined Esther. Esther denied feeling bad or having pain. Her vital signs were normal, and the nurse found nothing unusual on her examination except that her left ankle was swollen. Her ankles were usually somewhat swollen, but after comparing them, the nurse decided the left was larger. The nurse did not see any bruises on Esther's skin. The doctor examined the ankle and, acting on a hunch, sent her for an X-ray, which showed a recent fracture.

Walter was a big, powerful man when he was admitted to residential care. His wife thought he declined after admission, but the facility thought the changes were just part of his adjustment. He lost appetite and weight, and he stopped moving about and preferred to sit all day in one place. He seemed less alert and mumbled more incoherently than he had at home. He fell several times, which led to a physical therapy consultation. Walter had had polio as a child and in the weeks just before admission had often threatened his wife with his cane. The facility had taken away his cane, leg brace, and heavy boot so that he would not hurt other residents, but the physical therapist pointed out that the loss of these supports led to his falls and that the distortion of musculature caused him pain.

Pain is common in older people. Many alert older people tolerate high levels of chronic pain without complaint. (Those who moan and groan are in the minority or in severe pain.) Add that to the fact that people in long-term care often have other illnesses that cause pain. When you add dementia to these problems, you find many confused people whose confusion is made much worse by their pain.

At first the staff thought Mrs. Joho was "sundowning." Every afternoon she became more irritable and resisted moving and walking. Then staff members noticed that after lunch she tended to sit quietly in one position for a long time. Like many people with dementia, she did not change her position often. The staff guessed that she was getting stiff, sore muscles from sitting and began reminding her to shift her position.

There is no evidence that people with dementia do not experience pain. They may not say they are in pain, or they may fail to rest a painful area, but researchers find that they experience pain in the same way as others.

There is also no evidence that Alzheimer disease causes pain. The disease occurs only inside the brain, where there are no pain-sensitive nerves.

Pain hurts: suspect pain when you see any of the indicators of excess disability. Suspect pain when the person is reluctant to move; is restless or irritable; is combative when touched or moved; cries; whines; holds a part of her body; or whose facial expression or body language indicates pain.

Check for pressure points, abdominal distention, postural distortion, stoop, a change in gait, tight clothing, oral infections, sores on feet.

If the person cannot report pain accurately or says "yes" and "no" indiscriminately, remember that pediatricians have the same problem. A characteristic of some people with dementia is to answer the previous question when you ask the next one. Take a little time to chat between questions to eliminate this response.

Put your hand on the body part and ask, "Does it hurt here?" Ask about no more than three sites; come back in a few minutes and ask about three more. If you are not sure, ask about the same body part several times over half an hour. A consistent answer usually means pain.

Watch facial expressions. You can usually learn to recognize the change in expression when the person you care for is in pain.

Try giving the person a mild analgesic. If behavior improves or complaints diminish, consider pain likely. Have a physician examine the person.

Treat pain as serious, and report it promptly. Don't expect the person to remember to rest a painful limb or to remember to keep using an ice bag. Keep repeating your reassurance. If appropriate, use ice bags, heat, massage, or rest (even briefly) even though the person doesn't seem to understand. As with illness, expect the person to be more tired, more confused, more stressed.

Use physical therapy consultations: a physical therapist can successfully reduce many kinds of pain.

Sometimes old age and the physical environment combine to create pain. Check to see if the person is sitting too long in one position, sleeping on a hard mattress, sitting slumped over in a way that would cause a backache, or squinting into the light. Brainstorm for more possible causes of pain. What would make you ache?

Administer pain medication wisely. Many people do well on nonprescription analgesics. Do not let pain build up between doses. Advocate for aggressive pain management for people whose terminal illness (such as cancer) causes severe pain. They cannot advocate for themselves.

Watch for allergies. People may have skin itching without a visible rash in response to laundry detergents, some prescription drugs, dry skin, or skin lotions. This explains why some people are constantly scratching themselves.

Know the person's diagnoses. Many illnesses cause pain, from cancer to constipation. Expect pain when a pain-causing diagnosis is present.

Overhead/Handout 3.8. How We Help

Ask the person if he experiences pain. Watch for behaviors, including facial expression that give clues. Never suspect the person of trying to get attention. Treat pain and give the person the extra care he will need in order to cope.

Overhead/Handout 3.9. Reactions to Medication

One aspect of medication is positive: it heals disease; it reduces symptoms; it allays fear; it reduces behavioral problems; it even treats the diseases of the mind. The benefits of modern medications are mind-boggling. In fact, many of the people with dementia we are now caring for would have died years ago without antibiotics and other drugs.

But all drugs have a negative aspect: they can cause side effects. Aspirin can cause bleeding ulcers, hand lotion can cause skin rashes; antibiotics occasionally cause anaphylactic shock and death.

> Ted's care created serious problems for his wife. He insisted on doing what he had always done, and he berated her for trying to help him. His physician had given him Haldol to calm him down enough that she could continue to care for him. Then one day he flew into a rage, grabbed her out of her chair, and slammed her into the refrigerator, shouting, "I don't, I don't want any. Don't you anyway." Then he stormed out of the house, and his wife had to call the police to bring him back. When the visiting nurse arrived, the wife was exhausted and distraught, and Ted was dozing in his chair. When she touched him, he jumped up, shouting. He seemed dazed and angry at the same time. The nurse was unable to even check his vital signs. Ted was admitted to a respite care unit to give his wife time to recover. The staff there eventually determined that he was severely constipated. Here the medication needed to treat agitation had the serious side effect of constipation. Ted's agitation diminished to his previous level once he was given a laxative and then started on a regimen to counteract the constipating effects of the Haldol.

Teacher: Ask for students' experiences of drug reactions (e.g., cold medications make people feel groggy; medication or skin cream rashes are common; various things trigger asthma).

Drugs go all through our bodies, not just to the spot where they are needed. This is true even of some medications we put on our skin. Although the body protects the brain somewhat, the brains of people with dementia will be exposed to many of the medications they take.

Older people's bodies process drugs differently. When the brain has been damaged by dementia, it is much more likely to react adversely to drugs. In general, older people will need lower dosages to have the same effect.

The drugs we use to manage behavior and to treat mood have many common and serious side effects.

Older people who take several drugs at once are at risk of drug interactions.

For people with dementia, all these factors come together to mean that they are likely to be further disabled by the drugs we use to help them.

The medication may add to the confusion of the person with dementia. Sometimes the doctor must prescribe these drugs, but she must carefully weigh the pros and cons and consider whether there is any other drug that would work as well.

People with dementia are often given drugs that act directly on the brain: tranquilizers, antidepressants, sleeping medications, and drugs to control behavior. Although these drugs can be helpful, they often make frail, vulnerable people worse. They can cause falls, aggressiveness, constipation, confusion, dry mouth, urinary retention, stiffness, restlessness, hypertension, and other problems. This sets up a vicious cycle: medication causes side effects, which require the use of other medications, which increases disability.

Direct care staff members, who see the most of the person with dementia, must watch for drug side effects the person cannot report. The pharmacologist should monitor for the uncommon side effects of each medication because these frail patients are so vulnerable to side effects.

Overhead/Handout 3.10. How We Help

Because the use of medications is so common in people with dementia, caregiving staff members must always *suspect* medications as a cause when they see a problem that might be excess disability.

Direct care staff members, as well as nurses, must *know* when a person with dementia is taking more than one medication because these people are more vulnerable to medication interactions.

Whenever a new medication is added or a dose changed, direct care providers need to know, so that they can *monitor* the person for change—either side effects or the desired improvement. If the person does not improve as the physician had expected, the physician needs to know this. Ineffective drugs must be stopped and a new intervention tried.

Behavioral symptoms can be so frustrating that staff members are often desperate for a medication that will help. However, it is important to *recognize* that behavior-modifying medications have powerful side effects, which can set up a vicious cycle leading to worsened function and increased medication.

Overhead/Handout 3.11. Sensory Deficits

Teacher: Help students relate to sensory loss by talking about the impact of the sensory environment on them: dim light, glare behind the instructor, smeared printouts, noise in the classroom will all make students feel tired and irritated. Ask if the students need more light to thread a needle—all eyes need more light as they age, yet facilities often have poor light. In a discussion, help the students be more attuned to the ways in which the environment they work in supports or impedes sensory function. Because it is unlikely that students will be able to move a wall or turn off a furnace, ask them to look for ways they can modify the environment to make it work better.

Cognitive impairment multiplies the effect of the sensory loss. The person with a dementia may not know she has a sensory deficit. The person with dementia may not understand the need for adaptive devices such as hearing aids and glasses. Adaptive devices may be annoying: hearing aids can feel like a foreign object has been stuffed in one's ear; glasses can rub behind ears and, of course, get lost. Sensory impairments are difficult to recognize and diagnose, and interventions may be rejected by the person who does not understand them.

> Bill has a mild cognitive impairment. His daughter enrolled him in the adult day care center so that he could be with others and make friends, but this has not worked out. Bill refuses to participate in any activities, and he seems surprised and irritated whenever other participants approach him. He spends most of his time just sitting. He complains frequently. His daughter expected he would not have trouble finding his way around the well-marked center, but he often barges into the women's room by mistake, causing an uproar. During a thorough medical examination, the physician found that Bill needs new glasses. In a strange place he could not find his way around. He was able to adjust to his new glasses with frequent reminders to use them.

Any of the senses may be diminished in an older person. Aging eyes adapt more slowly to glare, need more light to see; disease may result in spotty vision or vision only in the periphery; poor vision may impair the ability to recognize people, see food, find one's own room. Glasses can distort vision if the impaired brain fails to compensate for the curve of the lens.

Hearing often diminishes with age. Certain pitches may be lost, particularly the higher pitch of women's voices; the person may hear a roaring noise or a high pitch in his head; background noise, vacuums, and showers may roar; people may seem to be mumbling. Hearing aids pick up background noise and can be annoying to wear. Hearing may be lost only to certain pitches.

People may lose subtle taste and need more seasoning in food; they may have a bad taste in the mouth; a dry mouth (a side effect of many psychoactive drugs) may make food difficult to swallow and cause dental problems. Food may taste like cardboard and stick in the throat. People may be unable to recognize that food is too hot.

A loss of smell affects appetite and pleasure. People may smell bad smells or strange smells when none is present.

Touch is a whole body feeling; it may be dulled or too sensitive; it may itch or feel crawly. The entire body may ache or burn (as in the flu). The sense of temperature may be impaired. People can burn themselves on hot water, food, and hot drinks. Always monitor the temperature of bath water and foods.

Overhead/Handout 3.12. How We Help

Use yourself. Tell the visually impaired person you are approaching her. Use touch only after she knows you are there. Show the person what you are doing. Sit close to the person. Sit beside his better ear.

Use adaptive devices (hearing aids, glasses). Encourage the person to use these devices but don't expect him to remember them or to know what they are for. Attach glasses or hearing aids to the person's shirt with a handsome cord. If all else fails, store the device and use it only part of the time, when you are with the person. Keep glasses clean and hearing aid batteries fresh. Be sure the prescription is current; out-of-date prescriptions for eyeglasses can make impairment worse and cause falls.

Make small changes. Use clothing, dishes, cups, activity supplies that are brightly colored and contrast strongly with the things around the person. Select pictures large enough for the person to see easily; seat the person with his back to the glare. Take the person to a quiet room to talk. Ask the person if she can see/hear. Tell the person what she is hearing or seeing ("That noise is the delivery truck coming"; "I am holding your orange juice"). Don't expect the person to know she is impaired or to compensate for her disability.

Change the environment instead of the person. Eliminate glare from windows, on tables, on waxed floors. Increase the amount of light in rooms. Aging eyes need more light. Increase the amount of contrast between doors and door frames, dishes and table, toilet and floor. Consider sensory losses when planning for safety.

Be alert for impairment in touch, taste, or smell. It is easy to overlook these in people who cannot report them, but impairments in these areas can make a big difference in quality of life.

Overhead/Handout 3.13. Balance Problems, Dizziness, and Tinnitus

Teacher: Most students will have experienced problems in balance and dizziness from alcohol intoxication, amusement park rides, or the flu. Ask them to recall the unpleasant feelings associated with these problems. Ask them what compensatory behaviors they used: holding on to things, not moving around.

People who feel off balance may refuse to walk or to do things.

Elderly people commonly have balance problems, caused by many different illnesses and arthritis or a side effect of many drugs. Just sitting motionless may make some people feel off balance when they stand up.

> Jorge got a mild cold and refused to do anything. He would not get out of his chair for meals, wet himself rather than get up to go to the toilet, and complained constantly. The staff thought his uncooperativeness could not be explained by his mild cold and encouraged his wife to get him up and walking around. Jorge fell and broke his shoulder. His cold had led to unsteadiness and dizziness.

Often people with dementia have no way of describing to us their feelings of dizziness or poor balance, and a physical exam may not reveal the problem. It is easy to overlook possible balance problems because the causes are so common: dizziness or unsteadiness are side effects of so many drugs and illnesses that we forget to watch for them. Often we overlook evidence of balance problems, as well. People with balance disorders develop compensatory behaviors, which they cannot maintain after they develop a dementia. Families often do not know that a person has a balance problem.

People who are unsteady or dizzy are at high risk of falls. People who feel unsteady give up activities because they feel unsure, because moving about feels unpleasant, and because they fear falls.

These problems are so common that they should be considered in every person. Signs include reluctance to get up, holding on to walls or chairs, holding the upper back and neck stiffly, moving slowly, not turning the head, any illness that causes slight edema in the inner ear, nausea, or loss of appetite. Presence of medications should alert you to the possibility of balance problems. Be sure that glasses prescriptions are not causing the problem.

Tinnitus is a fellow traveler of balance disorders. Cognitively intact people report that ringing in the ears can be so unpleasant that they seek medication, surgery, and even suicide to escape it. Expect balance disorders whenever a person complains of tinnitus, and expect tinnitus in anyone with a balance disorder. Assume that this symptom causes severe suffering. Loud noises such as in the shower can trigger tinnitus, which can last for hours.

Overhead/Handout 3.14. How We Help

Change the person from lying or sitting or standing slowly; move people slowly; encourage touching or hanging on to things; be sure there is adequate light (people with balance problems use their eyes to help them). Change medications; treat balance problems with medications. Reduce glare, bright lights, and sudden noises, which seem to make things worse. Use wing chairs so the person can steady her head. Let a person's stomach "settle down" before you offer food.

Exercise 2. The Role of the Direct Care Provider

Break up into small groups to discuss these questions. Introduce them by saying: We have been talking about a complex issue: illness, pain, medication reactions, sensory deficits, and dizziness. Whose responsibility do you think it is to monitor these matters?

Do you think you should know what signs to watch for? Or would it be better for you just to watch for any changes? Is it someone else's responsibility to watch for illness or side effects from medication? Does someone else see the person often enough to notice slight changes?

How do you find out what the potential side effects are of any drug the person you are caring for is taking? How are you going to learn to recognize signs of illness?

To whom will you report your observations? Will this person be able to act? Will you feel comfortable reporting things when you might be wrong?

Will you receive feedback? Do you want to be told what was happening with the person, or is this not part of your job?

If you want to change the way these things happen, what could be done without taking up too much time?

Exercise 3. The Impact of Excess Disability

Break the group into pairs: assign each person one item causing either sensory loss or pain from Exhibit 3.1. Each partner will tell the other:

1. In what way would the quality of my life be diminished if I . . . (fill in your assigned impairment)?
2. In what way would my ability to carry out my daily life be diminished if I . . . ?
3. How would a cognitive impairment make that disability greater?
4. How would . . . increase my risk of accidents?
5. If I also had a cognitive impairment, how might . . . make me agitated, angry, depressed, withdrawn, or moody?

Clinical Experience

As a small group or as individuals, identify a client and make a plan. Describe the problem you think might be caused by excess disability. Ask yourselves: Are there symptoms that fluctuate or are unstable? Does the client's health status indicate a possible excess disability (check the chart)? Might the person be in pain? Might medications be contributing to his difficulties? Does he have a sensory deficit that might be contributing to excess disability? Make a plan for a simple intervention that can be carried out in your setting within two weeks. Obtain the assistance of your supervisor to carry out the plan. Report to the group about what happened.

Section 3.3. Factors That Influence Excess Disability in People with Dementia

Objective

The student will learn the compounding effect that the impairments of dementia (memory, language, comprehension) have on the experience of additional illness, pain, medication reactions, and sensory deficits. This section emphasizes the range of potential causes of excess disability.

Information and Instructions for the Teacher

Many of these ideas have been presented in Section 3.2 and in Lesson 2. However, it is rarely easy to identify excess disability in people who cannot communicate or understand their distress. Sometimes even nurses and physicians miss some physical disability or are unable to identify its source. This section teaches the students how the cognitive disability interacts with the physical disability. The most effective way to teach this is to ask the class to discuss each point. Use Exercise 3 from Section 3.2, which is designed to make students more sensitive to this problem. Use Lesson 2 and Sections 3.1 and 3.2 as background. Ask questions that will trigger discussion: How might the brain damage (such as communication difficulties or inability to identify body parts) cause this problem? How could the physical problem make the person's thinking or ability to communicate worse? (The person who is in pain or tired from illness will not be able to function as well.) What examples of this problem have you seen? How might you get around it?

Use Exhibit 3.1 to remind yourself of potential causes of excess disability. It will be more successful to ask students to think of the range of things they have observed than to hand out this long list. Make suggestions from it to guide a discussion. Hand it out as a reference list for students who will become educators.

Use Overhead/Handout 3.10 for talking points. Use the text for additional information. Put it in your own words.

Lecture/Discussion Notes to Be Presented to the Class

Overhead/Handout 3.15. Detectives Wanted

The title "Detectives Wanted" is used to emphasize the problem-solving nature of this task.

The person with dementia may not know what is causing him distress. The person may become restless or distressed, cry, or refuse to do things without being able to tell you why. People may walk on fractures, feel weak or nauseated without reporting a problem.

Even if the person can usually explain where discomfort is or articulate her needs, the additional disability caused by the illness may make her unable to communicate this now.

Looking back over the disabilities in Section 3.2, what things might the person be unable to report?

To help the person tell you what is wrong, use the words the person might have used. For example, "feeling sick" means feeling nauseated to some; to others it means a general malaise. "A cold" means any complaint for some people. Check for appetite, for fluid intake, for not wanting to move. Check vital signs.

The person with dementia may not be able to localize her distress. A person may complain of pain "all over" when she actually means weakness, malaise, or localized pain. When a person reports pain "all over," this may signal a medication reaction or illness such as the flu that can cause a feeling of pain "all over."

The person with dementia may not compensate for the disability. She may not stop walking on a painful leg, not seek more light to improve vision, not turn the TV off to hear better or ask you to speak louder, not compensate for stiff muscles upon rising, and so on.

The same symptoms may mean different things at different times or in different people. It is risky to generalize even with the same person at different times.

While one person screams when she is tired, another screams only when she has a bowel obstruction; and a third becomes combative in both situations. The fact that there are symptoms may be more important than what the specific symptoms are.

The person with dementia may not know whether her distress is serious. A person may be truly distressed by minor problems that you know have no medical significance, whereas others may ignore serious conditions. Minor problems such as a gas pain or muscle cramp may be frightening or cause anxiety for the person who cannot assess what is happening. Use extra support and reassurance.

The person with dementia usually won't remember having already told you about her distress; nor will she remember that you reassured her. The person may complain every few minutes because she does not remember asking you before or being reassured by you. She may be frightened. She may not remember your instructions and keep walking on painful feet, for example, and keep on complaining. Complaining again and again is not attention seeking: it is a memory problem. Reassure her again and again; offer touch, eye contact. If possible, get her involved in something, but don't be surprised if she is unable to focus on anything beyond her distress. Advice such as "Just stop walking and watch your favorite TV show" will not be reasonable for her.

The person may not understand your questions or be able to make herself understood. Problems in using and understanding language often mean that you cannot understand what the person is trying to tell you. Rely on nonverbal communication. Never dismiss the client's efforts as meaningless.

The person with dementia often does not understand the need for the intervention (e.g., medication, physical therapy, glasses, hearing aid, staying in bed, soft diet, diabetic diet, disimpaction, restraints). Treatment is often experienced as a further threat or source of suffering.

No amount of explaining will help in the above situations because the person will have difficulty comprehending and remembering explanations. Reassure people over and over, repeatedly remind people to sit down or whatever relieves them, and accept the impact of these cognitive limitations.

Section 3.4. Information about Excess Disability and Delirium

Objective

Students responsible for diagnosis, assessment, referral, or treatment will learn additional background on causes and treatments of excess disability and delirium. This section may be used as independent study or as reference material.

Lecture/Discussion Notes to Be Presented to the Class

Many of the illnesses that underlie excess disability are chronic, and the medications that treat them contribute to excess disability. In some cases, aggressive treatment of an underlying illness is inappropriate because the treatment itself would contribute to the patient's suffering and disability.

Studies show that excess disability is common in people with dementia. It often contributes to behavioral and functional symptoms. Temporary improvement in cognitive function is observed in many patients, although permanent reversal of the dementia is uncommon. Treatment of excess disability is ongoing. As soon as one problem is identified and treated, another may appear. Often a person with dementia will have multiple causes of excess disability at once—when one is found, the task is not over. The clinical personnel must assume that ongoing judicious tinkering is necessary.

Staff recognition is only part of the task. Programs may have serious difficulty finding medical personnel trained to identify and treat underlying illnesses or the financial support for their time.

Despite these limitations, the search for excess disability, even when limited or incomplete, is worthwhile. The goal may not be cure but the improvement of life quality and the treatment of behavioral symptoms.

Excess disability may or may not include delirium. (A person limping because his shoe hurts him has excess disability but not delirium.) Delirium is characterized by a clouding of consciousness, impairments in attention, and a fluctuating mental state. (See Section 1.4.) It is commonly associated with illness or medication reactions and is thus associated with excess disability.

The Prevalence of Excess Disability

Studies report high rates of delirium in hospitalized patients. As many as 50 percent of some patient groups in acute care may have delirium. One study found that 96 percent of patients who had been delirious in hospitals were still delirious when discharged to nursing homes. Thus, patients transferred to subacute units will have high rates of delirium.

Causes of Delirium and Excess Disability

The most common causes of delirium are associated with circulatory, respiratory, infectious, and metabolic disorders. Expect delirium in the days or weeks following surgery.

The greater the number of medications, the greater the risk of delirium. New medications are always suspect. However, there may be a long delay (several weeks) before the side effects of new medications appear.

Old age and dementia, immobility, falls, gastrointestinal problems, arthritis, and restraints are risk factors for delirium or other excess disability.

Psychosocial factors such as isolation, loss, mood, use of restraints, and relocation may trigger delirium. Problems in vision and hearing may cause it.

If the underlying cause of the delirium is not treated, the outcome may be irreversible impairment or death.

The most common causes of delirium and excess disability were discussed in Sections 3.1 and 3.2. Following are a few causes discussed in the literature that are sometimes overlooked in dementia care.

Hypothermia. Age-related thermoregulatory control, underlying clinical conditions such as endocrine or neurological disorders, severe infections, circulatory disturbances, limited mobility, confusion, and certain types of medication place people at increased risk of hypothermia. Elderly people with dementia who live alone in social isolation; who have a low, fixed income; who live in substandard housing; and who have inadequate clothing or bedding are at risk. A preexisting mild confusion makes the person less likely to get help. Cognition will worsen rapidly with hypothermia. Symptoms of hypothermia include lethargy, confusion, cardiac arrhythmia, ventricular fibrillation, irreversible coma, and death. People in warm climates are also at risk on cold days.

Dehydration. Dehydration is common in people who forget to drink, people who are living at home, people taking medications, people with a medical illness, and people who do not like to drink water.

Malnutrition. Malnutrition is common in older people, including those who live alone, have no access to food supplies, and are no longer able to prepare food.

Oral Problems. Oral problems can directly cause excess disability or affect appetite and nutrition. The dry mouth caused by anticholinergic drugs for depression or agitation causes significant discomfort and compounds oral problems.

Constipation and Fecal Impaction. Individual patients may show behavioral changes after missing a bowel movement for only three days.

Excess Disability and Delirium May Be Chronic. Excess disability and delirium may both be chronic, and delirium from an acute illness may not fully resolve. Or the underlying cause may not be recognized and fully treated.

The Treatment of Excess Disability or Delirium

As a consequence of these factors, treatment requires three strategies:

1. frequent—in some cases daily—close monitoring of all people with cognitive impairment;
2. identifying all the threads of cause in a person with multiple illnesses; and
3. a complete record of the person's mental status over time. This identifies usual level of function, individual indicators of excess disability, and individual risk factors.

The nonmedical management of delirium in acute care is to reduce and simplify stimuli, provide reassurance and calmness, and provide one-to-one contact (for example, have a volunteer or family member stay with the hospitalized person). These strategies are discussed in detail in Section 11.5.

Overhead/Handout 3.16. The Use of Medication in Dementia Care

Use as few medications as possible. Both the physician and the nurse must monitor medications closely. Use nondrug interventions whenever possible. Do everything else instead of using medications to control behavior problems.

Watch for drug-precipitated delirium.

Know what the side effects are for each drug and watch for them. Report any changes you observe. In people with dementia, side effects may appear weeks after the medication was started. Consider this when a new symptom appears. Uncommon side effects seem to appear more commonly in people with dementia.

Go low and slow. Begin with lower-than-usual doses. Increase slowly, gradually, if necessary. Adjust the time of administration to the patient's symptoms. When using medication to treat behavioral symptoms, try to target the dose for the times of day when it is most needed and avoid the effects of the drug at times when the person should be active and involved. The level of some medications may increase in the body over days or weeks, resulting in a delayed overdose.

Consider drugs that have a short half-life and the fewest side effects. For example, choose a sleeping medication that does not stay in the body and make the person drowsy during the day.

Periodically reassess the person's medications. As the disease progresses, the person may no longer need the medication. Increased frailty may trigger side effects when the medication had previously been tolerated.

Choose a dosage form that can be easily administered. Is it easier for this person to take liquid or a pill? Use apple juice, orange juice, or any other food. Ask the pharmacist whether the medication loses potency if crushed or cut and not used right away.

Ensure that a responsible person administers medication. In home care, never leave a person's daily dose for her to take alone, no matter how able she appears. She may become confused later and put the pills down the drain or give them to the dog. Have a neighbor stop by to give her medication.

People with dementia may hide a pill in their mouth and carry it around, then put it down when you are not watching. They forget they are supposed to swallow it, and then forget what it is in their mouth. Watch to see that medications are actually swallowed. Tell the person to swallow or offer fluids.

Things to Remember about Psychoactive Medication

These drugs were designed to treat people who have symptoms such as hallucinations or delusions and other symptoms of schizophrenia or depression. They were not designed to treat the symptoms of dementia in frail elderly persons. Therefore, they must be used somewhat differently in this population.

In low doses these drugs can be helpful with *certain symptoms* of dementia such as agitation or irritability when these symptoms disturb the person.

They are sometimes helpful in situations in which the person needs to be treated quickly to prevent behaviors that place the person with dementia or others in danger.

These drugs may be nearly useless. If the target behavioral symptom does not respond to drug intervention, consider withdrawing the drug. These drugs usually don't help with behaviors that make sense to the confused person (such as agenda behavior). (See Section 11.2.) They should not be given in large enough doses to "snow" the patient so that she can't act out. At these doses there will be serious side effects. Target psychoactive drugs to symptoms that appear distressing to the person with dementia such as frightening hallucinations.

To be effective, the drugs must be used in combination with psychosocial modifications. They do not replace other interventions.

The side effects may be worse than the benefits. Some side effects may be fatal or cause irreversible harm. Other side effects cause discomfort severe enough to result in more behavioral symptoms.

It is easier to cause side effects than it is to get rid of them.

Many of these drugs are similar in their therapeutic effects. These drugs should be selected for their side effects in the light of the individual's needs (e.g., if a person tends toward constipation, use the less-constipating drug).

Exhibit 3.1. Some Potential Causes of Excess Disability

This exhibit lists conditions that may contribute to excess disability. It includes many that are easily ignored or missed because they are subclinical. Some of the items listed may seem trivial, but they are not trivial to the person who cannot get relief or to the staff member who must cope with a decline in function or an increase in behavioral problems. And remember, the person probably has multiple problems.

Use this list as a reference or discuss how one or two of these conditions might cause excess disability. A registered nurse will be able to describe the symptoms of these conditions to the lay student.

Headache
Crawly feeling in scalp or on skin
Stopped-up ears
Tinnitus (cognitively intact people report severe distress and suffering)
Buildup of ear wax (impairs hearing)
Dizziness
Sinus headache
Difficulty breathing, asthma
Airborne allergies
Sore gums
Oral abscesses
Toothache; canker sores; tooth sensitivity to hot, cold, or sweets
Burns, including tongue
Poorly fitting dentures
Disk disease; muscle spasm; stiffness in spine, all joints
Sore throat
Feeling of drowning (as in emphysema)
Shortness of breath (can be frightening; do not assume this is "psychological")
Feeling of weight on chest (may feel frightening)
Angina
Arthritis in neck, shoulder, hands, spine, hips, knees, feet
Gastric reflux
Esophageal spasm
Heartburn
Stomach pain
Nausea
Colds, flu
Pneumonia, bronchitis
Malaise and general aching from flu or fever
Hiatal hernia (pain)
Constipation (mental clouding and pain)
Diarrhea
"Gas pains" or bloating (can be very painful)
Urinary retention/frequency (needing to urinate every few minutes is a real feeling, not attention seeking, even when the person produces only a few drops of urine; look for drug side effect or illness)

(continued)

Exhibit 3.1. *(continued)*

Urinary tract infection
Itching, rashes on skin, rectum, genitals, underarm due to deodorant or lotions, herpes zoster, etc.
Unhealed sores
Tears in fragile skin
Fungal, yeast infections; skin tears in genitals; area beneath foreskin not clean
Burning from needing to clean skin in rectal, genital area
Hidden fractures or sprains in feet, ankles, wrists, hip; compression fracture of spine
Bursitis
Stiff muscles from lack of movement or poor posture in chair or bed
Muscle spasm
Feet distorted from wearing wrong shoes in past
Corns, bunions
Aches from poor circulation
Cold hands and feet; headache from cold ears
Dry eyes, cosmetics/shampoos in the eyes
Undetected ear infections, ear pain
Diabetes
Hair pulled too tight
Covers heavy on feet
Stuffy nose
Shaving nicks
Insect bites
Cracking and drying nailbeds
Bruises
Dry skin
Shoes that rub
Toenails cutting into flesh
Bras that ride up over the breasts
Clothing that binds or rubs
Sock stuffed into toe of shoe; other apparel or items worn inappropriately
Difficulty walking that makes people feel unsteady/afraid/painful/frustrated
Turtleneck giving feeling of choking
Rings that pinch
Allergies
Dry mouth; if fluids are withheld after dinner, person may be frantic, contributes to dental disease
Feeling cold: people who are older and less active often feel cold when staff members feel warm

Overhead/Handout 3.1. The Definition of Excess Disability

Excess disability is more disability than can be explained by the dementia alone.

Causes of excess disability:

- Illness
- Medication reaction/interaction
- Pain
- Sensory deficits (for example, vision or hearing impairment)
- Dizziness

The direct care provider is the best person to notice and report excess disability.

Overhead/Handout 3.2. Outcomes of Excess Disability

- More disability
- Decreased function
- Increased behavioral symptoms
- Falls
- Incontinence
- Risk of death

Overhead/Handout 3.3. Things to Watch For

Watch for change
- in irritability
- in ability or willingness to do ADLs
- in refusal to do things
- in mental function (drowsiness; lower level of alertness and less ability to focus; fluctuating ability over hours or days)
- at any time medications have been changed

Listen to complaints
- of pain
- of unhappiness

Overhead/Handout 3.4. How We Help

1. Watch for even slight changes in behavior or function.
2. Report these promptly.
3. Continue to observe the person for changes.
4. Never assume that worsened behavior or a decline in skills is a natural decline due to the dementia.

Overhead/Handout 3.5. Some Common Illnesses That Cause Excess Disability

Constipation

Urinary tract infection

Upper respiratory infection

Pneumonia

Oral abscesses

Overhead/Handout 3.6. How We Help

Check it out.

Get medical care.

Give tender loving care.

Overhead/Handout 3.7. Pain

Examples

Arthritis

Muscle cramp

Stomach pain

Compression fracture of spine

Cancer pain

Common Symptoms

Moaning

Increased agitation

Stubbornness

Refusal to cooperate with ADLs

Screaming

Overhead/Handout 3.8.
How We Help

Ask, explore for pain (sometimes people will not be able to answer).

Look for behavioral clues, including facial expression.

Take pain seriously.

Treat pain.

Give extra support.

Overhead/Handout 3.9. Reactions to Medication

Medications	*Common Symptoms*
Antipsychotics	Increased confusion Stiffness Falls Tardive dyskinesia Parkinsonian symptoms Constipation
Nonsteroidal anti-inflammatory drugs	Gastric pain
Minor tranquilizers	Depression Falls Increased confusion
Antidepressants	Dry mouth Difficulty urinating Depression/agitation Increased confusion

Overhead/Handout 3.10. How We Help

Suspect because side effects of medication are common in people with dementia.

Know when the people you care for are on several medications.

Monitor people for signs of excess disability when a new medication is added or a dose changed.

Recognize that medications can make behavior worse instead of better.

Overhead/Handout 3.11. Sensory Deficits

Deficit	*Symptom*
Hearing loss	
Needs hearing aid	Suspiciousness
Hearing aid unpleasant	Stubbornness
Profound loss, not responding to hearing aid	Hallucinations
Vision loss	
Cataracts	Reluctance to move around
Wrong glasses prescription	Fearfulness
	Falls
Taste	
Damage in the brain or at taste buds	Loss of appetite
	Eats only a few foods
Effect of medication	Seeks excessive seasoning
Does not recognize hot foods	
Complains that food tastes bad	
Dry mouth	Finds food difficult to swallow
Smell	
As above, closely related to taste	Loss of appetite
	Complains of bad smells
Touch	
Effect of brain damage	Does not recognize hotness
	Feels itchy or crawly
	Complains of achiness or burning
	Complains that being touched or clothing hurts

Overhead/Handout 3.12.
How We Help

Use yourself.

Use adaptive devices.

Make small changes.

Change the environment instead of the person.

Be alert for impairment in touch, taste, and smell.

Overhead/Handout 3.13. Balance Problems, Dizziness, and Tinnitus

Balance problems are common.

Balance problems are hidden.

Balance problems are dangerous and disabling.

Tinnitus causes suffering.

Overhead/Handout 3.14. How We Help

Be alert to the potential for problems in balance (clinging to things, reluctance to move, unsteadiness, illness, medications).

Allow the person to rest briefly when changing position from lying to sitting or standing.

Do not allow the person to sit slumped or twisted for more than a few minutes (leads to pinched nerves in arthritic neck).

Be sure that eyeglass prescription is correct.

Review all medications for side effects that cause dizziness or tinnitus.

Monitor balance when the person is ill (especially any illness that may cause edema or nausea).

Encourage the person to hold on to things.

Ask if the person feels dizzy or has ringing in the ears.

Avoid exposing the person to prolonged loud noise such as vacuum or shower (these exacerbate tinnitus).

Promptly correct noise caused by hearing aids.

Overhead/Handout 3.15. Detectives Wanted

The person with dementia may not know what is causing her distress.

The person may not be able to localize the site of her distress.

The person may not compensate for the disability.

The same symptoms may mean different things at different times or in different people.

The person may not know whether her distress is serious.

The person will not remember having told you and will not remember that you reassured her.

The person cannot understand your questions or make herself understood.

The person does not understand the need for the intervention (e.g., medication, physical therapy, glasses, hearing aid, staying in bed, soft diet, diabetic diet).

Overhead/Handout 3.16. The Use of Medication in Dementia Care

Use as few medications as possible.

Use nondrug interventions whenever possible.

Watch for drug-precipitated delirium (increased confusion).

Watch for drug interactions, side effects.

Use lower-than-usual doses; increase gradually if necessary (low and slow).

Adjust times of administration to patient symptoms.

Consider medication with short half-life, fewest side effects.

Periodically reassess the person's medications.

Choose a dosage form that can be easily administered.

Ensure that a responsible person administers medication.

Review the person's medications regularly.

Tailor medications to the individual; consider the side effect profile when selecting a medication.

LESSON 4

FACILITATING FUNCTION BY TREATING STRESS

Summary. This lesson describes the role of stress (physical, emotional, and environmental) in the behavioral symptoms of dementia. It teaches the student to recognize increasing stress, and it provides a repertoire of interventions.

Section 4.1. The Role of Stress in Behavioral Symptoms. Introduces the role of stress in behavioral symptoms, teaches the student to recognize increasing stress, and introduces strategies for reducing stress.

Section 4.2. Alleviating Symptoms of Stress. Further describes causes of stress and successful interventions. This section describes the prevention of and interventions for catastrophic reactions.

Section 4.3. Responding to a Catastrophic Reaction. Describes further interventions when a catastrophic reaction does occur.

Section 4.4. The Need for Stimulation and the Difference between Stress and Stimulation. Teaches the student to recognize the difference between noxious stressors and therapeutic stimulation.

Using the Sections

Introductory course:
- Section 4.1 required
- Section 4.2 select a few items appropriate to group
- Section 4.3 required
- Section 4.4 optional

Core course:
- Section 4.1 required
- Section 4.2 required
- Section 4.3 required
- Section 4.4 required

Problems You May Have in Implementing This Lesson

Many of the causes of overstress are common in institutional and home care settings. There is little the student can do to reduce the stress of showering a person if that person is already overwhelmed by background noise, an inhospitable environment, untreated health problems, and the like. If the staff members are trying to provide care in such an environment, aggressively look for ways to make environmental change.

The common assumption that the staff approach is the primary factor in behavioral symptoms is not always correct. Staff care may be appropriate, but the pressures on the staff and flaws in the physical plant may contribute to distress for the person with dementia. For example, well-trained staff members who clearly understand that time is lost when they try to rush people will rush people anyway when they themselves feel overwhelmed. It is psychologically very difficult to act slowly when we feel rushed or to act calmly when we feel stressed. Training will be more effective if leaders make the assumption that the staff members believe they are doing the best they can rather than criticizing them for failings.

Program design must include support and resources for the staff. People with dementia tend to focus their frustrations on the person who is caring for them and may calm down when a new person intervenes and the previous worker is out of sight. A staff member who is caring for someone who becomes upset should be able to quickly and informally trade tasks with a different staff member. This requires that all staff members accept that someone will substitute for them the next time. Quite often the staff member most able to step in is the supervisor or program director. Programs must be staffed well enough for this to be possible, and staff members must learn to be alert to their coworkers. In many cases, this means reprogramming for increased flexibility rather than for increased staffing. Stable staffing (often a problem) is important in the management of stress. During changes in staffing or times when the program is short staffed, people with dementia will be more likely to show evidence of increased stress. Recognize this and support the staff during such periods.

Distressed staff members should be allowed unscheduled breaks to calm down and may need extra support at times. Only a very unfeeling person could move directly from a distressing struggle to gentle caregiving for the next person. Sometimes staff members will receive serious bruises or scratches from people with dementia. They may shrug and say that it comes with the job. No one should have to have this happen on the job. In such an environment, there is little opportunity for the healing of human relationships to occur.

Because prevention is the key to success, schedules must provide time to discuss what happened and plan a preventative strategy.

Home settings can be stressful and not always subject to change. Family caregivers who are depressed and exhausted cannot be expected to readily change to care strategies that would be easier for the client. Part of the answer for people living at home may be to move them into a low-stress day care environment for part of the day. If the in-home worker is the only available respite and is entering a home where stress is already intense, the care plan must allow for this.

A key factor in any setting is for staff members to know the person they are caring for. If they do not know the idiosyncrasies and subtle cues of their clients and their clients are too distressed to be able to establish a trusting bond with the staff, there will inevitably be problems.

Few things are as overwhelming and frustrating as being asked to care for, or even keep control of, a group of distressed people with dementia. In this environment, even experts cannot figure out what to do next. Success with difficult clients requires that the staff members have gained confidence in their own skills by experiencing success. Start new staff members with people who are easier to care for. As staff members gain skills and confidence, they will be ready to meet greater challenges when the client's condition declines.

If you are training staff members who are already working with many distressed clients, assign them only a few clients so they have time to build trust and get to know them. Assign an experienced mentor to new staff members.

Working in a high-stress setting burns out staff members. It teaches them that an unpleasant workplace is inevitable with people with dementia and that they themselves have little power to change things. Classroom teaching will not, by itself, counteract this.

People with dementia are so vulnerable to stressors that it is unlikely that any setting will eliminate them entirely, and a few people seem driven by a level of internal distress so severe that most interventions fail. However, with good care, the overall level of catastrophic reactions can be contained. For example, on one unit, 16 clients with a history of combative behavior experienced no catastrophic reactions or striking out in one week. However, no shift passed during which staff members did not observe, and head off, incipient outbursts. It is important that the staff and management recognize this and set reasonable goals for the gradual reduction of catastrophic outbursts.

Section 4.1. The Role of Stress in Behavioral Symptoms

Objective

The student will learn the importance of stress—physical, emotional, and environmental—in the care of persons with dementia.

Background

Stress is a major cause of behavioral symptoms in dementia. This is the third of three factors influencing life quality and behavioral symptoms in people with dementia: the brain damage, excess disability and finally, the unique response to stressors characteristic of dementia.

These three factors are interactive: the brain damage alters the way the individual responds to excess disability and changes the nature of experienced stress as well as the person's ability to respond to stressors. Excess disability is itself an additional stressor.

Desperate caregivers often see medication as essential to keep people with dementia calm. However, there are as many good reasons not to use antipsychotics and sedatives as there are in favor of their judicious use. It is not possible simply to withdraw these drugs and expect the staff (or the person with dementia) to cope. It is essential that the transition to nonchemical strategies is made on an individual basis and over time, allowing the staff members to gain confidence in their new skills.

Information and Instructions for the Teacher

By now, your students have some idea of things that cause stress. Help them apply this knowledge in this lesson.

The lesson begins with examples of stress as a behavioral symptom. The first discussion is designed to help the student recognize what stress means through his own experience. Then the student learns that a cognitively intact person has much more resilience and ability to tolerate stress than the person with dementia.

Present the lecture in your own words and use the overheads/handouts for talking points.

Quite often the students will present clients whose behavior seems "impossible" to treat. If you find yourself suggesting various interventions that won't work for one reason or another, briefly discuss possible strategies, then let this topic drop. Instead of learning a list of ways to help, students are learning a new way of thinking. Encourage students to test new skills on the "easy" people. Eventually, often after the course ends, students will find easier ways to work with even the challenging people.

Novice staff members tend to look for one big cause of stress, which often cannot be eliminated (showers, going to the doctor). More often, a dozen stressors lead to the final blowup around the serious stress of showering or other activity. Encourage student problem solving to identify these "minor" stressors.

Solving problems requires accurately describing what is happening. The terms *agitated* and *combative* are vague and don't give staff members the information they need. Ask students to describe these behaviors in more specific terms. The students should include behaviors such as hits (name the target person), spits, bites (name the person), pinches, shouts, bangs (name what is struck), makes threats, cries, stubborn, refuses to do . . . , uncooperative (when), won't let you into her room, or won't give you something.

Material in this lesson repeats material in the previous lessons. Help your students to connect what they have learned previously to the problem of irritable or resistive behavior. The overheads/handouts in this lesson are also somewhat repetitive. Students need to hear and see key information more than once in order to learn it and to counter prior attitudes toward difficult behaviors. You may modify this material to suit the needs of your group.

Lecture/Discussion Notes to Be Presented to the Class

We have talked about how the loss of different mental functions affects behavioral symptoms. Then we talked about how illness and other disabilities affect function. In this lesson we will talk about the third major factor that affects function and behavioral symptoms: stress. Physical, emotional, and environmental stress are the cause of many angry outbursts, striking out, stubborn refusal of care, and similar behaviors.

Stress and stimulation are two sides of the same thing. Stress is the negative side. In people with dementia stress usually appears as a behavioral symptom or as crying or refusing to cooperate. Stimulation is the positive side: every person, whether that person has a dementia or not, enjoys stimulation. In fact, people with dementia need stimulation in their lives, and if their lives are too boring, they may become frustrated. We will address stimulation in Section 4.4.

Here are some examples of behavioral symptoms that are the result of too much stress for individuals with dementia.

In the midst of a craft activity Walter suddenly grabbed the scissors and began banging them against the wall. Soon Walter was completely out of control, waving the scissors and shouting. The staff members were afraid he would hurt one of the participants.

When her aide tried to dress Ann, Ann would first stubbornly refuse to get dressed, then grab the aide's hair. Sometimes she would strike out.

Joyce would sit quietly in the day room for a while and then abruptly start an argument with another resident.

Some people seem to remain angry and combative all day. Mrs. Waddell reported that her husband was shouting by breakfast time. He would grab her arms hard enough to leave bruises. He would stamp around the house, shouting at her in anger. Sometimes he hit her when she tried to get him to take his medicine. Sometimes he threw his food at her.

This kind of behavior is a frequent part of caring for people with dementia. It is exhausting for families and staff. In this lesson we will talk about what it is, what causes it, and what we can do to prevent or react to these behavioral symptoms.

Let's begin by not using terms such as "angry," "stubborn," "resists care." Terms that imply attitudes don't help us find ways to reduce these behavioral symptoms. Instead, we will think in terms of feelings of stress and the stressors the person with dementia experiences.

We're all familiar with stress in our own lives. (List some of the causes of stress experienced by staff members.) There are different kinds of stress. (On the flip chart, list physical, emotional, and environmental stressors. Ask the group to suggest some in each category. Below are some ideas. Remind the group to think of stressors of all sorts, not just emotional.)

Stress caused by physical feelings:

- having a headache
- being tired
- having a cold
- being up all night

Stress caused by emotions:

- not getting along with someone you care about
- being put down by your supervisor
- feeling angry or depressed
- having more work than you can finish

Stress caused by the environment:

- room too noisy
- not enough light
- too many interruptions

Our own experience of stress is that stressors add up. (Can you cope better with a headache if you were not also up all night and upset by your supervisor?) Our own experience of stress also tells us that there are mild and intense feelings of stress.

(Teacher: Ask the students to discuss how they react to stress.) What do you do when you feel stressed? Describe the behaviors that you see in yourself and other cognitively well people when you and they feel stressed. Do you argue? sulk? complain a lot? walk away?

Well people can rationalize the cause of stress (for example, "He's yelling at me because he had a bad day at work" or "It's not really my fault"). Or they can find a way to channel their stress (I'll go outside and have a cigarette or complain to my friend and then I'll be OK).

Now let's think about the person with dementia and how her experience of stress is different. The person with dementia experiences much more stress in daily life than we do. Imagine feeling embarrassed because someone else is putting your clothes on; needing to go to the bathroom and not being able to find it; not knowing where you are or what those noises are; feeling tired and not knowing what it is you are feeling. Just getting through the day is exhausting and stressful for people with dementia.

On top of the stress of just getting through the day, people with dementia experience many other stressors:

a. The confusion the brain damage causes creates stress: seeing or hearing people no one else does, anxiety or depression generated by the brain disease, the struggle to talk or understand.
b. Any excess disability is an additional stressor.
c. Things that frighten the person or that the person does not want to do (such as bathing or going to the doctor) are stressful.
d. Things the person does not understand (such as why his wife is now telling him what to do all the time) is another stressor.

In Lesson 2 we talked about how the damage to the brain affects the person. It is unlikely that the person with brain damage can rationalize or channel distress as you can. Because of the brain damage, the person with dementia is less able to cope with feelings of stress, even minor stress. We have talked about the person's impaired ability to understand or control frustration. Well people have a little voice in the back of their head that reminds them that they really do not want to yell at or hit someone. They can figure out the consequences of such behavior. People with dementia may have lost the ability to control their impulses. This means that if their impulse is to hit, they cannot keep themselves from doing that. In Lesson 3 we talked about the impact of excess disability. The brains of people with dementia are more vulnerable to the effects of excess disability. In fact, both the brain damage and excess disability are additional stressors.

The damaged brain seems more fragile—somehow more vulnerable to stress than our brains. Because of this, we use the term *catastrophic reactions.* A catastrophic reaction is an overreaction to a stressor, even a minor stressor. The person's reaction need not be catastrophic in the sense that it is violent: catastrophic means just an overreaction. Whether we call it a catastrophic reaction or "agitation," *things are different: the person with dementia cannot control his reaction.*

We might assume that people with dementia are not aware of all these problems. They often don't remember or know about specific events, but they probably do retain the increasing feelings of distress. We will talk more about this "retaining of feelings" as we continue.

Exercise 1. The Impact of Brain Damage and Excess Disability

Review a few of the disabilities discussed in Lesson 2. Ask the group how these alone would stress a person. Select a few examples of disability from Exhibit 3.1 and ask the group how even minor problems can stress these fragile people. Then ask the group for examples of how these will interact. (If you can't think clearly, have a headache, and someone is trying to shower you, these can all add up.)

Overhead/Handout 4.1. Examples of Common Stressors

Overhead/Handout 4.1 lists some of the common stressors for people with dementia. *(Teacher: Guide a discussion of ways in which these issues create problems for people with dementia. Ask the group for examples.)*

A common cause of stress is *cognitive overload.* Our minds work so smoothly that well people rarely notice this feeling, but the person with dementia may constantly feel overwhelmed. Having to think of several things at once, even listening to your explanation, remembering what will happen next, or trying to do several steps of a task means cognitive overload. Many people feel cognitive overload most of the day. Some tune out; others become angry and upset.

Imagine a world in which you *cannot figure out what is going on.* People walking around, someone doing something to you, going someplace—all can be upsetting because the confused person cannot figure out what is going on.

Because understanding language is one of the mental losses in dementia, *not understanding a request* often stresses people. Have you seen a person become more upset when you asked him to do something or when you tried to explain something?

Not being able to do things that were formerly automatic or the inability to do an old, familiar task is always stressful. Imagine how upsetting it would be not to be able to put your clothes on. (A zipper that jams can upset a well person!) Embarrassment at fumbling or failing can add to the stress.

Fatigue is a major factor in stress, even when it does not seem to the caregiver that the person should be tired. One caregiver said, "I'm doing everything for him. Why is he tired?" Consider the things we have just discussed. This may explain why he is tired. By the end of the day, fatigue may be making it impossible for the person to cope as well as he did earlier. This is one cause of "sundowning."

Imagine trying and trying—and your caregiver is trying to understand—but you can't explain that you are hungry or would like to be by yourself for a while. Or trying to tell a joke and being taken to the bathroom in response. You can see why the *inability to communicate* stresses people with dementia.

All these things add up to *frustration*. For the person who cannot control his expression of frustration, this may mean an angry outburst. The caregiver may be as frustrated as the person with dementia, but because frustration is "contagious," try to communicate calmness.

In Section 6.2 we talk about being patronizing. Although it is difficult to avoid treating a person who is so disabled in a childlike way, doing so emphasizes her disability and makes her feel worse. Even when she cannot understand words, the person with dementia can usually understand the caregiver's *nonverbal patronizing behavior.*

We talked in Lesson 3 about the impact of *not feeling well* on the person with dementia. Not understanding what is wrong or being unable to communicate her feelings adds to the stress the person feels.

Noise is tiring for most well people. Trying to listen in a classroom that is noisy or trying to concentrate when a machine is running in the background tires well people. For people with dementia, noise is particularly distressing because they may not be able to "tune it out," because they may not understand what the noise means, and because it interferes with their ability to think as well as they can.

All these thing we have described make people feel anxious, and the *anxiety* itself is stressful.

Well people are in control of lots of little things that they take for granted, such as where they have a snack or how they put on their clothes. People with dementia lose these routine kinds of control *and also are not in control of the major decisions* that are made about them. This is stressful. Often the impaired person will insist that she can manage just fine or will become angry over something that seems minor to the caregiver, such as who holds the TV remote control.

When people with dementia have some *unmet need,* such as needing to use the toilet, needing to rest, or being hungry, they may not recognize what the need is. They may not be able to communicate their need or even answer when asked if they need to toilet. They may just feel "not right." When a care provider knows each individual she cares for, she can often guess what the person needs and help.

Overhead/Handout 4.2. How We Help

The first step in helping is to accept that this behavior is something the person cannot control. It is not manipulative, mean, or deliberate. *But even though the person with dementia cannot prevent or control these behaviors, there is much that the caregiver can do to help.* This will make sense to you in most cases, but in some cases, these behavioral symptoms will still seem deliberate or manipulative. Such behavioral symptoms frustrate, anger, and discourage both family members and staff. Our natural impulse is to explain things, to argue, or to push the person to just get the task done and over with. But trying to get the person to make sense or stop doing what she is doing usually does not work. The most successful way to change the way the person acts is to use a different approach: we change the environment or change how we act.

The first step, always, is to consider how the brain damage is contributing to the problem. Can you find ways to *make fewer demands on the person's lost abilities* or to *take advantage of the person's retained abilities?* Second, ask yourself *whether the person is experiencing any excess disabilities?* Can these be treated? If not, can you help the person cope with them?

The most important and most successful way to help people *reduce the amount of stress people with dementia experience* and to reduce the number of behavioral symptoms is to reduce the number of stressors they feel. Section 4.2 focuses on this.

Once a person has become seriously upset, there

is little you can do to control his behavior. The situation is out of control. Therefore, *prevention* of a major catastrophic reaction is the only way to help the person—and help yourself avoid a crisis. Almost all of the rest of this lesson talks about prevention of overstress because once the person is experiencing a major catastrophic reaction, you have few options.

Take small steps. You will never completely solve the problem of stressors for people with dementia. In the best care situation possible, there will always be some agitation and an occasional outburst. There will always be the recognition that for some people a catastrophic reaction is not far away. Some people with dementia will challenge your skills to figure out how to help. With experience and with trial and error, you will become expert at heading off crises. Don't be discouraged if at first this seems impossible. At first, work with the easiest people. Don't start by discussing or trying to help the people with the most severe behavioral symptoms. Look for small steps to help these people.

There will be some causes of stress that you can't control: large, noisy units or poorly designed dining rooms and bathing areas. Avoid getting caught up in these problems. Focus on what you can do with what you have. You will be able to make a difference given whatever your situation.

Look for small gains. Do not expect that all will become peaceful on your unit or that your more difficult clients will stop their angry outbursts. Ask yourself if a stressful event was not so bad this time? Did you catch it earlier? Are they less frequent for a certain person? Is part of the day less stressful?

Identify the things that stress the individual. Use Exhibit 4.1 for more examples of stressors. These stressors will be different for each person. Many will be the common causes of stress that you have already discussed. Some will be the big things such as getting dressed or taking a bath. Some will not be easy to identify.

Here are some examples of the kinds of things that stress people and the ways in which staff members can make change.

> Joyce would sit quietly in the day room for a while after lunch. Then she would get into an argument with other people over whose chair was hers. She would insist that two or three of the chairs were hers, and no amount of explanation would help. Then suddenly she would strike out at another resident.
>
> One day a staff member sat in the day room and watched Joyce. He observed that when Joyce came into the room it was almost empty. As more and more people were brought into the room, Joyce became fidgety. Then the arguments would begin. Then she would hear the pager on the public address system.

The staff listed these stressors for Joyce: tired after lunch, more and more people coming into the room, uncertainty over which chair was hers, being disoriented and unable to control her confusion, and a voice (the PA system) emanating from the ceiling. The staff member noted that becoming fidgety was Joyce's warning sign that she was experiencing too much stress.

> Mike did well in day care until midafternoon. Then he would become very upset. One day he grabbed the stapler and banged it on the walls. The staff members were afraid he would hurt one of the other residents.
>
> The staff realized that as other people began to leave the center Mike was afraid he would be left behind. He was afraid he might be lost. Then one day a staff member thought to take him to the toilet. This calmed him considerably.

Staff members added needing to urinate and not being able to find the toilet to Mike's list of stressors. (Earlier in the day Mike could find the toilet, but by the end of the day, he might have been a little more tired and confused. This variation is one of the things that makes identifying stressors challenging.) Staff members noted that Mike's warning signs were increased pacing and searching for his coat.

What things would you suggest the staff try to help Joyce and Mike? Here is what their care providers did:

> After lunch a staff member took Joyce to her room for a rest. She took time to get her settled and remind her of where she was and that she was resting. She experimented with the amount of rest time she needed. Then she would get her up and reorient her carefully to the afternoon activity in a small group.
>
> Because several people got restless when the first group began to leave, the staff began taking coats out into the outer hall and helping people meet their families where the others noticed them less. The staff

members posted a discreet note to remind themselves to take Mike to the toilet.

Overhead/Handout 4.3. Ways to Help Reduce Stress

By this time, you will have many ideas for ways to reduce stress for people with dementia. Remember that the goal is to reduce stress before the person becomes so upset that she is out of control. Select one person known to you and list ways you can help. Look for things you can really do. Look for small things. Think about the individual, not about everyone. Pair up with another person and share your ideas. Overhead/Handout 4.3 lists some ideas for helping people with dementia. Can you apply any of these ideas to the person you are discussing? Exactly how will you do this?

This is a list of ideas. You won't be able to use them all, nor should you. As you work with people over time, review this list to remind yourself of ways to solve problems.

Section 4.2. Alleviating Symptoms of Stress

Objective

The student will learn to use appropriate interventions to reduce client stress.

Information and Instructions for the Teacher

Take time. Break this material into two class periods if needed. Use Exhibit 4.1 for additional examples of stressors. Do not hand it out. It is provided for teachers and for people responsible for diagnosis, assessment, referral, or treatment.

Lecture/Discussion Notes to Be Presented to the Class

In the last section we talked about the role stress plays in the lives of people with dementia. In this section we will expand our knowledge of the characteristics of distress in people with dementia. With this understanding caregivers can improve the quality of life for people with dementia, reduce behavioral symptoms, and enable them to function as well as possible.

Overhead/Handout 4.4. Characteristics of Stress

Demands on areas of lost function contribute to stress. So does not having the opportunity to do the things the person can do. This means we will look for ways to place fewer demands on lost functions (such as understanding words or finding one's way around) and give the person more opportunities to use whatever skills he still has.

Excess disability contributes to stress. This means we do all that we can to reduce excess disability or find some way to work around it.

Stress accumulates. A series of minor stressors is like an avalanche. Suddenly something will set off a catastrophic reaction. We help by recognizing the person's mounting stress and relieving it before it becomes overwhelming. It is difficult, if not impossible, to stop a catastrophic reaction once the person is seriously upset. Almost all successful strategies prevent the person's distress from reaching the levels described in the examples at the beginning of this lesson.

Think of the person's ability to cope with stressors as a traffic light with green (OK), yellow (warning), and red (stop) zones. *(Teacher: Copy Exhibit 4.2 onto the flip chart. As you speak, draw in a line of increasing anxiety as shown.)*

The green zone is where people feel comfortable. They are functioning as well as they can and are relaxed. This does not mean they are asleep or zoned out. They are alert, watching or participating; they may smile, talk, or walk around. They may participate in activities of daily living (ADLs) or other activities or watch others. They are calm and often seem happy.

As the person's stress increases, she may feel pressured, anxious, or irritable, but she will still be in control. This is her yellow, or warning, zone. She may fidget or appear restless. The person may begin to object to care, have more trouble focusing, begin to pace around, or withdraw from activities. This is your warning sign that you must take action to reduce her stress levels.

> George was in his green zone. He is very impaired, but he likes the song-alongs. He doesn't sing, but he leans back and smiles. But when the sing-along ends and the staff members begin to move people into the dining room, George becomes somewhat stressed. He is hungry, he needs to use the toilet, and he is confused by the group of people around him. Dinner is late, and George's stress increases when he has nothing to do. By the time the meal arrives, George is upset and begins throwing his food.

> At the beginning of the day, when Anna had slept well the night before, she was in her green zone. But the simple demands of getting up, being helped to dress, and having breakfast are enough to shift her into her yellow zone. Later, going to the activities group, Anna began shouting.

If the person's level of stress continues to increase, she will move into her red zone. She will be overly stressed, frustrated, angry, upset, and no longer functioning in a way that is usual for her. This is a catastrophic reaction. For example, George is throwing his food; Anna refuses to come out of the bathroom and is shouting; a man threatens the caregiver with clenched fists when she tries to stop him from going over the fence; a wakeful man has turned on all the lights, and his shouting is waking the other residents.

Sadly, many people spend their entire day shifting between their yellow and red zones.

What must it feel like to be stressed and anxious a lot of the time? Can anyone describe an anxiety or panic attack? How does it feel? The person with dementia is feeling all the unpleasant feelings associated with stress. He may feel angry, frightened, powerless, lost. Or he may feel nervous, confused, embarrassed. He may feel that he is shaking, his heart is pounding, and his throat is tight. He may not know whether this feeling is anger or nervousness. It is hard to think clearly when you feel this way. Some people with dementia have some of these feelings most of the time. Life must be very unpleasant. Caring staff members alleviate such feelings and help the person feel comfortable and at ease. Easing your client's distress is as important as stopping her from acting out.

The distress people with dementia feel has an effect on the staff. Staff members feel stressed in a stressful environment. Staff members *do* care how their clients feel, and they would like to help people with dementia feel less stressed.

When these reactions interfere with caring or the well-being of other clients, using medications to reduce them seems the only alternative. But as we discussed in Lesson 3, these medications create more problems.

It is difficult, often impossible, to stop a catastrophic reaction once it has reached the red zone. So the staff focuses primarily on preventing these.

You help by *learning to recognize each person's increasing stress and acting before it becomes severe.* Probably you already know that once a person reaches his red zone the person is out of control and that there is little besides restraints or medication that will help. Have you yourself ever experienced a time when anger or tears seemed to continue despite your efforts to stop? Imagine how difficult—impossible—that would be for a person with dementia.

Ask the members of the group to identify the behaviors that serve as warnings of increasing stress for clients they know. For a person whom you know, list the individual behavior that is her warning of her increasing stress. These indicators will be different for each person.

Most people with dementia experience multiple stressors.

> The staff members found that Joyce continued to explode on some days. After some trial and error, they realized that by midafternoon Joyce was a little hungry. They began offering her orange juice and a short timeout before she got upset.

Joyce's total list of stressors comprised the following: tired after lunch, too many people coming into the room, being disoriented, confused, the pager system, and needing a snack.

> By the time Mr. Brown had gotten his father to the day care center, both were exhausted. His father was banging on the car windows and shouting, "Let me out," and had been shouting for half an hour.

Some of Mr. Brown's many stressors included waking up wet and feeling embarrassed that his son was cleaning and dressing him. This was an affront to his dignity that he did not understand. By the time the dressing ordeal was over, both son and father were irritable. Then the father did not understand why he should go anywhere.

You will almost always have to search for multiple causes of a person's stress. This does not happen quickly. It takes trial and error, patience and determination. If the first intervention you try does not help, do not assume that it is the wrong intervention. Leave it in place and search for additional causes of stress. You will rarely be able to prevent all the causes of stress a person experiences, but you will usually be able to reduce enough of them so that the person does not overreact so often.

The person's tolerance for stress may vary from day to day. Everybody has good days and bad. These will seem more evident in a person whose coping skills are reduced on their bad days.

When it is impossible to remove the obvious stressor, reduce the overall stress burden. Sometimes staff members cannot remove the obvious stressor. For example, if the person is incontinent, he must have a bath even though this upsets him. Staff members then remove other things that add to the person's "pile" of stressors. Consider each possible cause of stress, no matter how minor. The goal is to reduce the sum of stressors enough that the person can tolerate necessary tasks. Change the time, staff member, noise level, number of people, place. Skip unnecessary tasks or activities.

> There was always a crisis around getting James to take a bath. He grabbed everything within reach, shouted, and eventually would hit staff members. The staff realized that waking in a place that did not seem familiar, not understanding the need for personal care, the morning bustle on the unit, thinking he needed to go to his office, and feeling rushed all added to James's feelings of distress. Nothing could be done about the activity level on the unit, and reorienting him did not help much, but when staff members gave up trying to dress him and let James move along at his own pace, encouraging him steadily, there was less crisis around the bath.

Once a person feels stressed over something, those *feelings of distress tend to linger* even when the person has forgotten their cause. A person may have no recollection of a frustrating morning but may unexpectedly become tearful in the afternoon over some small incident. Do not assume that forgotten incidents do not contribute to stress. This is probably a case of remembering feelings but forgetting facts, which we talked about in Lesson 2. Review the things that have gone on earlier. Did the person have a bad night? What happened during morning ADLs? Was arriving at day care upsetting? If bathing a person was upsetting, can you let the person have a quiet time before getting dressed afterward? Next time can you provide for less stress before a difficult task must be done? This often requires communication between shifts. This cumulative quality of stressors and the lingering effects of feelings may contribute to the behavioral symptoms known as "sundowning."

If you provide care by force or by restraining the person, the force or restraint increases the feelings of stress and will affect the person's level of function all day. In contrast, families of clients in day care often remark that the client is better in the evening. Nursing home, residential care, and day care settings that successfully reduce stress during the day find that residents can enjoy new, more demanding activities than before.

Stress can be contagious. Staff members often observe that one person in the group can upset others. Remove that person or lead the rest into a new setting while you allow that person to wind down. If a few people tend to show behavioral symptoms of stress much of the time, provide a separate small group area for these people. This creates a low-stress environment for those most vulnerable people at the same time that it prevents them from triggering distress in others.

Family members are often depressed, exhausted, and overwhelmed. Their distress can be communicated to the confused person as well.

Even when the impaired person cannot understand the cause of stress, the staff member's experience of stress is felt by the person with dementia. Trading jobs with another staff member is a good way to defuse this situation.

Not having anything to do can increase stress. Because we have been talking about creating a calmer, quieter, less active environment to reduce the stress people with dementia experience, being bored may seem counterintuitive. However, feeling useless or not being able to think of anything to do is stressful. People with dementia need to be involved in pleasant activities and ADLs adjusted to a level their minds can comprehend.

Feeling "put down" or talked down to is stressful—as it is for most people.

Catastrophic reactions are usually caused by immediate, obvious things, not by hidden, psychological things. Avoid assuming that the person's distress is linked to the past or to some deep psychological event. Usually the person's symptoms of distress center around immediate events. When staff members assume that some past event is the cause of the problem, they may be looking in the wrong place for a solution. *(Teacher: Use the examples in Exhibit 4.3 or select cases known to the group.)*

Some people seem to explode with little warning. It seems as if they move directly from their green zone to their red zone without any obvious warning. Although it may appear that the person has a catastrophic reaction with no warning, staff members can usually learn ways to help each individual. This may be either knowing in advance what will trigger an outburst or learning to recognize brief warning signs. For example:

> Wendy often dozed off in her chair. When she awoke, she would suddenly become upset.

Perhaps Wendy's momentary disorientation caused her behavior, or perhaps she was reacting to a dream. The staff learned to take a few moments to gently reorient her.

Some people move between their red and yellow zones most of the time. They must feel like they are having an attack of panic or rage all the time. This in itself is exhausting. Every approach to your client or every effort to get an ADL completed may result in yelling, hitting, or refusal to cooperate. Both the care provider and the client become frustrated and overwhelmed. Evaluate whether the environment, including a day that is paced too fast for the person, or multiple, cumulative stressors are the cause of this distress. Sometimes, however, the distress is part of the illness rather than caused by an external stressor. When it is clear that the disease is driving the person's suffering, *medication* may be an appropriate intervention. *(Teacher: See Exhibit 4.4 for people providing diagnosis, assessment, referral, or treatment.)*

However, the medications will do little to treat stress that is caused by other people, the environment, or the person's inability to cope with multiple stresses. To help the person cope with the environment, using medications requires enough to sedate the person. This leads to side effects such as constipation, which compound stress levels.

As the disease progresses, *the individual's tolerance for stress will change.* As the familiar tasks of daily living become difficult, the person may become more frustrated. Late in the illness, the person may not be as upset by personal care. Expect that the "pattern" will be highly individual, and be prepared to change interventions when they no longer work. In particular, medication to treat internal distress may be stopped once this stage has passed.

Exercise 2. Identifying Stress and Planning Interventions

Divide into small groups. Have each group select a client known to the small group. List the kinds of stress that are most likely causing behavioral symptoms for that person. Identify one or two interventions that can realistically be tried with this person.

Section 4.3. Responding to a Catastrophic Reaction

Objective

The student will learn strategies for intervention when a catastrophic reaction occurs.

Information and Instructions for the Teacher

Emphasize the importance of prevention. This was discussed in Sections 4.1 and 4.5. Do not blame staff when outbursts do occur.

It may be difficult for students to understand how to "stop whatever they are doing." Ask questions and discuss this concept. Lead your group to realize that this is the only safe option. Discuss when and whether staff members can trade jobs once a person with dementia has become angry with one staff member. Reinforce the material presented in Sections 4.1 and 4.2 if needed. Even mild outbursts are traumatic to the staff, the person involved, and other clients. Damage control is necessary. Staff members will feel angry, frightened, or distressed and will need time and space to recover. If they continue to care for others "as if nothing happened," their stress will communicate nonverbally to others, raise the stress level of the group, and set up another outburst. Discuss with administration how this can be accomplished.

Lecture/Discussion Notes to Be Presented to the Class

Overhead/Handout 4.5. What to Do If the Person Becomes Upset

There are fewer options on this list, which is one reason why it is better to prevent outbursts than to try to cope with them. *Stop whatever you are doing.* There is no other option. For example, if you are showering a person, take her out of the shower and wrap her in a warm towel. Finish up later.

Remove whatever set off the reaction, or remove the person from the problem. Try taking the person for a walk away from the setting. She may calm down.

Remove other people in the room, rather than trying to remove the upset person. This is counterintuitive, but it works. It is easier and safer to move a group into another area than it is to move a distressed and angry person.

Avoid arguing, explaining, or restraining.

Don't push, touch, or direct. At this point the person's ability to think and reason is gone, and these actions will only make things worse. Even a slight touch may be interpreted by the person as an attack. Never hold or restrain a person unless he is truly endangering his life.

If another staff member is around, *trade tasks.* Once a person starts to become upset with you, your presence continues to exacerbate the problem. She will see you as the cause of the problem, and your stress will be apparent to her no matter how hard you try to act calm.

Be calm, reassuring, and comforting.

Wait for the person to calm down. Give the person space, physical and emotional. Sit quietly near the person or stand out of reach if there is any possibility that the person will hurt you. If you cannot trade with someone else, *stay a little distance away* so that you can watch and be sure the person will be safe.

Many situations place the person with dementia, a staff member, or another client in danger. The major reason for preventing angry outbursts, reducing overall stress levels, and observing people closely is to prevent situations from escalating.

Combative Behavior

Hitting, pinching, biting, scratching, and similar behavioral symptoms are almost always catastrophic reactions. They are prevented by stopping the task or not pushing the person at the first sign of distress. Sometimes people who act aggressively in these ways are experiencing high levels of stress most of the time. It will require all your skills and multiple interventions to lower their stress levels and accomplish care goals at the same time.

Sometimes people with dementia strike out at each other. For example, an American and a German, both World War II veterans, often shouted and occasionally struck each other. Before concluding that this is a part of their history and therefore hopeless, look for ways to reduce other stressors in their lives and ways to give them other meaningful things to do.

What to Do after the Outburst: Reassure and Reassess

Reassure clients who observed someone who was upset. They won't recall details; say, "It's OK," "She's OK,"or "I took care of it."

Although the person who was upset may immediately forget the whole event, feelings may echo. Reassure the person that she is still accepted, that she is OK, that things are OK. "You and I had a discussion, didn't we, but I still like you"; "Well, we had a fuss. Let's take a break"; "Well, nothing's broken, and we're still friends."

The way to prevent another outburst is to know what caused this one and avoid its happening again.

Overhead/Handout 4.6. Questions to Consider Regarding a Catastrophic Reaction

Look for the things that happened just before the catastrophic reaction. These can seem insignificant: the way a plate was set down in front of a person; the way someone approaches a person with dementia. Use this set of questions to help determine what caused this catastrophic reaction. The best way to prevent another outburst is to identify exactly what caused this one and to share that information with the staff. *(Teacher: Ask the group to select a recent outburst they observed. Walk them through the questions and help them identify possible precipitants.)*

Overhead/Handout 4.7. Record for Catastrophic Reactions

Keeping a record of periods when the person appears to be stressed is a successful way to identify the cause of the distress for each individual. The record allows you to identify a number of possible clues to what triggers reactions. Use it (Overhead/Handout 4.7) and the list of questions regarding catastrophic reactions (Overhead/Handout 4.6) to help you recognize problems, develop strategies, and evaluate their approaches. Complete the record as soon as possible after the incident, and add as much detail as would be helpful to the next person who might need it.

Teacher: Working staff members may regard these records as more paperwork and ignore the information they produce. The following will keep the project manageable:

- *Teach the record keeping you plan to use. Ask the staff to try it with one person, and spend time analyzing the results.*
- *Do not make keeping these records a routine part of charting.*
- *Use the record or chart for only one person at a time and only until the problem areas are identified. In most cases, you will identify triggers in a week or less.*
- *Involve all shifts and everyone who is involved with the person.*
- *Ask the staff to write down specific details; never use generalized terms.*
- *Record outcome: Was there any change in the behavioral symptom?*

Exercise 3. Evaluate How You Are Doing

As a group, answer the following questions. Do this at any point in caregiving when your team is working to reduce agitated behavioral symptoms or catastrophic reactions.

- Did you have at least partial success preventing or limiting at least one outburst this week?
- What did you do that was successful?
- Which interventions are working best?
- Are you still not sure what is causing the outbursts? If so, ask someone to brainstorm with you.
- Does it seem impossible to make the changes you need to make? If so, ask someone to brainstorm with you.
- What is your next step?

Clinical Experience

As a group, select one person you know who becomes upset often. Do not select one of the more difficult clients. With the help of your supervisor, maintain the log or keep written notes about behaviors for this person for one week. Focus on identifying the situations that led up to an upset for this person. Also focus on the behavioral cues the person gives that he or she is becoming increasingly stressed. At the end of the week, use this information to make a plan to reduce this person's stressful periods. If possible, implement your plan during the second week, with your teacher's and supervisor's help, and report to the group what happened after a week of implementation.

Significantly reducing catastrophic reactions may take more time and require resources not available to you. Do not be discouraged. Look for small indications that you are helping: for example, that the person responds to you differently or that she is slower to become upset.

Section 4.4. The Need for Stimulation and the Difference between Stress and Stimulation

Objective

The student will learn to distinguish between therapeutic stimulation and stress. The student will learn to identify successful activities or tasks.

Information and Instructions for the Teacher

Do not overlook this short section. There is often confusion over protecting people with dementia from everything and protecting them from the things their impaired cognition cannot process. Without this section, the staff will remain confused about what "works" and what upsets people. Ask the students questions such as, When have you seen people respond to something they enjoy? How does this help their day? help you care for them? Activities are important in providing positive experiences for people with dementia, but most such experiences are a part of routine daily care. The next lesson, on ADLs, discusses this. Ask questions here about how small, brief, positive experiences can be introduced into daily care.

Lecture/Discussion Notes to Be Presented to the Class

Staff members tend to seek to protect people with dementia from any stimulation out of concern that the person will be overly stressed. However, stimulation and stress are very different. Stress results from things the person's impaired cognitive functions cannot process, however obvious or simple they may seem to us. Stimulation results from things that the person can still do or enjoy, no matter how simple.

Overhead/Handout 4.8. The Difference between Stress and Stimulation

The person's reaction to the task or activity will be different when she feels stimulated rather than stressed. This overhead/handout shows some examples of the different responses people have when they are stimulated instead of stressed.

Overhead/Handout 4.9. Stressful versus Stimulating Activities

Usually there are differences between noxious stressors and pleasant stimulation (a noisy facility versus a sing-along), but sometimes these are matters of degree rather than differences (helping to set the table versus trying to set the table alone). Often you can change a stressful activity into a stimulating one by simplifying it and paying attention to the person's response. This overhead/handout lists some examples of stressful activities that can be changed into stimulating ones.

Why is it important to create stimulation for the person with dementia? When simple changes can make an ADL enjoyable or at least tolerable for the person, he will be more likely to cooperate. For most of the dementia, the person still needs feelings of self-esteem, a sense of being in control of things, and opportunities to feel good about himself. Staff members put these good feelings back into ADLs and activities for the person. Doing so helps to reduce behavioral problems. Impaired people who don't feel they have any control or who don't feel good about themselves look for ways to create these feelings—usually by doing things that cause problems.

Having nothing to do also creates problems:

> Imagine that you sit in the doctor's office for two hours. You brought nothing to do, and there is no one to talk to. After a while you would become irritable from doing nothing.

A person can be stressed by boredom. People with dementia do nothing for long periods each day. Often behavioral symptoms are caused when people have no stimulation and do inappropriate things in an effort to stimulate themselves.

People with dementia need time to process information, but they do not need an empty life. An environment so calm that no one might feel stressed will generate behavioral symptoms in some people. How can you apply this information to the people you care for? Ask the members of the group how much of the day, when the people they care for are awake, are they doing nothing. How much of the time are their clients present in an activity without being engaged or involved in it?

Overhead/Handout 4.10. How We Help

Reduce as much stress as possible. When a person is moving between her yellow and red zones all day, she will be unable to respond to pleasant tasks or activities, even when these are very gentle and focused.

Individualize. Look for the balance between stress and stimulation that is unique to each person. Look for ways you can make things easier for some people in an activity that others find stimulating. You are probably already doing this by, for example, seating a more confused person next to a volunteer or aide while the rest of the group participates in a ball toss.

Try things. *Don't make assumptions about what will work.* Often people are stressed by things that the staff members think will be stimulating or are denied stimulation because the staff members fear it will be stressful. If you try something and it seems to be stressing the person, stop and do something else.

Modify the activity. Reduce the group size. Simplify the task. Use task breakdown (Lesson 5) and task assessment (Lesson 10). Change the time.

Reduce stress in other parts of the day.

> Mrs. F. had spilled part of her lunch on her dress. The staff decided to change her before her daughter came and found her "dirty." But Mrs. F. hated getting dressed and undressed. When her daughter arrived, she was tearful and irritable.

Next time, the staff explained to the daughter that the only way Mrs. F. would enjoy her visit was if she had time to relax before the daughter arrived.

Go slowly.

What stresses one person another will enjoy.

Sometimes what appears to be enjoyable will suddenly upset the person. If this happens, *do some detective work.*

> Jake loved to ride in the day care van. He always sat just behind the driver, stretched out his long legs, and gazed out the window. But occasionally Jake would balk. He would brace his arms in the van door and refuse to get on or off. Finally the staff figured out that on those days the driver had put some of her own things on "Jake's" seat.

Because Jake depended on routines to manage, he could not cope with changing his seat.

> Emma enjoyed coloring. Once she was settled with her markers and an adult coloring book, her pleasure was obvious. But after about 20 minutes, Emma would color faster and faster, demanding a new page before she had finished the previous one. She would get up and sit down and say she had to go home. At first the staff members could not figure out what was happening, but then they realized that although she loved to color, she quickly got tired.

> Herman enjoyed visits from his wife, his pastor, and his son. But when all three came at once, he would stay out in the hall and shout at them. Herman could enjoy one person, but three overwhelmed him.

Do very simple things. Sitting and watching the home care worker prepare dinner is enough pleasure for one woman. Tasting what the others prepared was just right for one man. Criticizing the staff member gave a sense of control to another.

Exhibit 4.1. More Examples of Stressors

Stressors that are a part of daily life
- trying to figure out what is going on here
- trying not to act foolish
- trying to still be me
- too many tasks or task steps to think of at once
- being ignored

Stressors associated with ADLs
- wondering when lunch is coming
- having someone else dress me (loss of independence, privacy)
- having someone take all my clothes off me and stuff me in a roaring shower
- too many people around

Stressors associated with the environment
- people rushing around
- noise
- caregiver behavior

Stressors associated with health
- having a headache
- medications
- not hearing or seeing well
- fatigue
- any excess disability

Stressors caused by emotions
- being afraid
- feeling anxious
- too much excitement
- feeling frustrated
- feeling lost and sad
- loss of self-esteem, loss of control

Interpersonal problems made worse by the dementia
- feeling put down, being controlled and told what to do
- not being able to make myself understood
- not being in control
- not understanding what someone is saying to me
- having someone else take over my familiar role in the family
- being rushed

Brain overload or underload
- too many things to do
- trying to do a task I can no longer do well
- having nothing to do, nowhere to go, nothing to think about, nobody to talk to
- needing to go to the toilet and not being able to do this without help

Problems in orientation
- not knowing where I am
- not knowing who others are
- not knowing whether I am safe

Exhibit 4.2. Levels of Stress

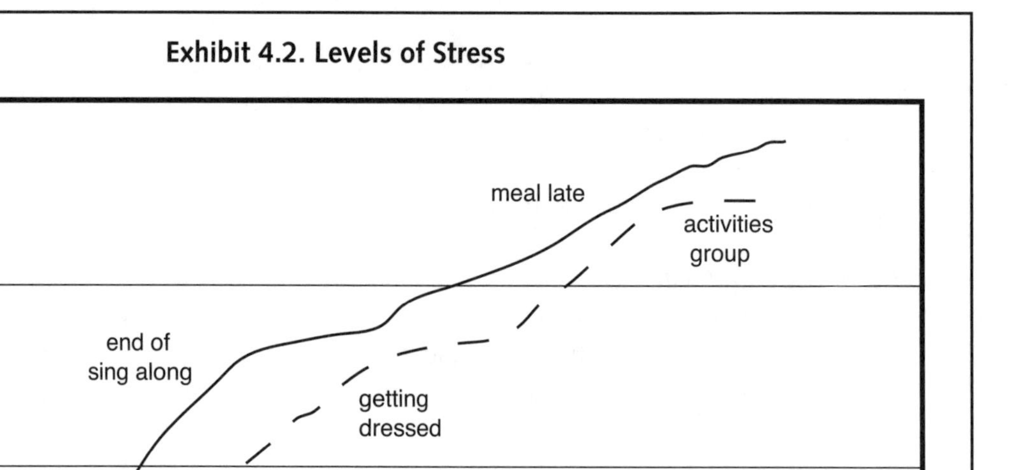

Exhibit 4.3. Sample Interpretations of the Cause of Catastrophic Reactions

Problem	Right Interpretation	Wrong Interpretation
Won't go to bed at night	Because she doesn't know where she is	Because her husband died in bed
Cries often	Because there is too much confusion in room	Because he is thinking about his long-lost brother
Fights getting into a shower	Because she is cold and shampoo burns her eyes	Because she has always had a water phobia
Won't speak to her sister	Because she does not know who the woman is	Because of a quarrel many years ago

Exhibit 4.4. The Effects of Medication

Medication may help:

- anxiety
- depression
- when agitation seems driven by the illness

Medication will not help:

- wandering
- being uncooperative
- agitation caused by the environment, health, or stress

Tailor the medication to the individual.
Start low and slow.
Watch for side effects.

Overhead/Handout 4.1. Examples of Common Stressors

Cognitive overload

Not being able to figure out what is going on

Not understanding a request

Inability to perform a task

Fatigue

Inability to communicate needs, being misunderstood

Frustration

Response to demoralizing or infantilizing treatment

Not feeling well

Noise, people moving around

Anxiety

Not being in control

Unmet bodily needs

Overhead/Handout 4.2.
How We Help

Make fewer demands on lost abilities.

Take advantage of retained abilities.

Identify excess disabilities.

Reduce amount of stress.

Prevent overreactions.

Look for small gains.

Identify the things that stress the individual.

Overhead/Handout 4.3. Ways to Help Reduce Stress

Reduce the number of things going on around the person or take the person to a quieter place.

Simplify the task. Compensate for lost abilities.

Don't rush the person.

Ask yourself whether you are understanding what the person is trying to tell you; don't ignore objections.

Give simple explanations more often.

Have the person rest a while before she overtires.

Ask the person if she needs to toilet, wants a snack, hurts.

Don't talk down to people.

Reassure people often.

Build a trusting relationship with the person.

Plan the day so that stress does not build up; do things at the person's best times.

Make the environment easier to understand.

Fill in when the person is groping for a word.

Take things one step at a time.

Maintain familiar routines but adapt if the person becomes upset.

Try things a different way when something upsets the person.

Accept odd behavior.

Tailor your strategy to the individual:

Know the person's limits and do not push beyond them.

Know what triggers outbursts.

If a necessary task like bathing usually upsets the person, consider each small step of the task: What can be left out? What can be simplified? What can be done differently? If you upset the person, can someone else try?

Overhead/Handout 4.4. Characteristics of Stress

Demands on lost areas of mental function contribute to stress. So does having too much done for one.

Excess disability contributes to stress.

Stress accumulates.

People experience multiple stressors.

Stress will vary from day to day.

When it is impossible to remove the obvious stressor, reduce the overall stress burden.

Feelings of stress tend to linger.

Stress can be contagious.

Boredom can increase stress.

Feeling that one is being patronized can cause stress.

Catastrophic reactions are usually caused by immediate, obvious things, not by hidden, psychological things.

Some people explode with little warning.

Some stress is part of the disease, and medication is helpful.

The individual's tolerance for stress will change.

Overhead/Handout 4.5. What to Do If the Person Becomes Upset

Stop what you are doing immediately, even if this seems difficult to do.

Remove the problem or remove the person from the problem.

Remove others rather than try to remove the person who is upset.

Don't argue; don't explain.

Don't push or direct the person.

Trade tasks with another staff member.

Be calm and reassuring.

Wait for the person to calm down.

Give the person space.

Get out of the person's way if she might strike or hurt you.

Overhead/Handout 4.6. Questions to Consider Regarding a Catastrophic Reaction

What did the person do just before he became upset?

Did he become stubborn, refuse to do something?

Become more restless, fidget more?

Flush?

Was there any other thing the person did that let you know that he was becoming upset?

What was going on at the time?

What were you doing?

What were you saying?

Were you trying to get the person to do something?

Were you feeling irritated or rushed?

Was a lot happening around the person?

Was something happening on TV?

What might have triggered this outburst?

Were you trying to get the person to do something she did not want to do?

Were you trying to get the person to do something she did not understand?

Was the person unable to make herself understood?

Was the person not feeling well at that time?

Could she not see well?

Could she not hear well?

Was the person unable to do something she was trying to do?

Were things too confusing? Too much to pay attention to?

Did someone talk to the person as if she were a child?

Does the person seem depressed?

Does the person spend more than an hour at a time doing nothing?

Did you argue or try to explain things?

Was the person tired?

Was it her bad time of day?

Overhead/Handout 4.7. Record for Catastrophic Reactions

Make notes while the incident is still fresh in your memory. Be specific. Do not use terms like "agitated." Describe exactly what happened.

Name ______________________________

Date ______________________________

Time ______________________________

Setting ______________________________

What did the person do? ______________________________

____

Who was there? ______________________________

____

What happened just before? ______________________________

____

What evidence of increasing stress did you see? ______________________________

____

How big a problem was this? (very serious, serious, not too serious, minor) ____________

____

Overhead/Handout 4.8. The Difference between Stress and Stimulation

Stress	*Stimulation*
Restless	Attentive
Picks at things	Alert
Looks or wanders away	Watching
Irritable	Smiles
Does not want to participate	Participates

Overhead/Handout 4.9. Stressful versus Stimulating Activities

Stressful	*Stimulating*
Large group of people	Small group of people
A hectic environment	A low-key, calm environment
Residents and staff moving about, people rushing	Relaxed laughter
Noise	Sing-along, piano playing
Action whose purpose is not evident to the person with dementia	Action whose purpose is evident to the person with dementia
A leader whose style is hyper or demeaning	A calm, supportive leader

Overhead/Handout 4.10. How We Help

Reduce stress.

Individualize.

Don't make assumptions.

Modify the activity.

Do some detective work.

Do very simple things.

LESSON 5

APPLYING SKILLS IN ACTIVITIES OF DAILY LIVING

Summary: This lesson is designed to put into practice the concepts learned in previous lessons. It will give the student the skills to devise interventions that work in her setting and with her clients.

Section 5.1. The Importance of Individualized Care and the Application of New Knowledge. Demonstrates the application of Lessons 2, 3, and 4 to activities of daily living.

Section 5.2. Implementing What You Have Learned about Activities of Daily Living. Encourages students to begin to plan care around the skills they have learned.

Section 5.3. Using Individualized, Social, and Emotional Contexts of Care. Discusses ways to use the care relationship and the setting to support activities of daily living.

Section 5.4. Suggested Interventions for Specific Activities of Daily Living. Discusses specific strategies for addressing sleep disturbance, falls, eating, and bathing.

Using the Sections

Introductory course:
- Section 5.1 required
- Section 5.2 required
- Section 5.3 use for suggestions; do not teach the entire section

Core course:
- Section 5.1 required
- Section 5.2 required
- Section 5.3 use for suggestions; do not teach the entire section

Special audiences:
- People responsible for diagnosis, assessment, referral, and treatment: all sections, including Section 5.4

Problems You May Have in Implementing This Lesson

Staff members most commonly complain that they do not have time to provide this kind of care. In programs with limited staffing, this will be true. In such programs, focus on what the staff member can do as she provides care. This includes talking to or interacting with the person as she feeds her, telling the person what is happening as she dresses her, and never treating the person as an object.

Often the way the staff members use their limited time will make a difference. For example, time spent reacting to a catastrophic reaction could have been better spent preventing it. Treating pain or an incipient illness early will save staff time struggling with a distressed client. These changes require teamwork and a committed administration.

Many programs have adequate staff to make a significant difference in activities of daily living (ADLs: eating, dressing, bathing, toileting, and walking). Other issues contribute to the perception that there is not enough time for different care.

There is pressure from all directions to accomplish the practical tasks of ADLs—getting people clean, fed, and dressed safely. Staff members know that these tasks must be accomplished. Because the outcomes are tangible and vital, completing them can override the need for compassionate care. Shifting the focus of care while still completing tasks requires time and commitment to change from management and supervisors. Simple issues must be thought out because they affect policy and regulations: Can Mrs. Jones eat breakfast in her nightgown? What if she is still in her nightgown at midmorning? What is the impact on the kitchen staff if Mr. Harris lingers over his lunch tray?

Under the daily pressure to complete tasks in limited time, staff members develop routines that they rely on, often without considering alternatives. Videotaping staff members providing care is an excellent way to help them analyze what they do.

In the classroom, help caregivers decide which changes in routines they can manage and how these will be accomplished. Do not let them blame others for time limitations. Do ask shifts to work together to plan the shift change, since a common practice is to leave some things for the next shift to do. Do focus on small changes. Many small changes take less time and help the staff succeed. Do point out small positive responses to caregivers. Expect client response to be gradual.

Caregivers provide the most intimate aspects of ADLs so often that this care becomes routine, but the client with dementia may experience it as an intrusion. Use role play and discussions in the classroom to help caregivers learn to do each task in an individual and personal manner.

Teach students how to get out of a grip and how to deflect a blow. Remind them not to wear earrings large enough to grab or clothes they do not want spoiled.

Section 5.1. The Importance of Individualized Care and the Application of New Knowledge

Objective

The student will learn direct care skills that apply their knowledge of cognition, excess disability, and stress. The important role of staff members in providing direct care is emphasized.

Information and Instructions for the Teacher

Teach Sections 5.1 and 5.2 as presented. Use Sections 5.2 through 5.4 as background material for yourself and when needed as students address plans for care.

In the previous lessons you introduced the students to three basic concepts: the impact of the brain damage, the impact of excess disability, and the effect of stressors on people with dementia. This section briefly reviews the impact of each. You may limit this review to a sentence or expand it as needed for your group.

Although previous lessons recommended ways to intervene, the focus of teaching now shifts to the application of this knowledge. This means that individual students/staff members will plan ways to adapt ADL care. Nonprofessional direct care providers are able to do this once they understand the basic issues. ADL care will always be planned jointly with supervisors and direct care providers. Staff skills improve with practice and as staff members gain confidence. The goal of this lesson is to help students apply and practice new approaches through ADL care.

Overhead/Handout 5.1 addresses three principles of ADL care. These are the most important points to teach in this lesson. This section also teaches task breakdown, which is essential to care.

This lesson does not specifically address other activities such as housework, gardening, using the telephone, preparing a meal, shopping—activities referred to as instrumental activities of daily living (IADLs). The same principles apply to them as to bathing, dressing, eating, toileting, and walking. If your students are caring for people able to do IADLs or parts of IADLs, teach them to apply the same problem-solving skills to IADLs. Task breakdown is especially important in enabling people to retain these activities and the self-esteem they provide. IADLs broken down into steps make effective activities (Lesson 10).

Lecture/Discussion Notes to Be Presented to the Class

In the previous sessions we learned how brain damage, excess disability, and stress affect the person with dementia. In this lesson we will apply that knowledge to ADLs: dressing, bathing, eating, walking, and toileting.

Optional Review

What are some of the ways the brain damage creates problems when we help a person with ADLs? As you list these, you will notice that the lost areas of mental function—such as not understanding or being confused—contribute to stress.

If we can do one thing to make ADLs easier and more pleasant, it will be to reduce the person's stress. Stress is the major cause of uncooperativeness, agitation, and anger around ADLs. Common stressors around ADLs are noise, too many people around, clutter, being rushed, being "done to," and not understanding what is going on. What are some of the things that stress people while you are helping them bathe? *(Teacher: Write the students' answers on a flip chart. Below are some ideas.)*

- not understanding why staff members are invading her privacy
- not understanding what is happening
- being afraid of getting her face wet
- thinking he already had a bath
- feeling cold
- feeling undressed in public
- the noise of the shower
- the strange-looking bathtub

If the person was stressed before you begin ADL care, this stress will carry over into the ADL task. Try to provide care at times when the person is relaxed. Schedule a relaxing activity or a rest before care that you know is stressful.

We've also talked about excess disability. One of

the most important aspects of care is that ADLs provide the staff with an opportunity to *monitor* the person for excess disability. For example, a staff person who knows her clients notices when a person's appetite is less, when she has had a bad night, when she seems unusually drowsy or irritable. This monitoring means that problems can be picked up quickly before they become large health or behavioral problems.

Second, the staff member can *compensate* for existing excess disability. For example, angry or combative behavior around dressing is often related to arthritic pain or other joint pain. Knowing this, the caregiver can move joints gently.

Give extra support on bad days: Like the rest of us, people with dementia have good and bad days. The consequences of bad days are more exaggerated when the person is cognitively frail. When the person is not feeling well, he will temporarily need additional support, need to have more done for him and fewer demands placed on him. These changes should be reviewed and lifted when the person feels better. Frail individuals may fluctuate between bad days when they will need more support and simpler care and good days when they can be more independent and functional. For example, a program should be sufficiently flexible to shower a person on her good days (or hours).

Overhead/Handout 5.1. Principles of ADL Care

All ADL care is either beneficial or harmful. It is never neutral or meaningless to the person with dementia. Why is this? Getting dressed, bathed, our teeth brushed is neutral to well people. It has to be done, but it is not as important to well people as seeing friends or receiving a good work evaluation. The things that matter the most to healthy people may be their social lives, sports, families, or studies. In contrast, for the person with dementia, ADLs make up most of the time the person is doing something meaningful. It is also one of the times that the person is doing something with someone else; the relationship, good or bad, that exists during this time is important because the person has so few relationships that he can understand.

Healthy people take things such as dressing and walking for granted. We do these things in order to do something more important. But when these tasks are all that is left for a person and the person can't do them well, they become crucial. This means that helping someone put on a sweater or walking a person to activities means more to that person than just getting a job done: it strengthens good feelings.

So it is in ADLs that we put back meaning and life quality for the person with dementia. If ADL care is rushed, impersonal, or done poorly, it makes the person feel more isolated, more incompetent, or less valued. This is why all ADL care is either beneficial therapy or harmful. This may seem like a strange idea because often people think that ADLs don't make much difference one way or another, but there is no neutral, unimportant part to routine daily care.

The sum of all the little things we do makes life quality better or worse. How we help people feel about themselves is not in something big that we do, such as celebrate a birthday in a big way, but in the sum total of all the little things we do. The person might not remember the birthday party for long, might even be upset by it, but as we discussed in the section on the brain damage, feelings tend to linger. Thus, good feelings about care linger and add up. The key is to think of all the little things that *add up* that make the difference. Feeling useless, feeling bossed around, feeling confused add up to anger. A smile from a staff member, successfully pulling up one's slacks, not being frightened in the shower add up to feeling good about oneself.

The staff person who provides direct ADL care is the most important therapist on the team. If ADL care—routine, daily tasks—become the most important thing in the person's life and are all that is left for the person to feel good about and if direct care providers are the people the person has the most contact with, then the direct care staff and the activity staff become the most important therapists on the team.

Exercise 1. The Importance of ADL Care

As a group, discuss the following:

Give some examples of people's behavior that indicate that ADLs are important to them (for example, becoming angry or trying to help you with a task). In the past, have you thought of ADLs as just getting a job done (neutral to the person)? Thinking back over the lesson on stress, do you now see this differently? Why? When have you observed that the way you provide care makes a difference? What specific things do you (or could you) do that are therapeutic?

Why might routine care be harmful (to identity, self-esteem, control)?

What sorts of actions might be harmful (rushing, ignoring the person, talking across the person, asking the person to do things she cannot do, being impatient)? Why?

Why is the sum of small things important? Give some examples from people you know. Think back over the lessons on brain damage. How do the losses people experience make the many small things more important?

Do you think you are the most important therapist on the team? Give some examples of how your care is so important to people with dementia. Do others on the team see you as the most important therapist?

Use Task Breakdown

Task breakdown is the process of helping a person with dementia successfully do or participate in a task or activity by making it a step-by-step process. People with dementia tend to become confused by the various steps in a task but can still do many things if we break the activity into its individual steps. Simplifying a task through task breakdown is different from making a task babyish.

We talked previously about some of the difficulties the damaged brain faces. Among these are remembering all the things involved in a complicated task, such as dressing, and deciding which step in the activity to do first.

The steps in getting dressed (first put on your underpants, then your bra, then your slacks, then your blouse) seem obvious to us (in fact, we can get dressed without thinking), but the dementia makes this increasingly confusing for the impaired person. Because one person ends up with all her dresses on at once and another with her bra on over her sweater, we end up taking on the job of getting the person dressed. But this makes the person feel useless or angry at being a failure when she can still get dressed with a little of the right kind of help.

This applies to everything the person does—all the ADLs, other activities—everything.

At first the person will need only a little help, but later in the disease the person will need much more. Task breakdown allows us to adjust for this.

Task breakdown helps the person retain dignity and a feeling of being in control of her life. Also, people are more likely to be cooperative when they are participating in the task themselves.

Teacher: It can seem as if task breakdown will take a lot of staff time. Have staff members test the intervention on only one or two people. Once they have learned it, busy staff members will find ways to insert partial task breakdown into their routines.

If the staff members feel that task breakdown is hard for them, list the obstacles they perceive. Time is only one of these, and task breakdown can save time. Staff members may feel that other obstacles include having to watch several people at once, feeling rushed, confusion over what the person can do, and problem behaviors that disrupt the task. Staff members may find writing out steps and advance planning unfamiliar at first. If so, try doing this as a group.

Steps in Task Breakdown

The first step should be done in advance:

Identify a task or an activity.
Write out each step. (This will take some practice in the classroom until the student learns to think in terms of steps.)
Mark the steps you think the person can do.
Mark the steps you will do. For example, as motor coordination is lost, people will lose the ability to button buttons, so the person will put on a blouse but will need a staff member's help to button it.
Before you try out the task, ask yourself:
- Is the person rested and calm?
- Is this a calm environment?
- Did I allow enough time for her to function slowly?
- Am I treating her as a friend? (Never do task breakdown in a degrading way.)
- Am I using touch, affection, appropriate humor?

The second step is to carry out the task:

Identify the first item to be used both visually (show it to the person) and verbally (name it).

Say what is to be done with it. Use clues that do not involve language (point, start the person's arm in motion).

Be patient. Many people work slowly.

Give positive feedback. ("That's right"; "That looks good.") Comment on how well the person looks. "Charlie, you look good in those pants." "Mabel, you've cleaned up your whole plate." Don't overdo praise so that it sounds false.

Repeat for each step.

The third step is done after the task is completed:

After the task is complete, review your plan. (This is essential. The first time we do this with a person it is easy to incorrectly estimate what the person can do.)

Mark the places the person had trouble.

Divide this step into simpler ones. Example: on the first try, you told the person to put his feet in his pants, and he got upset. Next time break this down. Say, "First put this leg into this pant leg." If the person still becomes upset, try holding the open leg right by his foot.

Are there any steps you did that the person might be able to do? If you break things down sufficiently, perhaps the person can be even more successful than you anticipated. Did you make things too simple for this person?

Do you need to change the environment? More light, quieter?

The final step is to try out the modified tasks. If you still have problems, ask for suggestions from the family and your co-workers.

Section 5.2. Implementing What You Have Learned about Activities of Daily Living

Objective

The student will learn to put new skills into practice.

Information and Instructions for the Teacher

This is a classroom activity to be carried out as a group exercise. The guidelines below give the instructions. Use Sections 5.3 and 5.4 to help you. If your group is having trouble, teach selected items from Section 5.3.

Begin by discussing several clients as a whole group. Then use any of the following methods to encourage the group to consider more case examples.

a. Divide the students into small groups to discuss cases, then discuss their plan in the large group. If students work in small groups, circulate among them and provide information.
b. Ask small groups to role-play the problem and then their planned interventions.
c. Ask students to make a plan and implement it to determine how well it works and how much time it takes.

If your students feel that they can do little to change the status quo, go directly to Exercise 2, complete it, and then return to this activity.

Expect that the group will discuss several clients. The more clients that are discussed, the clearer it will be to the student that change can be made.

Lecture/Discussion Notes to Be Presented to the Class

Overhead/Handout 5.2. Guidelines for ADL Care

By this time you have many skills in caring for people with dementia. In this lesson we will focus on learning to apply these skills in real life. We will plan ways to provide ADL care for people you know. We will discuss our ideas. Use the guidelines in Overhead/Handout 5.2 as you make plans. Whenever you plan for care in your clinical setting, use guidelines 3–11.

Teacher: Once the steps in Overhead/Handout 5.2 have been completed for an individual, review with your class how to incorporate them into making a care plan according to your facility format.

Exercise 2. The Role of the Direct Care Provider

Teacher: This is a difficult kind of discussion to lead. Although you do not want it to turn into a "gripe" session, you must take students' concerns seriously, even if they do not seem so to you. Keep in mind that the objective of such a discussion is help the group identify ways to make some changes. Let these ideas come from the group. You may have to advocate for your class or ask an administrator to participate in a discussion.

As a class, discuss the following:

Doing ADLs this way may be asking you to make a major shift in the way you provide care. Perhaps you have concerns about this. If so, let's discuss them in the classroom. What you say here is confidential and will not affect your job. But concerns are real and need to be talked about. Here are a few concerns staff members often have. You may have others.

Should you be the one who is responsible for making a new plan for doing an ADL? Is this part of your job? Do you want to be responsible for making a new plan for a person? Who has the ultimate responsibility for the plan? *This course does not ask direct care staff people to make care plans independently; they will contribute to the care plan as part of the team.*

How will you find time for the change in the way you care? Will you be able to get someone to cover for you or to trade jobs if your client becomes angry with you?

Probably you have routines that make it possible for you to get through your heavy workload. What will changes do to your routines? Can you accommodate these changes in routine? Might you be able to change your routines without ruining the day?

Will other people let you make changes in caregiving? Your supervisors? Your co-workers? Other departments? Family members? Who is responsible for problems here?

Is it fair to try changes on just one person? Suppose you and your co-workers decide to take more time with one person's bath so that she does not become terribly upset. Is this fair to the others, or should nobody receive better care because you cannot give everyone more time with a bath?

Are there other issues that you think will prevent you from using these techniques?

Clinical Experience

Try your plan with one of the people you have discussed. Plan ahead how you will do this and when. How much time did you spend? Were you interrupted by other demands? If necessary, ask other staff members to cover for you, just for this person. You might try making your own videotape: care for the person in the usual way and the next time care for him allowing him as much time as he needs. The video will tell you how much the difference in time is and will show you ways you had not thought of to get the job done. If you cannot use videotape, ask someone to time you. Carry out your plan for a week. How successful was it? What problems did you encounter? *(Teacher: follow up on this experience. Help your students improve their plan and address obstacles.)*

Section 5.3. Using Individualized, Social, and Emotional Contexts of Care

Objective

The student will learn a variety of strategies for care.

Information and Instructions for the Teacher

This is a long series of ideas. They will not be retained as well if taught as written. Students tend to remember and use these ideas best when a specific idea is emphasized as an applied part of a plan. Teach these as needed; they build on suggestions presented in previous lessons. An effective way to use them is to offer them as suggestions as the group carries out Section 5.2. You may use Overhead/Handout 5.3 as a reminder list for students able to work independently. Be sure you yourself know these suggestions well and use them throughout the course.

Lecture/Discussion Notes to Be Presented to the Class

Overhead/Handout 5.3. Suggested Interventions

Individualize each task or activity. Learn the person's history. Does the person prefer to bathe or shower? Does she hate certain foods? Did she consider showering a task to be gotten done or an opportunity for self-indulgence and fragrant soaps? As much as possible should be learned around the time of admission. Talking to families may provide a wealth of information, but little history is available for many people, and families may not know things. Close observation of the person is a reasonable substitute. Add what you know about the person now: he likes this, he dislikes that.

Try talking about the person's history as you care for her. Even if you are sure the person is too ill to take in what you say, it is something to talk about that says to the person that you are there with her.

Select the person's best times for ADLs. Postpone a shower until afternoon if a person is in better spirits then. Hold a tray until a person wants it.

Be flexible. Flexibility includes flexible scheduling; staff routines that allow a person a few more minutes in bed while the caregiver helps someone else; a caregiver who can be jolly with one person and slow and gentle with the next. Flexibility includes stopping a task or activity if it isn't working; it means figuring out a unique way to interact, reassuring family members when something has not been done "on time" or backing off for a while if the person becomes upset with you.

For example, when things got tense on one unit, the activity director would take a few restless people for a ride. This seemed spontaneous, but the van was always kept ready; the activity director had checked out a few places to go; teammates helped people to the toilet and into their coats.

Flexible care does not necessarily take more time. Here are some examples of flexibility on a unit where each staff member had to provide all morning ADLs for seven people.

> Betty had three people to get up. All three knew her. The first, Alice Frank, was quite impaired and did not like to wake up. She wanted to curl up under her blankets. Betty knew that Alice understood almost no words, so Betty used many nonverbal cues. She sat on the edge of the bed and helped Alice swing her feet over the side and sit up. Putting her head close to Alice's, she said, "I brought you some orange juice, Alice." She had found that the juice helped Alice wake up. She put her arm around Alice and held the cup. Once Alice was up, Betty's genuine affection would help both of them through changing Alice's clothing.
>
> Janice was not as impaired as Alice and was sensitive to the slightest patronizing behavior. Betty spoke to her cheerfully and commented on the sunshine as she opened the curtains. She did not sit on the bed, but when Janice's muscles seemed stiff, she said, "Would you like a hand?" "Breakfast is ready," she said to prompt Janice to keep on getting up. "I'll just run those to the laundry for you," she offered, tactfully not mentioning that Janice's clothing was soaking wet.
>
> James was considered by the staff to be combative, and no one but Betty could get him up without a fight. James remembered the days when he had commanded a ship, and he liked to keep women "in their place." Betty humored him on both counts. She did not open

> the curtain because she had found that the sudden light disoriented him. Instead she stood at the foot of the bed and called to him. When he opened his eyes he asked, "Who the hell are you?" "Just Betty, sir," she said. "It's eight bells and I'm officer of the day." "Get the hell out of here," he said. "Yes, sir," she said, but she knew that standing just to one side was enough. "I brought your coffee, sir," she said. She left him sitting on the side of the bed with his coffee while she started his bath because he needed the time to awake fully.

Betty knew that James would urinate and soak the bed, but that had been planned for. Rushing him into the bathroom usually led to his striking out.

Many tasks of personal care are done in private. It can feel threatening or invasive when another person takes these over. It may not feel right to have someone in the room, standing so close, or touching you. The person with dementia may not understand his need for care. Find ways to do your work without making the person feel that you are intruding. For example:

- step behind a door;
- dry a person off with the towel serving as a screen; or
- have only one familiar person do a task.

Some people like to be touched; others prefer hands off. Some like to be hugged; others are reserved. Respect these differences, and modify your approach with each person. Avoid coming up behind people and touching them. Tell the person who you are and what you are going to do; avoid invading personal space unnecessarily; emphasize privacy; build trust with each person slowly.

Protect the person from embarrassment and from feeling stupid and clumsy. Help the person save face. Take time to persuade the person rather than make him do something. Being pushed around makes most people angry and resistant, but most people will cooperate if you give them the chance to feel as if the decision were theirs.

There are many excuses you can give a person for cooperating: "You want to get cleaned up for church." "This is the only day we have water for baths." "We're doing all the wash today, so could I please have your dress?"

Rewards work only if the person can remember the reward. Rewards that are immediate and concrete are best. Say: "See how nice your hair looks." "That ice cream was good, wasn't it?"

Remind the person of the goal of a task.

White lies may help when they share the person's reality or support the person's dignity and autonomy. Use them sparingly. Remember that the person may recall whatever white lie you told him!

Ask for the person's help, or give the person a task to do.

Avoid telling the person that "anyone" might do that when the person has just made a mistake that obviously "anyone" would not do.

Offer help tactfully, and provide the person with an excuse for agreeing.

For example:

> Ruth refused to use incontinence wear. Her caregiver got out three thick diapers along with Ruth's clothing in the morning.
>
> "I'm not going to wear those," Ruth announced.
>
> "Just in case," offered the caregiver.
>
> "No."
>
> "Well, how about just two?"
>
> "I'll wear just one, if you insist."
>
> Ruth feels as if she won.

Never talk across a person, never ignore the person while you provide care in silence, never give long explanations the person can't remember, and never rush the person.

Use personal trust and extra support.

When the person is anxious and is unable to understand what is happening no matter how hard the caregiver tries, the caregiver can build a trusting relationship and use it to accomplish difficult things (even medical procedures). Sometimes the best strategy is to give no information, just reassurance. Promise and keep your promise.

- "I will stay right here with you."
- "I won't let anything happen."
- "I know what's going on, and it's OK."

Focus on the person you are caring for and respect him for where he is now. Treat the person as a friend, never as an object.

If a person is racist, sexist, or demeaning, accept that it is too late for him to change.

Never be patronizing.

Use humor and affection. People with dementia often have trouble comprehending jokes, but retain a sense of humor when they are not overly stressed or depressed. They will enjoy a spontaneous chuckle over immediate events. Never laugh at the person's mistakes; laugh at your own or about the situation. Let the person know that you like her. Let her know what it is that you like about her, but avoid treating her like a baby. Smiles and chuckles are a good indication that the care you are giving is working.

Enable. Let the person do as much as he can. Letting the person do as much as he can of each ADL supports feelings of competence and self-esteem. Simplifying, working step by step, and using task breakdown and task analysis make it possible for the person to be involved.

Sometimes the staff members do not know how much a person can do for herself when she is not stressed. After you reduce the stress for the person over several weeks, explore whether she can do a little bit more (but don't push her; she will not grow through the effort; you are only releasing her current potential). Look for things that even very impaired people can do: hold the washcloth (which also keeps their hands from grabbing things), hold a spoon, smooth down her skirt, or indicate yes or no.

Use caring and support. Know when this is enough. Doing too much encourages feelings of uselessness and frustration.

When a person is very distressed or very impaired, many of these strategies will not work. They just need to be cared for in a comforting way.

Know when you are doing the best you can:

> Mrs. Liu was very impaired. Despite the best efforts of an excellent staff, she threw her food. She did not understand what food was anymore. She probably no longer was able to associate opening her mouth with feelings of hunger. The staff offered her small bits of food, never a full plate, and fed her in a place where thrown food would not land in other resident's meals.

Use cues. As the person has increasing difficulty figuring out what is happening, we help by increasing the visual, auditory, tactile, and smell cues. Cues are focused and relevant, unlike noxious stimuli, which are often general and irrelevant. Cues focus on things the person needs to know and not on general background information such as traffic in the hall. The brain damage idiosyncratically affects the person's ability to use cues, however, so the staff may need to experiment and to remind people to attend to cues, such as saying, "Smell the coffee, Myrtle. It's breakfast time."

Do not use cues separately from daily life or as an activity. Cues provided outside daily routines can be seriously disorienting. For example, nothing in Myrtle's life experience helps her make sense out of sitting in an activity group and smelling things in bottles.

Use multiple cues that all point to the same thing: the taste of food, its texture, utensils, an attractive table, good smells from the kitchen. Tell the person the beginning, the middle process, and the end of the task as you do them. Repeat often. For example:

- "I'm going to help you shower now."
- "I'm unbuttoning your dress."
- "I'm running warm water for you."
- "Feel the water. Is that right for you?"
- "Now I'll wash your back."
- "You are all finished with your shower now."
- "This is the activity room. Mary is making muffins."

Vary the number of cues and repetitions to find what works. Too many cues will make some people anxious.

Orient people often. Because people forget quickly, tell them again in a few minutes. Say:

"This is the dining room. This is your table. Your friend Betty will join you soon."

Orient people to the next task when you are finished.

> An activity director took a group off the unit for activities they enjoyed, but the group was more agitated when they returned to the unit. When she reoriented them to unit activities (lunch) and unit staff members, they settled comfortably.

Show the person what you will use. ("Here's your razor.") Let the person hold or touch it. ("It makes a noise.") Turn it on.

Use uniforms to give certain cues. For example, nursing uniforms are cues that some people can understand as a reason why you are performing personal care. They are disorienting to others. Uniforms give cues that one is in an institution, which many programs wisely avoid. Try slipping a lab coat on to see if it facilitates a specific intimate task for an individual.

Use ordinary social/interpersonal cues. Being dressed up is a cue that one is going out. Conversely, wearing a bib is a cue that one is childish and messy. Attractive smocks do the job and send more appropriate cues. A homey environment provides cues for ordinary behavior, whereas an institutional environment provides cues for illness behavior.

> One facility had a handsome sitting room that was seldom used. However, someone went in regularly and turned out all the inviting lights.

Here the cues were not quite what the interior designer had planned. For this group, the room was too "nice" to use, and lamps turned on were a cue to conserve electricity and turn them off.

Use touch. Touch can communicate affection and guide a person. Touch the person's body part lightly to encourage him to use it. Touch the back of the knees to help a person sit. Touch the arm you want to go in a sleeve. Confirm that the person perceives this as helpful and not as invasive. An occasional person will perceive touch as invasive or misinterpret touch as sexual or threatening. Base your approach on the individual's response.

Use imitation. Show the person by doing. People will try hard to do what you are doing. Be sure the person is paying attention to you.

Use reminders, lists, signs. Some people can use written cues such as a sign on the door that says "Take your key," labels on the dresser drawers (blouses, socks), a letter from family saying when they will return or where the person's money is kept, calendars recording simple schedules or planned visits. Such cues are important for people who can use them and confusing and frustrating for those who cannot. Some people will be able to read the written cue but be unable to act on what they read. Some people are reassured to have a note even when they can't read it.

Use diversion. Diversion and distraction are cues that help the person do something else. Some people have difficulty changing sets, and distractions enable this. In general, divert motor behaviors with motor activity (something to hold) and divert verbal activities with verbal tasks such as singing. Ask the person to do something with you or to help you. Diversion is useful in routine care, but when the person has a powerful goal of her own (such as "I have to get home to my children"), it will only irritate her.

Use predictability. People with dementia are sometimes reassured by having things done in the same way in the same sequence. A sense that things are going along in order helps a person feel in control even when she cannot remember exactly what will happen next. Flexibility means the care provider is able to adapt to the person; predictability means meeting the person's need for sameness.

Create context. Make bathrooms, toilet areas, bedrooms, day rooms, and dining rooms seem like the appropriate setting. That means making them seem like home to the impaired brain. Programs with limited resources have demonstrated that the creation of context can be accomplished with a few cans of paint and staff behavior rather than an expensive building.

It will be easier to get hair washed in an area that looks like a beauty parlor. Giving medicine in a public area is an "institutional" cue. Pajamalike clothing reinforces a "sick" role. Unappetizing smells discourage eating. One's things in one's room remind the person that she lives there. Use familiar styles of clothing that remind the person of dignified roles.

Make the goals of a task obvious. Many people are more comfortable knowing what the goal of a task is: we wash our hair to look nice (show her how nice she looks in the mirror when you are finished); the craft project is a gift for the administrator who is expecting a baby). If the goal is not immediately obvious, you will need to keep reminding the person: "We're on our way to lunch." For some people late in the illness, awareness of goals may be irrelevant.

Plan ahead. Successfully using these strategies requires advance planning. Do you have the supplies you will need to do a different activity? Is the place available? Will others help you or cover for you? What will you do if problems arise with one member of the group? Think about what cues and reminders will work with an individual. If something does not work, what else could you try?

Section 5.4. Suggested Interventions for Specific Activities of Daily Living

Objective

The student will understand detailed assessment and interventions for ADLs.

Information and Instructions for the Teacher

This material is intended for reference. Use it for an in-service focused on one ADL problem; when a specific difficulty is identified by the resident assessment or when it is observed in care; or when a behavioral symptom centers around an ADL. Some interventions are the opposite of other suggested interventions. What works for one person will be different from what works for another.

Lecture/Discussion Notes to Be Presented to the Class

Sleep Disturbance

People with dementia appear to have more disrupted sleep patterns with less deep sleep time. This would point to a basic change caused by the disease. Caregiving programs, however, report success in improving sleep patterns. This is likely to be an area in which care strategies can influence disease patterns. Following are points to be considered:

- Older people may need fewer hours of sleep, yet many settings put people to bed early. Encouraging the person's natural bedtime and wake time may be more successful.
- The person may have slept too much during the day. Are medications making the person drowsy? Has the person had adequate daytime stimulation? Programs report that people who are more involved during the daytime sleep better. Providing fresh outside air and exposure to morning sun are also helpful.
- The person may wake because he needs to be toileted or is wet. It is helpful to toilet immediately or to change promptly when the person rouses. Avoid waking the person to change him. This can lead to increased confusion and behavioral symptoms.
- Environmental problems that might not bother a younger person may disrupt the sleep of an older person. Have one person spend a night in your facility: What did he notice?
- Darkness may be an issue. Are rooms too dark or nightlights too bright? Does light leak from the hall? Did the person grow up in a very dark rural area or in a well-lit city?
- Noise may be disturbing. Are there outside traffic, hall traffic, a public address system, television, and staff voices outside the person's room? Does a cleaning crew arrive in early morning banging equipment and loudly reminding each other to be quiet?
- Be alert for sleep apnea.
- Arthritic pain, restless leg syndrome, and muscle cramps may wake people. Try a mild analgesic.
- Avoid using sleeping medications. They are less effective and have more side effects than environmental interventions. When these are necessary, choose medications for their side effect profile and select those with a short half-life.
- Sleep disruption for families caring at home is so serious that it can result in illness, depression, and exhaustion for the caregiver. More aggressive use of sleep medication may be called for.
- It takes a long time for interventions to take effect. Make change slowly rather than abruptly withdrawing medication, and expect several weeks to pass before you see any improvement.

Falls

Falls are a major hazard for people with dementia. It is probably impossible to prevent all falls and still maintain as active a life quality as desired. A well-considered compromise may be wiser. Facility policy with input from family members must provide guidelines for the staff.

As a group, people with dementia fall more often than others, and about half of these falls result in injury; a significant number result in hip fractures.

The neurodegenerative changes in the brain in combination with the physical environment are the primary causes of falls. Concurrent illness and age-related issues are also significant. Many medications increase shuffling, tripping, stiffness, falling, and inattention to the environment. When a person is unsteady, medication should be reviewed. In combination with the increasing apraxia, older people often have problems with vision or dizziness and comprehending the environment. Lost peripheral vision and poor hearing also contribute to falls. Malnutrition, common among people with dementia, is a contributing factor in falls.

There is a difference between helping the person to walk about (or use a wheelchair) independently and preventing falls. A good program focuses on maintaining independence and using remaining mobility as part of a safety program. Think in terms of enabling ambulation rather than preventing falls. Ask how this person can maintain quality of life by continuing to ambulate—safely.

Quiz yourself on your knowledge of falls by using Exhibit 5.1.

Individual Assessment of the Risk of Falling. The first step in intervention is to record all partial or near falls (tripping, staggering, slumping). These provide essential information with which to identify individual risk factors. They often occur before a serious fall and serve as a warning sign, but only if recognized and recorded. Regulatory agencies that penalize documentation of partial falls prevent the program from identifying risks. When charting patient falls and near falls include: When, where, doing what, blood pressure, tired, stressed? With whom? Assess the risk of injury during a fall (presence of osteoporosis, floor surface, risk of hitting objects as one falls).

Review how the person interacts with her environment (how she goes to the toilet, gets out of bed, uses a walker, and what her agenda was when she fell).

Prevention of falls include

1. neurological and physical therapy assessments of balance;
2. expert pharmacological management;
3. mild exercise/skill maintenance;
4. effective identification and treatment of Parkinsonian symptoms and depression; and
5. environmental modifications that support vision.

Interventions. Physical therapy consultations are helpful in facilitating ambulation and preventing falls.

Make falls less dangerous: use lower beds or chairs and resilient flooring. Pad surfaces, eliminate items the person might fall against; use shower stools, grab bars. Creating a dementia-safe physical environment involves removal of objects that cause the person to trip or fall. The environment should be familiar, well lit, free of glare, and easy to see, with distinct color contrasts that define steps and other obstacles. Smaller spaces are easier for people to process. Falls occur in bathrooms and dining areas where people slip or where seating and grab bars are inadequate. Unnecessary distractions, even noise, can increase a person's risk of falling or tripping.

Change staff behavior: never turn your back on an unsteady person; do not rush the person; find alternate ways to manage behavior with fewer neuroleptics; use physical therapy consults to assist staff members in learning to support and transfer people safely. If a person falls but is not injured, let him calm down before getting him up; then give him step-by-step instructions to get up as you assist him.

In a residential care, day care, or nursing home setting, it is tempting to modify the environment to the needs of the most impaired people and in doing so sacrifice the independence of those less impaired. For example, a facility with a lovely, secure atrium determined that no one could go outside independently because some might fall. A better policy would be to adjust activities so that more functional members of the group can enjoy the freedom of going outside at will.

People with dementia may shuffle or have a slow gait. Check the floor surface; ensure that shoes fit and that shoe soles are not slick. Confirm that medication is not the cause of the shuffle. Provide a level floor surface and improve lighting. Rushing a slow-moving person will increase the risk of a fall. Never push or pull a person.

If a person tilts to one side, forward, or backward, review medications, and assess the person for arthritic or muscle pain. Try offering your arm for support. For some people the tilt is part of the dementia. Assess how steady the person is and do not limit activities if the person seems able to do them.

If a person develops a limp, assess for pain, shoe fit, skin problems, irritant in the shoe, corns, blisters, or binding garments. Limping can cause muscle pain, which leads to behavioral symptoms.

If the person used a cane, walker, brace, or other assistive device before he became impaired, he may continue to use it. If he begins to use the device later in his dementia, he may be unable to learn to use it correctly.

Preventing an unsteady person from walking may have the unintended effect of increasing his risk of falling. Once he stops walking, balance and muscle strength decline, and the person may fall while being cared for or when he does stand up. Regular exercise and physical activity may help reduce the risk of falls. Loss of mobility may contribute to the reduction of bone density, increasing the risk of fractures.

Almost any illness can increase a person's risk of falling, and a fall should be considered an indicator of possible illness. Upper respiratory illness causes imbalance or dizziness for many people, yet the person with dementia may not be able to tell you that she feels unsteady. Dehydration will contribute to falls. After an illness or fracture, encourage the person to resume walking. Some programs report limited success in helping people who have had a hip fracture to resume walking. Other programs have had significant success. One factor seems to be a longer period of physical therapy. Regaining mobility after illness or a fall probably increases the chances that the person will not deteriorate as rapidly.

Nonambulatory people can fall during transfers and ADLs. Some people who are no longer steady will try to get up and walk. When walking must be restricted, use devices and strategies that discourage rising rather than more restrictive restraints. Increase positive social interaction.

Some people will remain ambulatory until a few weeks before death. Some will stop bearing weight and may draw up their legs when supported to walk. Assess for illness. Do not try to get this person to walk. This can injure staff members. Provide passive exercise to prevent contractures.

Nonambulatory people may slump in their chair. Slumped and twisted positions may be painful and lead to calling out or striking out. A physical therapy consult is helpful in determining how to use pillows to support the person.

Mealtimes, Eating, and Nutrition

Despite the efforts of staff and family caregivers, many people with dementia are malnourished or at risk of malnutrition. This is as true of people with dementia living in residential or nursing home care settings as it is of people living alone. Malnutrition affects the person's overall health and thus contributes significantly to behavioral symptoms as well as health problems. The person's increasing problems with motor skills, perception, ability to focus long enough to eat, distractibility, and depression challenge the caregiver. The physical environment and demands on the staff add to the problem.

When other, obvious interventions have failed, a consultation with a nutritionist can result in significant improvements.

For most people, mealtime has been a social time: family life, gatherings, and festivities focus around food. But the large dining areas with many people, confusion, and noise are incomprehensible and stressful for people with dementia. When the staff members feel pressure to get enough food into a person, the focus on a social experience is further lost. In the home setting, the tired and stressed caregiver also focuses on the task rather than the social experience. Finally, the behavioral symptoms make a social experience seem impossible. Thus, many of the successful interventions revolve around reducing stress in the dining setting, replacing the social cues, and improving environmental cues.

For those who have the option to modify or build a building: programs report that small dining areas (seating fewer than 15) for people with dementia result in fewer behavioral symptoms; these programs find that clients eat better and may gain weight in these settings. Small areas are less noisy and encourage social opportunities. Some programs have provided an even smaller, more private space for seating a few people with behavioral symptoms related to eating.

Flexibility is important. People with dementia seem to benefit from six small meals each day rather than the traditional three large meals. Snacks provide an excellent opportunity to meet nutritional and social needs not met at mealtime. Snacks should be available at all times including early morning and late night. Some people are early risers and become hungry and irritable before breakfast is served, while others are late risers and would naturally awaken after breakfast is served. Much irritability is prevented by accommodating these natural rhythms. If possible, have juice, toast, coffee, cold cereal, and milk available for early risers and for those who awaken at night. Be able to hold meals on the unit for those who eat slowly or dawdle. Flexibility also takes pressure off the staff to feed everyone or have everyone ready for a meal at once.

The social nature of mealtime is usually restored through serving the person with a small enough group that she is able to relax and by staff interaction with the person. Try sitting down and staying at the table with a small group, visiting with the individual as you feed him. Talking with the person while you feed her is low key, slow, and undemanding. Smile, look directly at the person. Never ignore the person you are helping or talk across people.

Some people have problems initiating eating. Sometimes a person can feed himself but cannot start the process. In such a situation, staff members may begin total feeding too soon. Lay a utensil and plate in front of the person and begin feeding him. He may pick up a utensil and attempt to feed himself once he has eaten a little. If so, encourage him and stop total feeding each time he begins to feed himself.

Some individuals do not use food utensils correctly or can no longer use them at all. Assess joint problems, consult with the occupational therapist, reduce distractions, feed the person when she is not feeling stressed. Assess whether medications are contributing to tremor or stiffness. Build up handles for people with joint pain; use plate guards or cup guards if they do not further confuse the person. Experiment with different utensils. Use finger foods (many foods can be adapted as finger foods, and messiness must be accepted). Be sure that the person can see her food. Increase lighting and use plates that contrast with the food. When people spill foods, try a spill-proof cup. Fill the person's glass only part way.

Some people do not recognize food as food or do not connect feelings of hunger with a desire to eat. They may not understand your invitation to go to a meal or become confused almost immediately. Many become restless if they must wait for food to be served. Increase sensory cues such as food smells. Try an activity program in which people immediately smell and eat what they prepare.

Pureed diets are particularly unappetizing. Pureed foods can be reformed to provide shape and texture.

Depression often reduces appetite. Treat depression if possible; offer small snacks frequently, and increase social cues. Medications sometimes reduce one's appetite or cause dry mouth. Review medications, offer sips of liquid between bites, serve soups or stews with more moisture content. Concurrent illnesses or pain reduces appetite. Abrupt decline in appetite signals a need to review for illness or pain. Try medicating for pain before mealtime. Use diet supplements.

If the person says she can't afford to eat or has no money, try saying something like, "Your daughter already paid."

If the person refuses to go to the dining area, review the possible causes listed earlier. Reduce the group size and noise. Change your approach; don't ask in advance; use different or more frequent cues; provide foods in the person's favorite place (own room, hall, or day room).

If the person fears being poisoned, avoid trying to reason with the person; the fear is not amenable to reason. Medication may be helpful. Eat some food yourself from the same plate (this is a violation of health codes, but it works); monitor for adequate nutrition; try a different staff member.

People who are very restless may leave the table before finishing, pace, or be too restless to sit down for a meal. The problem may be overstimulation. Reducing noise or group size is most effective. Be sure that the person was not stressed before the meal or when walking to the dining area. Be sure that the person does not need to use the toilet and that he is not in pain. Reduce the number of food items. (This can be done by setting a full plate nearby and transferring a small amount of food at a time to a plate the person can reach.) Restlessness or inability to sit still may be caused by the disease itself or by certain medications. Monitor this person for weight loss; this level of activity and anxiety burns many calories. Increase calories with diet supplements. Prepare finger foods and walk with the person while carrying the food and offering a bite at a time. Trade off and space this task through the day and evening.

Bathing

Bathing, while necessary, often seriously distresses the person with dementia. (See Exhibit 5.2.) The trauma of bathing may echo throughout the rest of the day, making it difficult for the person to enjoy other activities and increasing the person's irritability. There is a risk of accidents and falls during bathing and of injury to staff members.

The primary purpose of bathing is to maintain cleanliness, prevent odors, and preserve skin integrity. If incontinence occurs, areas exposed to urine or feces must be cleansed promptly and thoroughly to protect the skin. However, if bathing distresses the person, the entire body need not be washed each time, and the method of bathing can be modified.

In the residential or nursing home setting the pleasures of bathing often are overshadowed by the demands of the task. Relaxing in the bath, reading or eating, and (for women) applying lotions and scents and using pretty accessories may have been a lifelong pleasure that with skillful cueing can be used to help people relax.

Safety First. The physical plant, staff stress, and the stress the impaired person feels combine to make bathing a high-risk area. Following are steps to ensure safety:

- Eliminate slippery surfaces; clean spills immediately.
- Use grab bars, safe equipment, adequate light.
- Reduce staff feelings of being rushed, stressed.
- Work slowly.
- Plan bath in advance; lay out all supplies.
- Have a second person available.
- Do not bathe people who are frightened or combative. Help them to relax; bathe them later.
- Prevent other confused people from entering bathing area.
- Review all near accidents for ways to prevent them in the future.
- Never turn your back on a person in the bathing area even to reach for supplies.

The Bathing Area. The bathing area must be private. Only staff members involved in the bath should be present. The area should be well lit and quiet. Visual contrasts should be used to delineate areas. Ample towels and supplies should be within easy reach of the staff members so that they do not need to turn away from the person with dementia. Nonslip surfaces and grab bars, shower stools, and seats for dressing and resting are necessary.

Feeling cold is common in older people. Although the room may seem hot to the staff members, the person with dementia may feel cold. The room should be cozily warm. Some programs report that a towel warmer and larger towels, far from being a luxury, are excellent ways to comfort and reassure an anxious person.

Showers should be large enough to allow the caregiver to reach the person easily; they should drain well and be easily accessible. Encourage the person to use grab bars and the shower stool.

Methods. When possible, use the method most familiar to the person with dementia. Select a time of day when the person used to bathe or that best suits his present daily routines. It is reasonable to bathe some people early in the morning, some in the afternoon, and some before bedtime.

Allow ample time for each bath or shower. Working slowly reduces the risk of accidents and allows the staff members to reassure and comfort the distressed person.

Wash hair separately in the beauty parlor if the person is distressed by the bath.

Wash sensitive areas early and quickly. This way it is not necessary to complete the bath if the person becomes upset.

Caregivers can select among varied options for bathing:

- Showers can be used for some people.
- Easy-access tubs are useful for people who have difficulty walking into a shower and standing. Use them also for slow, relaxing baths.
- Bed baths are used for people who are distressed by showers or tub baths.
- Wash only essentials. This means washing only the face, underarms, and areas exposed to urine. This can be done using a basin in the person's room, with the person seated on a bath chair. It is often less distressing than a full bath.

Causes of Problems. Most bathing problems are caused by overstimulation, intrusion into personal space, and anxiety. Overstimulation can result from not knowing what is happening, why clothes are coming off, where one is going; the number of people involved; noise. Some aspects of bathing can be perceived as intrusions into personal space: being undressed; being touched; having a staff member standing close by; having the staff member do very personal tasks. Finally, overstimulation and feeling intruded on can create anxiety, as can feeling afraid of what will happen, of getting soap in one's eyes, of falling.

Exhibit 5.1. Reasons for Falls

Test yourself. Which of the following increase the likelihood that a person with dementia will fall?

- The person has already fallen within the year.
- The person functions reasonably well physically but is difficult to care for.
- The person does not exercise.
- The person is a man.
- The person has Parkinson disease or Parkinsonian symptoms.
- The person uses antidepressants, antipsychotic drugs, diuretics, or vasodilators.
- The person has problems of balance.
- The person has impaired vision.
- The person has recently been admitted or transferred.
- The person has limited opportunity to walk around.

(According to studies of falls, all increase the risk of falling.)

Exhibit 5.2. Strategies for Bathing

Bathing often is one of the most difficult tasks facing caregivers. Both the staff member and the person with dementia often end up wet, angry, and exhausted. However, simple interventions often make things easier. This exhibit lists potential problems associated with bathing; each problem is followed by one or more suggested interventions. Identifying the cause of the problem, if possible, helps in designing a successful intervention. For example, some people fight getting to the bathing area or getting undressed or balk at the suggestion, but they calm down when the bath begins. Others fight the bathing process itself. Suggested interventions often work for more than one problem.

Problem: Person fights the bath itself. The primary causes of problems are overstimulation from noise, the demands of the task, being overstimulated just before the bathing task, too much going on at once, and being confused. People often feel rushed, naked, frightened. They may feel that they have lost autonomy and control of the situation and that their personal space has been invaded. Agnosias prevent the person from recognizing the setting, no matter how many cues are given.

- Reduce stress. Reduce stimuli. In home bathrooms reduce number of objects in the room. Reduce noise, number of people involved; limit your instructions to the person.
- Never turn your back on the person. Have everything laid out in advance. Use paper and pencil to plan every step in advance.
- Avoid rushing the person; allow enough time to work slowly at the person's own pace.
- Bathe at the person's best time of day. Provide a low-stress activity or rest before the bath time.
- Use a hand-held shower hose for best control.
- Use task breakdown and task assessment.
- Use personal reassurance and trust.
- Conceal your own feelings of frustration or need to rush.
- Once a person becomes distressed by the bath, her anxiety and fear may increase with each bath. Switch to basin or bed baths or wash only necessary areas for a week or two.
- Find ways for the person to retain a sense of being in control. Give him a washcloth to hold, ask him to hold the grab bars, ask him to wash part of his body. Offer help tactfully: "I'll wash this side, you wash there."
- Use attractive dressing gowns. Wrap the person snugly in warm towels.
- Do not work silently. Talk gently to the person; tell him what you are doing one small step at a time; remind him to experience sensory cues; tell him what will happen after the bath. Never talk to another person while providing care.

Problem: Person fights getting to the bathing area or getting undressed or balks at the suggestion but calms down when the bath begins. The person may not understand your request or know what "bath" or "shower" means.

- Don't bring the subject up until the person is in the bathing area. Simply say, "Come with me."
- Pause to chat on the way to the bathing area (admire wall decorations).
- Don't transport the person in a chair or stool. Let the person walk at her own pace. Encourage her one step at a time instead of pushing her to get to the bathing area.
- Undress the person in the bathing area.

Problem: Person has impaired hearing or sight.

- Increase color cues.
- Reduce noise.
- Try showering the person with or without hearing aide.

(*continued*)

Exhibit 5.2. *(continued)*

- Try with and without glasses (don't get water in his face).
- Monitor water temperature.

Problem: Person says she has already bathed. Since bathing was a lifelong routine, the person is likely to assume she has already bathed if she can't remember. She may be uncertain how to bathe or what is involved, may not understand what you want. She may be embarrassed to be asked about such an intimate activity by a person she perceives as a stranger or outsider.

- Post a calendar in the person's room and clearly mark bathing days and times. At the beginning of the week, ask the person if she would rather bathe "Monday or Tuesday"; write her choice on the calendar and then negotiate "morning or afternoon." Do the same for the rest of the week. This gives the person a sense of control. You can then point out that she agreed to this. You may try it with people who are too impaired to really understand the plan. Keep your word.
- Try not bringing the subject up until the last minute.
- Use a note from the physician saying that the person is to have her bath on certain days and times. Read it to her if she can't read it.
- Ask the person in such a way that she does not have to offer excuses or feel that she has forgotten something as important as personal hygiene.
- Don't argue back; don't embarrass her. Give her an excuse for a bath:
  A family member drew the bath and then pointed out how wasteful it would be to let all that hot water get cold.
  A day care worker pointed out that if a woman had her bath at the center the "water company would not know and therefore could not send a bill."
  Try saying, "I have to wash the clothes now."
  "Your family is coming to visit" often does not work because it requires that the person retain the abstract thought of a later visit. Experiment until you find the right excuse for each person.
- Take advantage of old habits: in areas where people traditionally did not use a bathtub or shower, some programs have tried hip tubs.
- Bubble bath, fragrant soaps, luxurious towels, and similar items can be promoted as a spa.

Problem: Person is depressed, tired; has concurrent illness; has delirium.

- During these periods, modify the bathing procedure to avoid establishing a habit of fearfulness. Reduce stimuli, use basin or bed baths, bathe only part of the body if person tires.

Problem: Person resists being undressed. Person may not understand goal of bathing or may be modest.

- Use towels for privacy.
- Reach under clothing or under towels to wash.
- Reach around the shower curtain to wash a person who needs privacy.

Problem: Person is confused when a family member tries to bathe her; does not understand why a stranger is bathing her.

- Replace the family member with a staff member or another family member of the same sex.
- Try wearing a nursing uniform; alternatively, try not wearing a uniform.
- Try having a family member step into the shower with the person.

(continued)

Exhibit 5.2. *(continued)*

Problem: Person is upset by being bathed at an unfamiliar time.

- Learn about old habits; use cues that remind person of past habits.
- Adapt facility schedules to fit old habits.
- Undress the person in the bathing area, not in his room.
- Link bathing to time of dressing or undressing.

Problem: Person is upset by the bathing area. Institutional areas have strange smells, lack privacy, may be cold and drafty, may appear dirty, may remind the person of old, dirty public bathing areas.

- Eliminate negative cues and enhance appropriate cues, provide visual boundaries, use color. Provide adequate lighting: poor light creates shadows that some people perceive as dirt.
- Avoid visibly dirty linens.
- Conceal drains by painting them to match the floor.

Problem: Person complains that room is cold, that she feels cold.

- Feeling anxious may make the person feel cold; reduce anxiety.
- Older people often feel cold when caregivers do not.
- Dry the person quickly and thoroughly.
- Use preheated towels.

Problem: Person is distressed by noise of shower, noisy room, background noise, activities of others in area. The noise of the shower can exacerbate tinnitus or cause dizziness in many people; this can last for several hours after bathing and can lead to falls. Institutional bathing areas absorb sound poorly; large rooms echo and therefore seem excessively noisy. The presence of others in the area is a cue that this is not a private bathing area.

- Remodel the area using sound-absorbing materials; eliminate noise from adjacent areas, background noise; turn off fans.
- Limit the presence of others in the room when bathing this individual.
- Review medical history for tinnitus, dizziness, drug side effects; ask if the person has tinnitus or feels dizzy.
- Monitor for falls during and after bath.

Problem: Person is distressed by unfamiliar hoists, stools, shower hoses.

- Use another bathing method.
- If the person never used a washcloth, do not use one.
- Touch the person, hold his hand, reassure him.

Problem: Person is afraid of water, complains that water is too deep.

- Use no more than an inch of water in the tub.
- Let the water out of the tub after the person gets out.
- Don't use the tub.

Problem: Person fights having hair washed.

- Use beauty salon/barber shop environment.

(continued)

Exhibit 5.2. *(continued)*

- If a person's hair must be washed in the shower, never get soap in her eyes; keep her face dry, let the person hold a dry cloth over her face: tipping her head back may cause dizziness or balance problems.
- Use dry shampoo.

Problem: Person has difficulty stepping over rim of shower, stepping into tub (apraxia).

- If possible, design the shower without a rim or build a mini-ramp into the shower area.
- Use a specialty tub.
- Use touch to cue the person; touch him behind his knee to cue him to step up.
- Request a physical therapy consult if the person must continue to use home bathtub.

Problem: Person is unsteady, fall risk; fears falling.

- Never turn your back on the person.
- Use a fall risk assessment plan.
- Have a second staff member present to steady the person.
- Ask the person whether she feels dizzy.
- Document near falls, slips; note causes, exact situation.
- Use tub/shower seat / bench.
- Use hand-held shower hose.
- Use nonslip surfaces and mats.
- Repeatedly remind the person to hold grab rails.
- Use a specialty tub.

Problem: There is a new caregiver; task routines are changed.

- Don't change what works; new caregivers should learn from prior caregivers what works for each client; be reassuring.

Problem: Person grabs at things (grasp reflex, fear of falling, desire to help).

- When someone has a grip on the staff member, both are at increased risk of falling; stop working, move slowly, do not pull away or shout, use the call bell to get assistance.
- Give the person something to hold; remind him to keep holding it.
- If the person grasps your wrists, do not jerk away; gently ease out of her grasp.
- Fasten up your own hair so it is out of reach.
- A little soap on your wrist or shampoo on your hair will make it easier to slip out of a person's grasp.

Problem: Person washes only one area (perseveration).

- Accept the behavior.
- Occasionally remind the person to wash elsewhere; use motor cues.

Problem: Person urinates or defecates in shower or bath.

- Some people have a long-standing habit of urinating in the shower; the shower becomes a cue; you may not be able to prevent this.
- Showering a person in a commode chair may trigger incontinence.
- Use a shower seat with an opening, a hose to clean up, latex gloves.

(continued)

Exhibit 5.2. *(continued)*

- Toilet the person just before bathing.
- Time the bath for after the person has a bowel movement.

Care after the bath

- Repeatedly reorient the person ("Now we'll get you dressed"; "I'm taking you back to your room").
- Be sure the person is completely dry, including genital area.
- Help the person relax; provide quiet activity.

Overhead/Handout 5.1. Principles of ADL Care

1. All ADL care is either beneficial or harmful.

2. The sum total of all the little things we do makes the quality of life better or worse.

3. The staff member who provides direct ADL care is the most important therapist on the team.

Overhead/Handout 5.2. Guidelines for ADL Care

1. Select one person at a time.
2. Select someone whose care is reasonably easy but with whom you have some problems. Do not select someone who is very difficult to care for. If you care for a person who is functioning well, select an IADL, such as preparing a simple lunch. If you select a person who has difficulty with simple tasks, select one small part of an ADL.
3. Identify one issue or one part of one ADL. Do not select a large project. For example, select brushing teeth rather than all of morning grooming; select changing a person who is wet rather than the complete dressing activity; select eating lunch rather than all the tasks involved in eating a meal.
4. For this person, identify the areas of impaired function that cause problems in this task.
5. For this person, identify areas of spared function that you might be able to take advantage of in carrying out the task.
6. Identify any excess disability that will complicate the task and any way you can help the person (for example, if the person does not see well, you will give more verbal cues).
7. Identify sources of stress that complicate the task and ways to counteract this (for example, you might plan to work more slowly with a confused person).
8. Plan an intervention, using task breakdown if appropriate.
9. Plan for small changes and small interventions.
10. The intervention must be realistic and possible in your setting. Consider whether you could obtain permission to carry out the activity, whether another staff member might cover for you while you try it to see if it will work, whether you could videotape the task once to see how much time it takes. Are there other ways in which you can reasonably modify your setting to try the task a few times?
11. Describe how you will know whether the plan, if you carried it out, would help the person (for example, the person would be able to sit still during her meal or get her teeth brushed without becoming angry).
12. Present your plan to the rest of the group.

Overhead/Handout 5.3. Suggested Interventions

Individualize.

Select the best time of day.

Be flexible.

Enable.

Use cues.

Use touch.

Use imitation.

Use reminders, lists, signs.

Use diversion.

Use predictability.

Create context.

Make the goals of a task obvious.

Plan.

LESSON 6

HELPING THE PERSON BY ENRICHING COMMUNICATION

Summary. Communication is a vital aspect of human life, yet dementia greatly limits communication. Loss of the ability to communicate frustrates both the staff and people with dementia and impedes care. It makes the person with dementia more isolated and destroys important relationships. This lesson discusses ways to strengthen and sustain communication.

Section 6.1. Verbal and Nonverbal Communication. Teaches interventions that support expressive and receptive aphasias. This section covers the use of nonverbal communication, which often is retained longer.

Section 6.2. Avoiding Patronizing Behavior. Teaches staff members how to avoid patronizing behavior. Patronizing behavior on the part of caregivers is subtle and difficult to avoid as language is lost. Patronizing the client seriously damages his self-esteem and leads to anger or withdrawal.

Section 6.3. Information about Assessing Communication. Identifies information that will be useful in communicating with the person with dementia.

Using the Sections

Introductory course:
- Section 6.1 required
- Section 6.2 required

Core course:
- Section 6.1 required
- Section 6.2 required

Special audiences:
- People responsible for diagnosis, assessment, referral, and treatment: all sections, including Section 6.3

Problems You May Have in Implementing This Lesson

Students enjoy the insight into their own lives, but some will need a basic introduction to the concepts of body language.

The biggest pitfall is to assume one is an expert. The study of human facial expression and nonverbal communication reveals that this area is complex. Illness and cultural differences make it more complex. For example, people with Parkinson disease show little facial expression. Teachers and students should approach their observations with caution, "It appears that he is angry," or "It seems to me that she is sad."

Communication is highly individual. Staff members must work consistently with the same people to learn to communicate with them. This means that staffing should be planned to allow for this. Backup staff members should have some experience with each individual before working with her.

Staff members may have been taught to treat people with dignity and respect but may not know how to implement this. If you can use video, even if only of the staff and not the clients, this will help students recognize concrete ways to treat people with dignity. Patronizing treatment can undo staff efforts to raise self-esteem and therefore is a destructive force in care. Patronizing behavior can be very subtle, and thus the educator and other experts may inadvertently seem patronizing. While educators and staff members may have difficulty recognizing subtle patronizing behavior, it is not at all difficult for the impaired person!

Section 6.1. Verbal and Nonverbal Communication

Objective

The student will improve his ability to use the client's remaining verbal skills and will become more aware of nonverbal communications.

Background

The loss of language (aphasia) is part of most dementias. It may be abrupt, as in the case of stroke, or gradual, as in Alzheimer disease. It may be retained longer than other skills, as in alcohol-related dementia. Expressive or receptive language skills may not be lost at the same rate, so a person may understand more than he can say or may talk well but understand little. It is easy for caregivers to be mislead and assume that both skills are lost in parallel. Language impairment is often not a good indicator of the degree of loss of other functions. This, too, can trip up caregivers. Caregivers tend to overuse verbal language with people who are aphasic. This can overwhelm and upset some people.

Students are already expert in nonverbal communication, which is acquired early in life. Use this section to validate what students already know. While the concept of nonverbal communication is new to some students, others will have had experience with it. Urge more sophisticated students to observe more subtle behaviors. People who are "good" with people with dementia are tuned in to body language: both their own and that of the ill person.

It is difficult to "act out" nonverbal communication in the classroom because people feel awkward. Worse, even experienced people unwittingly send nonverbal clues that say, "I am acting: I don't really mean this."

People may be largely unaware of some of their own nonverbal signals. Focus on increasing self-awareness in this lesson.

Information and Instructions for the Teacher

Use the overheads/handouts as teaching points. The text will guide your presentation. Teach this material as discussion. Stop frequently to ask the students how they can apply these ideas and which of their clients would respond. Use examples you are aware of and ask for examples students have observed. It is not necessary to teach all the suggestions in these lists: select those that are relevant to your group. It is important in this section to teach students to be aware of verbal and nonverbal communication. Their ability to communicate well with people with dementia will follow naturally.

Videotape students interacting with clients. (See Chapter II.) This will help them become aware of their own nonverbal messages and those of the people they care for. Encourage the students to critique the films in the classroom.

Select a movie or soap opera that shows emotions, gestures, facial expressions, and body postures. Preview the film several times to identify the most effective sections. Write down the stop and start times. Before going to class, preset the film at the point you wish to start it. Show the film without sound. Show only two or three minutes of film to study facial expressions or body language. Longer units of film contain too much material to analyze. Stop the film and discuss what the class observed. Observe still sections or repeat the film as needed. Ask the students what emotions are expressed and how they know that. Confirm their opinions by playing the tape again with the sound. Do not use films about how to care for people with dementia. In many of these, performers send double messages or show patronizing behavior, which you do not want to reinforce.

If you use film or videotape, use less of the lecture notes. Use the notes to guide you in a discussion of the film or video.

Lecture/Discussion Notes to Be Presented to the Class

Overhead/Handout 6.1. Ways We Communicate

Human beings spend a lot of time communicating with each other. What methods do people use to do this? *(Teacher: Ask the students to name these, list on flip chart.)* Include the following:

- Talking
- Listening
- Hand gestures
- Facial expressions
- Eye contact
- Tone, volume, pitch of voice
- Body posture
- Touch
- Pointing
- Singing
- Writing
- Reading

Teacher: Ask the students to give an example of each of these techniques.

When we use written or spoken words, we are using *verbal language* (talking, listening, reading, writing). When we use gestures, facial expressions, touch, posture, or tone, volume, or pitch of voice, we are using *nonverbal language.*

Dementia often damages the brain's ability to understand and use spoken (verbal) language. When a person has a stroke that affects the language part of the brain, the person may suddenly be completely or partly unable to speak or understand what others are saying. In diseases such as Alzheimer's, these abilities are lost slowly and gradually over time. People who have had a stroke may recover some language skills. There is little evidence that people with Alzheimer disease can relearn language skills. Because it is the basic process of talking, not the ability to form words, that is lost, many people with dementia will not be able to use storyboards or sign language or to follow instructions.

The loss of communication is devastating to people with dementia. It accounts for much of their rage, terror, withdrawal, and grief. As relationships are lost, the person loses identity. People depend on verbal language to organize thoughts. As language is lost, the ability to think with words is lost. The loss of language is also devastating to family relationships and creates obstacles to care.

The brain seems to process nonverbal language differently, and for many people with dementia nonverbal communication abilities remain and last longer. Caregivers help the person by identifying and using what verbal language skills remain and by learning to use more nonverbal communication. This lesson will discuss ways to take advantage of remaining verbal skills and to become more aware of nonverbal communication.

Exercise 1. The Importance of Communication

As a class or in small groups, discuss these issues:

Imagine being in a situation in which you don't know what others are saying or what they are thinking. How would you feel? Suppose you could not communicate with others. Discuss just how important being able to communicate with others is. Have you been in a setting where everyone else was speaking a language you do not understand? What must it be like for the person who can't make any sense out of what you are saying but realizes that she is missing something? If you could not communicate, how could you have a relationship with another person? Is communication essential to all our relationships with others? with pets and babies?

Overhead/Handout 6.2. Making Yourself Understood with Words

As the dementia progresses, most people will have increasing difficulty understanding what you tell them. This is frustrating for caregivers.

Consider this list of strategies. How can you adapt them to individuals whom you care for?

Be sure the person can hear you and is paying attention. Look to see if she is paying attention, take the person to a quiet place, look directly at her, remove distractions, reduce the stress she is experiencing. If the person has a delirium, do not expect more than a few seconds of her attention.

If you have taken her hearing aid out because she loses it, give it to her when you communicate with her and then put it away. It is upsetting to be hard of hearing and have someone shouting at you as she does something personal to you.

Speak slowly, and use a low pitch. Do not raise your voice.

Support your words with nonverbal clues.

Say less. Give less information. Reduce explanations and reasons. Ask questions that can be answered with a yes or no. Know how much the person can process. Some people can take in only three or four words. Some remember the last of a sentence, others only the first.

Try not using open-ended questions, such as "What do you want for dinner?" or "How do you like your room?" Such questions force the person to search for words to reply to you.

When you give complex information, the person may be unable to register more than a small part of it. For example, when the staff member said, "Let's get you dressed for breakfast. There's a movie after breakfast, and it's one of your favorites," what the person with dementia heard was, "Let's get you."

Speak slowly, but speak normally, *not as if you were speaking to a child.* This is difficult and takes practice. Say a few words and wait for the person to think about these. Then say a few more. Watch to see if the information is registering.

If the person does not understand you, *repeat exactly what you said once.* Then say it differently. The person may be misunderstanding you.

Sometimes people don't hear things correctly. For example, when the staff member said, "Would you like to go to the party?" what the person with dementia heard was, "Would you like to go potty?'

What will you do if your accent is different from that of the person with dementia?

Tell the person what to do, not what not to do. Being told what not to do is frustrating to a person who cannot remember even obvious "right" ways to do something. "Don't do that" sounds like a parent scolding a child and irritates many adults. For example,

Wrong: "Don't pound on the chairs with the croquet mallet."

Try: "Let's go out and hit some balls."

Wrong: "Don't put your legs through your sleeves."

Try: "Can I turn that around for you?"

Overhead/Handout 6.3. Understanding the Person's Communications

Look at the person's body language and facial expression. *Listen* carefully.

Stop what you are doing. People deserve to be heard even if not understood. Sensing that you are giving her your full attention will make the person feel less stressed and may improve her ability to communicate.

Sit down so you are at eye level with her. When a person is upset, she may wind herself up more and more as she talks. If this happens and you are not able to understand her, continue to give her your attention but distract her. Offer to talk about it again in a few minutes. The person may be better able to communicate when she is rested.

When some people with dementia speak, the first few words are meaningful. Then the person rambles on, getting lost in his words and taking you with him. If this happens, listen closely for the first few words and react to them. If you are sure the person is lost in his own words, gently remind him of what he started to say.

Some people take a long time to speak. Wait. Ask the family what the person is saying.

The nature of the brain damage is such that many people cannot point to what they want. If pointing does not work, do not push it.

Focus on context more than on content. Focus on right now. Expect the content to be about current issues, needs, or statements. People with dementia are often trying to express immediate social ideas just as we do: "I like your hair"; "I want someone to sit with me." Most people do not go around talking about their distant past to everyone. Do not assume that the person is talking about some long-past trauma.

> A woman insisted that her husband was cheating on her. The staff member assumed she was talking about a painful past episode and reacted accordingly. Then one of the staff members noticed the husband walking in the garden and holding hands with a young woman.

Think about the whole message: body language, expression, and tone of voice. What is the general drift of the conversation? Think about what is going on around the person, what has just happened. The person with dementia is usually speaking to the context she perceives.

Ask if you understood. When a person says something but you don't know what, ask him to say it again. If you are still lost, be honest and say you can't understand. If possible, find someone who knows him well and can find out what he needs.

People with dementia often struggle to find a word. Fill in the word for him, but be sure that is what he meant. Leaving him to struggle to make himself understood increases his stress and lowers his performance level.

Nouns may be lost before other parts of language. For example, the person may say, "You were sweet, honey, to do it and I want to tell you. They all did and I did too." There are no names of things in this statement. Spoken correctly, it would say, "You were sweet, Ann, to bring me this orange. And I want to say thank you. They all liked their oranges and I liked my orange, too."

Another person said, "I have one. I have it here. They made me a, a small one. I feel like one of those, you know." Corrected: "I have my house key. I have it around my neck. It makes me feel like a child (to wear a key around my neck)."

People with dementia may talk around a subject when they can't find words. If you ask a person to name a watch (as you do when you conduct a Mini-Mental State Examination [MMSE]), he may say, "It's one of those and it's round and it's if you want to know when you should." A man who was usually seated in the dining room with three other people was alone on one occasion. He asked, "Isn't there supposed to be, supposed to be, one of them, here with me?" When you hear such sentences, recognize that the person is almost saying what she means. *Ask her if she means* . . . [fill in the blanks for the person who is groping for a word].

Some people substitute a word when they can't find the correct one. Asked what she wants for lunch, a woman might say, "round balls." Instead of saying, "You really don't want to eat a ball," guess that she might mean meatballs.

It is essential that you *know the person* you are communicating with. Much of the time you will be guessing what the person is saying, but it is an informed guess when you know the person's usual concerns and pleasures. (This is one of the reasons for taking a good history on admission. Without a history, the staff may be trying to help someone but have no clue about what she is saying.) For example:

> A man was talking to a visitor who did not know him. He was earnest and working hard to make her understand him. She replied, "Oh my. That must be hard for you." At that moment a staff member who knew the man came by. "He's telling you the story about the three walruses and the sex machine. He loves that joke. (We learned this from his family.)"

A person with dementia may be able to understand more than she can express, or vice versa. When this happens, the staff may not realize what is happening. It is easy to assume that because the person has difficulty expressing herself she cannot understand you or to assume that because she communicates well she also understands you. Consider the people you care for: Have you observed examples of this?

A person may have good language skills but serious impairment in other areas. When this happens, the staff may overestimate other abilities. A person may be able to tell you that no, she does not want any dinner, without understanding at all what dinner is or that it relates to her feeling of hunger. Other people may have serious difficulty understanding or making themselves understood but still be cognizant of many things. For example, a person may not understand anything you told her about her bath and may be unable to object, but this does not mean that she does not understand where you are taking her or that she does not like bathing.

When you can't understand a person with dementia, *don't lie* and say that you do. Say that you care but you don't understand.

Using Nonverbal Communication

As the ability to speak and understand words is lost, many people with dementia retain their ability to communicate nonverbally (through expression; eye contact; posture; tone, pitch, and rapidity of voice; gestures; and touch). Whenever you are having difficulty with words, focus on nonverbal communication.

Staff members who are skilled in understanding and using nonverbal methods of communication can often figure out what a person wants. They are able to maintain nonverbal relationships with people with dementia. This nonverbal communication helps to sustain connections, identity, and self-esteem.

Enabling communication is rewarding to staff members because people with dementia visibly brighten up when they understand or are understood. Staff members already have good nonverbal communication skills and can use these creatively to help the person with dementia. The things you will learn in this lesson focus your communication skills on those with dementia.

We use nonverbal language all the time, without

thinking. For example, we might say of a child, "I can tell just what he is thinking" or "My wife's feelings are written on her face."

We change our facial expression, posture, the tilt of our head, or the position of our hands to emphasize our words. Much of the time we are unaware of our nonverbal language, but because it becomes critical for communication as people lose verbal skills, we can improve it.

We sometimes contradict ourselves with our body language. All people, including those with dementia, tend to trust our nonverbal expression over our verbal statements. Imagine a small boy who has been told he has to rake the yard but does not want to. Even as he says, "All right, I'll do that," you can see that he does not want to. Imagine you are cleaning up a person who has had diarrhea. You are trying hard to be kind because the person is embarrassed. But your face says, "Oh, yuck." What will the person understand? How will he feel?

Overhead/Handout 6.4. Learning to Use Body Language

Facial expressions convey emotions. Most people "read" and "speak" them easily. Emotions expressed in the face seem to be similar all over the world. You can learn to improve your skills in recognizing them.

To experiment with facial expressions at home in private, watch yourself in the mirror and think about a time when you felt a certain emotion. Imagine yourself in that situation (perhaps you were angry with someone). What slight changes do you see in your face? a frown, a tight mouth, narrower eyes? Try slightly raised eyebrows, wrinkled nose; try a big smile and then a tiny smile as if you were hiding the smile. Can you see the changes in your own face?

Practice watching other people's faces. Watch for movement around their eyes, mouth, and forehead. You can usually tell when a person is happy or sad. What else can you see?

People with dementia may have a "flattened affect"; that is, their face does not show much. Parkinson disease and certain drugs have this effect. If you watch closely, you will see a hint of a smile or frown. Close attention will reveal many expressions that might otherwise be overlooked.

Why are people who smile often considered likeable? If a person has Parkinson disease and therefore rarely smiles, might people incorrectly think he was always grumpy?

How does your face communicate to the person with dementia? If you fake an expression, your face may give away the deception. Do not use exaggerated expressions because they don't look sincere. When you communicate with a person with dementia, focus on that person and let your face naturally express how you feel. Instead of thinking about your expressions, which will make them seem fake, ask others in the group what your face shows.

Eye contact helps establish the relationship between two people. It can be positive or negative. It can help to hold a person's attention, or it can seem dominating and controlling. Lovers gaze into each other's eyes for a long time, but gazing too long at others is staring. Angry parents who want their children to do something may "stare them down."

Are there ways to use eye contact to avoid embarrassing a person or to comfort the person? Does this help some more than others?

In addition to facial expressions, we communicate by using the rest of our body: the way we stand, hold our shoulders, head, and arms. *Body movements* express emotion, affection, and who is dominant in the relationship.

Think of several ways to express affection with your body. Describe how people walk when they are happy.

What would you do to communicate "I'm listening"? What does walking away, acting restless, or watching something else convey?

Standing over or above the person often signals that you are controlling that person. If the person is in a chair, how can you counter that signal?

Watch the person with dementia. What behavior indicates that she is paying attention to you? that she is becoming angry? Select someone you know and identify the smallest body signal that he or she is growing angry.

What are the body signals that she has stopped listening? is tired?

What does the position of the head and feet tell you about depression, pain, dizziness? (People who are dizzy often hold their head stiffly.)

Listen to and use tone, pitch, and rapidity of speaking voice. The sound of a person's voice, even when the words are not understood, can be soothing or upsetting. Tone expresses feelings. You may not be able to describe or perfectly imitate feelings expressed in voice tone, but think about how you recognize them.

Think about the sound of happiness in your friend's voice over the telephone. Does she sound "bubbly"? Can you hear fatigue over the telephone? What about sadness? What do you mean when you say a person "sounds awful" or "sounds better today"?

Can you hear a tone of disbelief? of authority? Can you hear frustration, affection, or confusion in the tone of voice the person with dementia uses?

What is a high-pitched voice? a low-pitched voice? Sometimes we raise the pitch or volume of our voice when we talk to people who are hard of hearing or have a dementia. Might they perceive this as demeaning?

It may be easier for a person with a hearing problem to understand a lower-pitched voice.

Gestures include pointing, tapping a plate, raising your hand to say "Stop," or waving to say "Come on." They include walking away from, walking toward, shrugging shoulders, spreading your hands. Some gestures are easy to observe; others are subtle.

How do you say, "Come here" or "Eat that" with gestures? Can you do this rudely or kindly?

Ask the family which gestures the person uses and which ones she understands. What gestures does she use to tell you to stop? that she has had enough? What gestures would make the person angry? Gestures vary from one culture to another. If there are people of varied cultures in the group, discuss these variations. Ask families about gestures that might be insulting in their culture but not offensive in yours.

People use *touch* frequently in all forms of nonverbal communication. It may be the form of communication that people with dementia retain longest. Our use of touch is complex and varies with the culture we grew up in. Discuss:

Using hands only, how would you touch a person to make him stay in one place? to reassure the person that she is safe?

How does a person with dementia use her hands to communicate her fear to you? to ask you to stay with her? to tell you to leave her alone?

Can you touch a person as if she were an object instead of a person?

What is the difference between seductive touch and washing a person's private parts?

What does a hand on a person's knee mean? affection? seduction? restraint? reassurance? Or could it mean any of these, depending on the context? Can the person with dementia get the context wrong? Choose any form of touch and evaluate all its possible meanings.

Some people like a lot of touch; others don't like to be touched. How much touch do the people you know prefer? Do you touch all the people you care for about the same amount, or do you treat them differently? Do you touch people you don't like more or less? Which is better for the person?

Might the person with dementia misinterpret your touch as aggression or restraint?

In some cultures, people stand close to each other. In other cultures, people stand farther apart. For example:

> Mey always stood too close to the nurses. They interpreted this as aggression, but where Mey came from standing close was friendly.

Exercise 2. Role Play

Use role play to understand messages. Select a person known to you whose communication is difficult to understand. As best you can, and without exaggeration, act out what she does that you don't understand in front of other staff members. Imitate the person's face and other body language. Copy what the person does: do not say what you think the person was feeling. Ask the group members to tell you what they think you were communicating.

Clinical Experience

Select a person who is having difficulty with communication, and make a plan for improving communication with this person. Try this approach for one week.

Section 6.2. Avoiding Patronizing Behavior

Objective

The student will be aware of patronizing behavior and will learn alternatives.

Information and Instructions for the Teacher

It is essential that students understand the concept of patronizing behavior and learn to avoid it. Patronizing behavior is a subtle but constant stressor and probably contributes toward behavioral symptoms in people with dementia. Staff members at all levels, including supervisors and management, tend to be patronizing.

The first step in reducing patronizing behavior is for the student not to think of the person with dementia as diminished or less human. What works best is for everyone to know and come to respect even the most severely impaired person. Each lesson in this text addresses this.

Use films of staff members at work to identify patronizing behavior.

Groups vary: some staff members will be working to reduce the use of overtly babyish behavior and pet names such as "honey," whereas others will talk across people. Some will have learned that they engage in such patronizing behavior but may be unaware of more subtle mannerisms. Target your training to your group. Videotape people providing care and ask staff members to critique each other as they continue to refine their skills. Supervisors should participate as well.

Staff members rarely mean to be condescending. They are unaware of their nonverbal behavior. In teaching this concept, avoid making staff members feel as if they are "to blame." Patronizing behavior is in some ways a common response to severe impairment and must be "unlearned."

Teach this in your own words. Go slowly. Avoid pointing out past patronizing behavior a student might have used. This will make the group defensive. Let ideas come from the group, or use yourself as an example.

Lecture/Discussion Notes to Be Presented to the Class

Patronizing behavior is using words or gestures in a way that is condescending and that makes others feel put down, treated like a child, or devalued. It is as if you are making yourself sound superior to the other person. The person with dementia probably will not be able to say, "Don't treat me like that!"

We convey patronizing behavior with our body posture, the expression on our face, our tone of voice, and our words.

> The CEO sat in on a lively discussion of patronizing behavior toward nursing home residents. At the end, he got up, put his hand on the woman teacher's shoulder, and said, "Great! You girls carry on." He had no idea why the class burst into laughter.

Even when we have no intention of being patronizing, our face or tone of voice or posture may make us seem this way. Patronizing behavior can be very subtle. Often we are trying to be kind or supportive, but we come across to the disabled person as patronizing. Sometimes what we do seems patronizing to the ill person but not to us.

Treating the Person as If She Were a Child

When people can't hear or understand, when they wander away and can't take care of themselves, it is human nature to treat them the way parents treat children. However, people with dementia know they are not children. They are adults, and they react negatively to this treatment.

Dementia profoundly affects verbal language, reason, and memory, but it usually has much less impact on the ability to interpret body language. People with dementia are often alert to patronizing behavior and react to it. The postures and tone of voice that people use with children and *the staff behaviors that the person with dementia perceives as put-downs are some of the most damaging environmental factors in dementia care.* These are factors that can be changed.

Some people with dementia take offense. They become angry, restless, or upset. If they feel put down much of the time, they may be chronically stressed and have frequent catastrophic reactions. (Of course, the person is not aware of—or in control of—her reaction.)

Other people with dementia take their cue from you. When people around them apparently think they are babies, they become like babies: passive, docile, whining, or clinging. They may be easy to care for, but they have given up on themselves too soon.

The problem is that it is difficult to learn to change.

Avoiding Patronizing Behavior

Nicknames. Do not call people by pet names such as "honey" or "baby." Never say, "Mary is my baby." Call people by their first or last names or by a lifelong nickname.

Putting People on Hold. Don't ignore people or keep them waiting a long time; don't tell them you will do something but then not do it. These are powerful messages that say, "You are worthless." People with dementia are unable to figure out that you are busy, and because they have no sense of time, telling them "I'll be right back" has little meaning. They can only respond to the feeling of being ignored. Try taking that person with you while you finish a task.

Posture. Patronizing behavior is more often communicated with our posture and hands than with words. Get on eye level with the person. Sit down beside the person. Try to look like you are not rushed. Give your full attention to the person for that short time. When people want you to stay with them for a long period, apologize. Come back to them soon.

Voice. Listen to your tone of voice. People naturally talk in a higher pitch to babies. This is great for babies because it gets their attention, but it sends a message to the person that you are treating her like a baby.

Touch. Pay attention to the way you use your hands. The way we touch others always sends a message. Think about ways you have been touched that you don't like.

Some People with Dementia Appear to Like Being Treated as Babies

For some people, being treated like a baby is one coping mechanism in response to their disability and the treatment available—they do get attention this way, but it still damages self-esteem. Staff members need to continue to provide loving care but with more respect.

Staff members may argue that using interventions for children helps severely impaired people. Ask them to discuss how these interventions are different from put-downs. For example, having a baby doll seemed to comfort Mary. Staff behavior toward Mary is what makes the difference. A staff person might patronizingly say, in a high-pitched voice, "Have you got your baby doll today?" or in a normal adult-to-adult voice, "Mary, do you want to take your doll with you to lunch?"

Using a similar example may help the staff understand the difference in staff behavior. "John enjoys his model trains" is different from "John, are you playing with your little trains?"

It takes a lifetime to learn this skill. Teaching staff members to treat impaired people as adults needs to be reviewed regularly.

Exercise 3. Recognizing Patronizing Behavior

The best way to recognize patronizing behaviors is to film yourselves. Rent a video camera and take turns filming each other as you provide routine care. Be sure to film your instructor and nursing director as well. As a group, review the film in the classroom. You will spot a lot of put-down behaviors of which you were unaware but which were creating a negative, stressful environment for those you care for. Many of these behaviors are not intended to be a put-down—they are just the way you do things. Study the film and try to eliminate the things that the other person may interpret as patronizing.

To protect client privacy, film the client's back or leave the client out of the video—film staff only. Destroy the tape immediately after viewing it. Get permission to use video. If you cannot use video, take turns observing each other.

Section 6.3. Information about Assessing Communication

Objective

The student will understand assessment and intervention techniques for communication.

Background

This section reviews assessment data that staff members will have obtained for each person and suggests ways to make the data useful in facilitating communication.

As is true of other functions, language impairments vary with each individual. Assessment will often identify areas in which communication can still be accomplished. This section lists only a few types of questions that can be used to assess the individual.

The assessment information is useful only if everyone knows it. Use posters or staff meetings to exchange information about an individual.

It can take several weeks for the staff to get to know a person well enough to communicate effectively, especially if no history from family is available.

Use Exhibit 6.1. (Delirium, deafness, drugs, and disease are described in Lesson 3.) Distance refers to the distance the person is from a group leader or speaker. In general, people with dementia tend to focus more successfully on people who are close to them.

Lecture/Discussion Notes to Be Presented to the Class

Observation

Chapter V discusses observations of the client that will help communication.

Not all communication problems are due to the brain disorder. As you evaluate communication, ask yourself questions like the following, which will help you separate hearing difficulties, clarity of speech, and comprehension.

- Is the person delirious? having difficulty focusing? If so, treat the underlying problem to the extent possible.
- What is the nature of any hearing loss? Are low tones better understood? Does a quiet room help? Find the distance at which the person seems to function best.
- Are dentures poorly fitting or are there other oral problems that make it difficult to understand the person, or are these problems discouraging the person from trying to speak? Correct the problem or improve it as much as possible.
- Are medications or disease (e.g., Parkinson disease or depression) making the person appear apathetic or to have flattened affect? People with Parkinson disease often show only slight facial expressions. By training yourself to watch for these, you will better understand the individual.

Neuropsychological Assessment

Ask the neuropsychologist to explain how neuropsychological data can assist you in communication. For example, a person with poor language skills can appear to be more impaired than she actually is, and a person with good language skills may conceal disabilities that lead to frustration and unrealistic staff expectations. The neuropsychological testing will help you identify such unevenly retained abilities.

The Mini-Mental State Examination

The MMSE is a useful tool for identifying common communication problems. Using it will help direct care staff members. (See Chapter VI.)

Information from Families

Useful information can often be provided by family members. Several questions can be asked about the person's background:

Does the person have a prior history of hearing or language problems?
What/who does the person talk about or ask for?
What words do the person and his family use for

specific tasks? (for example, toileting? pain? fatigue?)

What signals, verbal and nonverbal, does the family use to get through tasks?

If the person speaks a second language, what familiar words do you need to know? Ask the family to make a tape of commonly used non-English words and their translation. Ask the family to speak slowly and clearly.

Information the Staff Members Learn and Share

The following are questions the staff can use for assessment:

How many words can the person process before his attention or his ability to understand is lost? How quickly does the person tire?

Does the person communicate better when only one staff member is present? When she is rested?

Does the person communicate better at certain times of day?

Is the person's accent adding to the problems?

Do the first few words the person says make sense before the person rambles on?

Do some staff members have better success than others?

Is the person being stressed by the effort to communicate?

What clues can you gather from body language, facial expression, tone, and eye contact?

Does interrupting the rambling help or frustrate?

Does filling in words help or frustrate?

Are your gestures understood?

Can the family understand the person's message or reach the person?

What nonverbal behaviors cue the staff that the person is upset?

What nonverbal cues that staff members use help?

Does the person answer indirectly or vaguely? Can you make sense of this?

Use of Communication Tools

A communication board, a board with pictures on it that identify needs and that the person can point to, is helpful for some stroke patients. American Sign Language is important for people who learned and used it before they developed a dementia. People with dementia may be able to use reminder notes for part of their illness. However, in Alzheimer disease what is lost is the ability to use language in any form. Therefore, communication boards and sign language will usually be useless after the early stages. Using them may frustrate the person.

Music can be used to communicate. Words to songs are often retained long after other words are lost. Occasionally a person will be able to understand or communicate needs through singing. Certainly most people will enjoy music and singing for most of their illness.

If English is a second language and if the person has Alzheimer disease or a related disorder, it is likely that she is losing the ability to communicate effectively in any language. Ask the family how well the person communicates in the primary language.

In general, nonverbal body language is the only communication system that remains strong for much of the illness.

The Use of Language Varies with the Disease

The specific changes in verbal language vary with the disease. Thus, diagnosis is important in understanding how to help each person. People with Alzheimer disease often have trouble with the names of things early in the illness and gradually lose all spoken language. People with Parkinson disease may understand and speak longer. The loss for people with multi-infarct dementia will depend on where in the brain the strokes occurred. People with Korsakoff syndrome may speak fluently despite severe memory loss and may confuse the staff into thinking they have more function than they do.

Curse Words

Occasionally a person with dementia will rely heavily on curse words. For some of these people, cursing is something they never did in the past. All of us learn curse words as a child, and most of us quickly learn from our mother not to use them again, but they remain stored in the brain. Perhaps curse words are stored differently in the brain. As the ability to communicate is lost, curse words may be the only words the person can find. This is not intentional, and it is not "bad." It is the result of the brain damage.

You can ask the person politely not to use those words, but she will use them next time. Anticipating the person's frustrations and reducing her stress may help. Singing may divert some swearing. The best treatment for cursing is to accept this as an unfortunate part of the dementia over which the person has little or no control. Help the staff and family to accept this.

Exhibit 6.1. Seven D's That Block Communication

Delirium
Deafness
Distance
Distractions
Dentures
Drugs
Disease

Overhead/Handout 6.1.
Ways We Communicate

Spoken or written words

Facial expression

Eye contact

Posture

Tone, pitch, rapidity of voice

Gestures

Touch

All communication is two-way:

Receptive (what is understood)

Expressive (what is communicated)

Overhead/Handout 6.2. Making Yourself Understood with Words

Be sure the person can hear you and is paying attention.

Say less.

Speak slowly.

Use body language.

Never be patronizing.

Repeat yourself once, then say it differently.

Tell the person what to do, not what not to do.

Overhead/Handout 6.3. Understanding the Person's Communications

Stop, look, and listen.

Focus on context, not content.

Ask if you understood.

Focus on right now.

Know the person.

Try, don't lie.

Overhead/Handout 6.4. Learning to Use Body Language

Be a good observer/user of facial expression.

Use eye contact.

Use and observe body language.

Listen and use tone, pitch, and speed of speaking voice.

Make gestures simple and meaningful.

Use touch appropriately.

LESSON 7

HELPING THE PERSON BY SUSTAINING RELATIONSHIPS

Summary. For the person with dementia, loss of memory and loss of communication gradually destroy the person's relationships with others. However, the person's need for relationships is not necessarily lost. This is nowhere better stated than by the woman who said, "I don't know who I belong to." Loss of relationships contributes to depression and behavioral problems, such as searching for lost family.

Section 7.1. Family Relationships. Discusses the impact of the disease on relationships and on the need of the person with dementia for connections to family. (*Family* is defined to include unrelated people with close ties to the person with dementia.)

Section 7.2. Friendships with Staff Members. Discusses how staff-client friendships, because they occur on a day-to-day basis, help the person with dementia who has lost or forgotten other relationships. These bonds also facilitate care.

Section 7.3. Friendships between People with Dementia. Discusses ways to sustain the fragile relationships that may form between clients.

Using the Sections
- Introductory course:
  - None
- Core course:
  - Section 7.1 required
  - Section 7.2 optional; use only if you have time and resources to implement in the care setting
  - Section 7.3 optional; use only if your setting facilitates such interactions

Problems You May Have in Implementing This Lesson

While direct care staff people must communicate closely with families about care, they must at the same time be protected from the family's grief and anger. Hands-on staff members cannot be placed in the role of social worker or therapist, but they must learn to relate successfully to family members. This balancing act is the responsibility of management. Have a plan in place to support direct care providers. They and the families must know what the facility's policies are and how to use them.

If serious problems arise through the behavior of family members, management must take the responsibility to set limits that are in the best interests of the staff and other clients. Long-term staff demoralization can result when a family abuses or accuses the staff. Management should consider a last-resort policy of discharging a client to protect the well-being of all clients and staff members.

Section 7.1. Family Relationships

Objective

The student will understand how family relationships are important for the person with dementia. This section focuses on ways to sustain these relationships.

Background

An extensive literature describes the impact of dementia on the family and the family's experiences and distress. This section focuses on the needs of the person with dementia for ongoing relationships with others. It does not address the therapeutic support of families.

When further information about families is needed, use the videos and other materials provided by the Alzheimer's Association or other sources that are sensitive and compassionate toward the family. Address negative staff attitudes toward families only if needed. If staff members raise concerns about problem family behavior, address these, but balance them with discussion of other families who cope well and relate well to staff members—as the majority do. Many staff members are or have been family caregivers as well. Draw on this experience.

The experiences of care providers will differ considerably depending on whether the person with dementia is living at home (home care and day care) or in a group facility. Focus your teaching accordingly.

Administration and social work play a major role in establishing policy, in setting the tone of relationships with family members, and in protecting staff members.

Help students focus on the reality that the disease, not family, destroys relationships. Whatever the family's history, the disease has a profound effect on relationships. The capacity for relationships, positive or negative, changes as memory, communication skills, and behavioral symptoms change.

Information and Instructions for the Teacher

This section presents information about a spectrum of needs and issues. Of necessity, much of this material is presented briefly and may seem like a list of ideas. Select those that apply to your setting and your students' needs.

First, select the information that is relevant to your facility or program. Your social worker will be a part of this process. Because this section raises issues of agency policy (for example, to whom do family members complain?), be sure these issues are clear before beginning to teach.

Second, select the information that your students will need to interact with families. This will depend on the setting (people living at home or people living in residential care or nursing home care settings), facility policy, and the degree of involvement families have with your clients.

Students need to learn the following basic information: facts (versus myths) about families; that families are partners in care; that the disease, not the family, is at the root of problems the staff members see; the things families need from the staff and the things the person with dementia needs from the family; and agency expectations regarding the relationship with family members. Your group will also need other materials. Use details and examples from your own experience. Present the material you select as discussion, asking the students how they might apply these ideas and whether they can be applied in their setting.

For some materials, such as the list of suggestions for successful visiting, you might let your students know that these are available, without teaching it as lecture.

Lecture/Discussion Notes to Be Presented to the Class

Everyone has connections, relationships with others: family, friends, co-workers, even people we dislike. People vary in the kind of connectedness they seek: some have many family members and friends; others have only one friend or a pet; still others stick with seemingly unhappy relationships. But all relationships matter. Having relationships with others is a part of being human, but as memory for others and for past times is lost and as the ability to communicate is lost, people lose their connections with others.

Helping people with dementia feel connected helps reduce depression and modifies behavioral symptoms. In this lesson we will talk about the connection of people with dementia to their family (this section), to staff members (Section 7.2), and to other people with dementia (Section 7.3).

A definition of family: In this text, *family* means those people who are important to the person with dementia. The term as defined here may include traditional nuclear families, siblings, unmarried couples, gay couples, nonblood children, and friends who function as close relatives might. For the person with dementia, the key is those people she thought of as family.

Whom do you treat as a client's family in your work? For example, in what situations would you treat as "family" a man raised as a son but not adopted? Whom does your program define as family? When does the legal definition matter? Establish a definition of family that is appropriate for your needs.

About Families

Use Exhibit 7.1 if your students have stereotyped ideas about families.

Because families often seek placement when they are exhausted or ill or when the primary caregiver dies, staff members frequently see people with dementia who have few family members who visit. Also, the difficult family members stick in the memory of providers, so it seems as if families often are difficult.

However, the studies of families consistently remind us that the majority of families care for the person with dementia well and for a long time. Dementia can often last 20 years—as long as it takes to raise a child. Because the diseases destroy the mind, the ability to act reasonably and to communicate, the caregiver loses the valued relationship. Even so, most caregivers manage as long as they can. Caregiver exhaustion, desperation, illness, or death is often what leads families to seek outside help. Moreover, not everyone has the emotional and physical resources necessary to cope with this devastation. Nevertheless, studies of families repeatedly point out the strengths and resourcefulness of families and their ability to adjust and work with paid providers. The quality of care the agency or facility is able to provide (resources may limit this) and the ability of the paid providers to accept and understand family members are all that is needed to make the partnership between staff members and family members work in almost all cases.

Exhibit 7.2 provides additional background on responding to the emotional needs of families. *(Teacher: Teach and discuss those items that are important to your group, or refer to this material when topics arise.)*

Families are our partners in care. They affect the life quality of the person with dementia. But dementia has two victims: the person with dementia and the family caregiver. This means that the paid provider must work with family members, learning from them how they care for the person, sharing care plans, and encouraging family involvement. At the same time the family member—as the second victim of the disease—is suffering and may not cope well; he may need support or understanding. This situation creates an ongoing challenge to families and professional care providers alike.

It is the disease, not the family, that devastates relationships. Behavioral symptoms and the losses of mental function, memory, and recognition are far more important factors than family history or family "dysfunction" in the difficulties experienced by families of people with dementia. You will be most successful in working with families if you relate to them in the here and now. Although it may be appropriate to refer them for counseling, assuming that families' behavior is caused by their history distracts you from the powerful feelings of grief, anger, and pain that families face when a person develops a dementia.

Overhead/Handout 7.1. What People with Dementia Need from Their Families

Each person with dementia will have different needs based on the history of the family and the severity of the illness. As you work with families, remember that everyone—family members, the person with dementia, and staff members—deserves compassion.

Most people with dementia need the following things from their families:

- *Affection, love* (usually demonstrated by visits, hugs, touch). Families who are caring at home are sometimes so overwhelmed by the tasks of daily living that they will need help to find time and energy to do something pleasant with the impaired person.

- *A sense of belonging.* Even when the person no longer remembers the family members, she may still feel that she belongs to someone because these people are supposed to be her family.
- *Adequate care and supervision of the person who is living at home.* The time may come when the family caregiver cannot provide needed care or supervision. The family may need help to accept this.
- *Visits, contact with the outside world, stimulation, fun.* When the person lives in residential or nursing home settings, the family provides a contact with the outside world. Most important, because staff members are busy with the tasks of daily care, families provide time for pleasure.
- *A way to sustain roles.* Even when the person does not remember family members, the contact helps to sustain the sense that she has *the role* of a spouse, a grandparent, etc. Show families how to do this by suggesting appropriate activities.
- *To relate to them as they are now* (for example, accepting that the person is unable to remember people in the family or tires quickly). This may be difficult, if not impossible, for some families. Accept the family members' difficulty and refer them to a support group.
- That family members *take responsibility for the person's care, safety, and finances*
- That family members *relate to the staff so that care is effective*

Overhead/Handout 7.2. What Families Need from the Staff

The single most important thing that families need and want is that you provide good care for the person with dementia. They hope that you will see the relative as a unique person and that you will care for that person with love and respect.

Each family is unique. However, the Alzheimer's Association provides information about what families need in residential homes, nursing homes, home care, and day care. Families also need the following:

- *Good communication with caregiving staff members.* Families need to know care providers well enough to trust them. They need to know whom to talk to for information, whom to complain to, and to whom to give information that will help in care.
- *Understanding rather than criticism for their coping strategies.* Although most families cope well with the emotional burdens of a person with dementia, some react with denial, withdrawal, anger or other behaviors that are not helpful to the staff or the person with dementia. They need time, understanding, and support. Counseling or support groups help, but caregiving staff members cannot undertake this task. Staff members need patience with and acceptance of those who cannot change.
- *Information about your program, about the disease, about helpful resources such as the Alzheimer's Association.* They need to know about support groups or counseling and how to plan ahead.
- *Recognition that their options are limited.* Financial support for adult day care, home care, and residential or nursing home care is limited. So is financial support for health care and counseling. Families face other demands beyond the needs of the ill person (such as the health or financial needs of other members of the family), as well as limitations on their own physical and emotional resources. Every family must make choices, and often there are no "right" choices. For example,

A sister stopped visiting. Both of her parents had had Alzheimer disease, and she could not handle the pain of seeing another family member with the illness.

A family kept a grandparent at home even though the family members' ability to care was inadequate. They had decided to save their limited funds for a son's education rather than for nursing home care.

How do you feel about these family members' decisions?

- *The feeling that there is a balance between what they retain control over and the help the paid care providers give.* When the ill person lives at home, paid care providers are often frustrated by their inability to make even simple changes that would benefit the client. In residential settings, families are frustrated because almost all the control over the person's care is in the hands of the staff. The issue of who controls care can get in the way of successful staff-family interactions. It is addressed in part by agency policy and in part by direct care providers who listen to the family members and respect their position.

Exercise 1. Discussing the Roles of Staff, Family, and Agency

Teacher: You may choose to teach the remainder of this section before doing this exercise.

As a class, discuss the following issues: Determine the roles of those in the class in meeting these needs (Overheads/Handouts 7.1 and 7.2). What does your agency expect from you? What resources do you have? How do you work in partnership with families? How do you take care of yourself? As a group, define guidelines for how you work with families.

Planning Ahead Helps Relationships with Families

Planning ahead for care helps families know what to expect and how to interact with the program staff. Unfortunately, this is often not an option. Some clients enter care with little or no available family. For many families, the need for care arises urgently, leaving little time for planning. Family caregivers are overwhelmed with the basic issues of admission and cannot absorb any more information. They may also be too overwhelmed to provide much information about the client.

There are some ways you can help:

- Be sure that your policies are clear and well documented, so there is no internal confusion.
- Plan when and how each issue will be discussed with the family and which issues can be covered gradually over the first few weeks rather than immediately.
- Program policies should include admission policy, procedures for obtaining a history, procedures for giving family information about the facility and care practices, the family's role in care planning, how families will be frequently informed about the client's status, late-stage planning (including at what point a person can no longer be cared for in your setting), what the facility expects from the family, visiting policies, whom the family should talk to, complain to, and get information from, client safety, financial issues, and client privacy.
- Internal policies should include how the staff will respond to depressed or distressed family members. A policy should be in place to protect direct care staff people from family behaviors that interfere with care or distress the staff.

Overhead/Handout 7.3. Strategies to Facilitate Interactions between the Facility and the Family

Give families written information to read later. Be prepared to repeat information and to provide it orally, in written form, and on video.

Offer a short "welcome" orientation course for families that allows time for a discussion of facility policies, responses to family questions, and a presentation of basic knowledge about the nature of dementia. You can talk about ideas for successful visits and to whom to turn for information. Some families may be so exhausted that they do not come. Encourage them to join a later group. (Studies have shown that the first year after placement is as stressful for the caregiver as the year before placement. Knowing this helps staff members accept family issues.)

Refer families to support groups. These may be run by facilities, the Alzheimer's Association, or other groups. Good ones are an excellent way to help families deal with their emotional needs and to learn skills in working with paid providers.

Ensure that the families know what your program offers, what is expected of them, and what your policies are. Many conflicts are avoided when programs are up-front at the beginning. For example, if your policy is to tolerate odd behavior (someone half dressed, wandering around, or wearing someone else's clothes), tell the family members that each client has the freedom to be herself but that this also means that they may see others doing the same. If your policy is not to re-dress someone who has spilled on her clothes and does not want to change, help the family to understand that you choose to respect such choices.

Encourage families to replace valuable wedding rings with less expensive rings and to select clothing that will hold up if staff members wash it. This does not mean everyone should wear jogging suits, but staff members should not be burdened with caring for cashmere suits. Ask families to anchor personal items with Quake-Hold or Blu-Tac. Original photos can be replaced with copies.

Be sure that the family members agree with your policy regarding the balancing of safety and freedom. For example, do they understand when you will or will not restrain people to prevent falls?

Establish who does which tasks. For example, in home care should the paid provider do housework? Or in residential care or nursing home care, who maintains clothing? An open discussion, with both parties present, mediated by the social worker, will usually clear the air.

Respect and accept the care skills families have found to be effective. Confusion is common when family members give the staff instructions about how to care for a person. Information from a family member is invaluable. The family member has often figured out, by trial and error, how to accomplish a difficult task. Care providers must listen to such advice and treat it with respect. Providers also need to remind themselves that the family members want you to care for the person as they themselves would in a perfect world. Family members cannot always recognize that the care provider has several people, not just one, to get dressed and fed. Here, too, a mediated discussion will usually be effective.

Overhead/Handout 7.4. Facilitating Family/Client Relationships When the Person Lives at Home

When the client lives at home, the paid provider has limited control over what happens in that setting. However, staff members can take many steps to facilitate relationships, such as the following:

1. *Teaching the family caregiver* about dementia and clearing up misunderstandings about the client's capabilities. Referral to support groups is important.
2. *Sharing strategies for care* with the family caregiver. For example, when day care or home care staff members discover a way to reduce a catastrophic reaction or facilitate personal care, this can be tested by the paid care provider and then taught to the family caregiver.
3. *Interpreting the meaning of behaviors* for the family. For example, "She may not mean to scold the children all the time; she may not remember that she spoke to them a few minutes earlier."
4. *Being alert to problems of safety,* the potential for abuse, and the risks that occur when the family overestimates the ill person's abilities.
5. *Observing when the family caregiver is ill, exhausted, or otherwise unable to care* effectively and guiding the family toward a change in the care plan. Caregivers are prone to chronic illness and depression and may ignore these in order to continue to care.
6. Listening to caregiver frustrations. A staff member, often not the direct care provider, can listen to the caregiver and provide counseling or *referral to therapy if appropriate.*
7. *Encouraging the caregiver* to use the time during paid care for rest and personal recovery. Perhaps the caregiver wants simply to stay home and sleep when the home care person is there. Families often need encouragement to take time for themselves for pleasure or sustaining friendships.

In addition, the home care or day care facility can *be knowledgeable about residential and nursing home care* and can help the family get on waiting lists and make financial plans.

Facilitating the Transition to a Residential Care Setting

Some programs tell families not to visit for the first few days or weeks after placement. This allows people with dementia to "adjust," they say. This cruel strategy breaks the heart of people who cannot remember why they have been abandoned, although they may be more docile out of despair. Grief and loss after a move are normal.

When she was placed in a nursing home, one woman refused to eat or to get out of bed. She begged her family to take her home and cried for hours after each visit. The family was devastated by guilt. Nevertheless, the staff encouraged the family to keep visiting, and staff members frequently reassured the woman that her family would visit again soon. In time, she settled into the facility.

Look for strategies to help the person understand that her family member will come back. It is painful for everyone when the person begs to be taken home, but helping the person through this transition is part of care. It helps if the person can feel a connection with one staff "buddy." In some programs, this person visits before placement in day care or residential care. Allow the person to set her own pace for becoming involved in the new setting, and be alert to the possibility of depression. The family and staff will need extensive support through the transition to placement.

Some programs feel that it is "bad" for families to visit every day. If the person is not overly stressed (visibly upset) after the visit and appears to enjoy it, it is probably good for him. Family members are adults and can decide for themselves whether this is how they want to spend their days. For people who have lived together for decades and have been caregivers for years, there may be nothing to do at home, and frequent visits work for both parties. You may decide with some families to plan a gradual reduction in time at the facility once the adjustment period is over.

Visiting plans should be individual and may change over time. The person's needs for relationships will change as the disease progresses. Suggest more successful things families can do: talk gives way to touch; memories give way to just being together. Several visitors become too many, or things families and clients did together become too difficult.

Also use Exhibit 7.3 when appropriate.

Not Visiting, and Not Visiting on the Holidays

Some caregivers are burned out by the time of placement, or there is a history of family conflict. Neither visiting nor not visiting is wrong. If the person with dementia misses the caregiver, remember that she also often misses deceased individuals who will not be visiting. Deal with the person's search for the absent person in a similar way.

Walter's wife was 53 when he placed her. He had been caring for his four daughters, ages 5 to 14, and running a large farm. The family had cared for Walter's wife almost since the last child had been born. No one made the long drive to the facility for about two months. The daughters refused to visit: they were deeply distressed and dealt with this by becoming very active in school. Then Walter began to visit about twice a week but was upset by his wife's disability. After one visit, he revealed to the social worker that he had "met someone." She encouraged him to talk about this with her by phone. One Sunday he brought two daughters, the friend, and his mother. The friend was a warm woman who had taken the girls into her heart. The family explored with the social worker their feelings about adultery and "living together."

Teacher: Ask the students as a group or small groups to discuss whether it is wrong for a caregiver who feels confident in the quality of care you give to "get on with his own life"? Was Walter wrong to "abandon" his wife?

Successful Visits

Families may not know how to visit or how to make the most of their visits. Visiting in a facility involves different activities than those that are a part of providing daily care at home. Use the following suggestions with families.

Help families to realize that now that the burdens of daily care are in competent hands, their job is to provide pleasure, memories of old roles, love, and companionship. The purpose of a visit is to provide pleasure to *both* parties and to reinforce relationships and support roles.

When families participate in the care plan, help them to make their visits a planned part of care.

If the person with dementia is upset and restless during a visit, suggest staying a shorter time. For families who travel a distance to visit, suggest they try going out for coffee and coming back for a second visit.

Suggest visiting at a different time of day, a time when the staff knows the person is at her best.

Have only one person at a time visit. If several people come at one time, they may take turns with short visits.

Don't expect people with dementia to remember things (pictures, other family members, events).

Don't push the person to do things she cannot do.

Staff members are often more aware of declines and can make suggestions such as, "Instead of asking him where his room is, walk there with him and point out his things."

Suggest that families routinely check to see whether the person was upset after a visit. Because all aspects of care matter and visits are therapeutic, this is a way for families to participate in care. But never blame the family for upsets.

Suggest an attractive area where family members and the person with cognitive impairment can walk. Remind families that pointing out things to see, smell, and touch (including murals, the fish tank, or outside items) is a good way to make conversation. Recommend safe walking areas, and show families what you do to avoid falls.

Some facilities have an ice cream parlor or a coffee shop where the visitor and resident can "go out for a bite." Some have an arrangement so that the resident can "host" and pay for this outing. Such a visiting corner need not be elaborate.

Suggest that families give personal care: doing the person's nails, giving a shampoo or back rub. Be sure that families understand that this is not a money-saving strategy but that doing something familiar together is a more meaningful visit than trying to have a conversation with a person with language problems.

Suggest activities such as making a door decoration or room decoration with the impaired person. Encourage families to select items that relate to the person and to use pictures that have meaning for her. The family should discuss the objects with the resident as they are assembled. Don't rush; this can take several visits.

Ask the family to make a memory book with the person with cognitive impairment—a photograph album with small items and pictures that may trigger memories. Be sure the pictures are accompanied by orienting information about them for the staff to use; pictures should be as large and clear as possible. Use a large-print typewriter or hand-write labels in large print.

A treasure box can provide fun. This is a box (perhaps fishing tackle box for a man, jewelry box for a woman) that contains old familiar personal treasures. Or try a rummage drawer—fill a dresser drawer with items the person would normally have used.

A sorting box might be filled with buttons, bits of lace, or nails and screws. Have the family get this out only for visits.

A grandchild box is filled with toys that grandchildren would use to play with. The person with dementia can then play with the children when they come to visit. Some residents might fiddle with these toys themselves, but this box of toys *must* always be referred to as "for the grandchildren."

Some families have written a letter reminding the person of her history, the story of her life. "I met you when you worked at McCrory's and I was home on leave. We used to hide behind the railroad tracks and talk and cuddle for hours."

Suggest that families write a letter to the resident reminding him of the last visit or keep a log of all visits. This is very useful for letting the staff know what went on and reassuring the person of the next visit. "Mom, I came to see you Sunday. We sat outside and fed the squirrel. . . . I will see you again next Sunday at 3:00."

Suggest that families do a task *with* a resident such as sorting clothes or mending. Remind families that tasks should not be used to test how much the resident can do.

Urge families to avoid discussion topics that the person can't remember, such as "You remember Aunt Martha? Well, she . . ."; "What have you been doing today?"; or "How have they been treating you?"

Invite families to potlucks so they can meet each other and get acquainted with residents and staff members.

Encourage families to help a relative sustain old roles. Family members must assume many roles, but for part of the illness the person with dementia can still maintain the semblance of old roles. For example, consult the person for advice. Children trigger grandparent roles even in very ill people.

> One woman was so impaired that the staff had to help her hold a baby. But she still remembered to lift up her blouse as if to nurse the child.

Clinical Experience

Select one family and develop a plan that will be more therapeutic for the person with dementia. Look for small interventions: for example, suggest to the family a new visiting strategy or refer the family to a social worker.

Section 7.2. Friendships with Staff Members

Objective

The student will learn to see herself as a therapeutic instrument in care.

Information and Instructions for the Teacher

This section spells out a concept that has been presented in every lesson: the individual relationship between staff members and the impaired person. One program calls the staff "enablers" instead of aides. This term aptly describes the role of staff members in relation to the person with dementia. Teach this as discussion, emphasizing what staff members are already doing. Friendships between staff members and people with dementia are possible only when the staff members are well supported and the person with dementia is not overly stressed. In such a climate, friendships will occur spontaneously. *They cannot be forced.* Do not expect or require them. Funding sources and regulators do not reward—or even recognize—such relationships or their value. Thus supervisors must praise the staff. Do not teach this to those who are already stressed or not able to give time and emotional contact to people with dementia. People with dementia decline and move on or die. Thus the offer of friendship is always accompanied by loss. This will burn out staff members unless they are very well supported. Teach them to identify what they already do and the ways people with dementia are already responding. Point out the value of these interactions: trust gets a bath done, friendship wins a smile from a complainer.

Lecture/Discussion Notes to Be Presented to the Class

Staff members often observe that people with dementia know that they know certain staff members and trust them. (They may also know whom they dislike.) This quality allows the staff to sustain relationships with even very impaired people. The staff members whom people with dementia see regularly matter to them, either positively or negatively. The impaired person may never learn a name, consciously recognize the person, or correctly understand the relationship, but through the entire course of the disease, caregivers provide a major part of the human bond with the impaired person. When the impaired person has few visitors or cannot remember family, staff members provide the only human ties, and these are essential.

"She's the one," the man told his wife, pointing a shaking finger at an aide.
"Is she your friend?" asked the wife.
"Yeah. She's the one."
"What's her name?"
"She never told me."
Of course, she had told the person many times. Instead of focusing on this, focus on the fact that the man remembers the feeling of relationship.

Whenever the director came into the unit, the same group of women were always sitting outside the nursing station. The director began bringing pictures of her children and passing them around. Although the women never learned who she was or to expect her, in some way it became clear that they knew that they knew her.

Relationships with staff members may be the most valuable thing in many people's lives. These relationships are in the here and now—they don't require memories of the past or expectations for the future. They are relationships in which the staff member adjusts himself to make the friendship work and accepts the impaired person as she is. They are rewarding for the ill person and often for the staff as well. The client's ability to interact can be surprising.

One woman was behaving in a way that embarrassed the unit director during a visit from an official. Of course, the unit director said nothing about her discomfort, but one of the other residents suddenly walked over to her and patted her on the shoulder. "You'll be OK," she said to the unit director. Such moments allow the person with dementia to feel "whole" and valuable.

Friendship with an impaired person may speed

his recovery from an illness. It may also make it possible for a staff member to provide care that the person previously perceived as threatening, and it may enable the staff member to stop a person from dangerous or disruptive behavioral symptoms. In these types of situations, the staff member is an anchor for the impaired person in a terrifying world.

A bond of friendship is a gift of oneself. It is not part of the job description. The gift of friendship is voluntary.

These are therapeutic friendships. The staff members establish them because of their benefit to the client. They are largely one-way. Staff needs for friendship and emotional support are met elsewhere. It is inappropriate to expect recognition or understanding from people who are struggling with basic coping. However, you may be surprised by the effort people with dementia make toward you. This is their way of contributing and giving a gift, too.

These friendships take time to build. You and the person have to get to know each other. Interact with the person while you are providing care. Take 15 seconds whenever you pass the person in the hall. Give the person clues that you are her friend: "I like you," "You have a great sense of humor," "Mary and I are buddies" (if Mary thinks this is true). Remind people of the continuity of the friendship: "You and I did the laundry yesterday."

Any friendship is about trust. You must help the person with dementia begin to trust that you will not let her make a fool of herself and that you will not make fun of her. The person with dementia must trust that you did do the laundry together yesterday, that you will get her to dinner on time, and so on.

How can people who can't remember who you are learn to trust you? It works, although it is difficult to explain. Emotional bonds may still function in the absence of cognitive memory.

Connections are more difficult in home care and day care if the staff member is seen less frequently. The client may not establish any sense of connection. This is an important reason for consistent staffing. Greet the person with reminders of who you are and where he is, establish routines (coffee first, then getting dressed), and end your day with verbal or written reminders (or both) of when you will see him again (even though he won't remember).

You adapt these friendships to fit the person. Mary may like to be cuddled and touched, whereas Alice likes you near but doesn't like to be touched. Some people constantly complain or act out: an enabling staff member accepts the person anyway.

Not every client will like you, and you will not like every client. This is normal. If possible, one person who is a good match with the ill person should be the person's buddy. This one person might even be a nonclinical staff member or a volunteer.

Staff members find their own style for friendship. Some hug, others smile, and still others have a great sense of humor.

Exercise 2. Building Bonds

As a group, discuss the following issues:

List all the ways group members have observed offers of affection or friendship from people with dementia. Look for the little things. For example,

> A man approached a staff member and handed her a piece of paper. "You keep this," he said. She understood that in his mind this was a gift, and she thanked him.

Discuss how you will find the time for this. Friendship is usually facilitated during frequent quick moments and during activities-of-daily-living (ADL) care rather than in longer or more formal periods, partly because the dementia makes it difficult for the ill person to sustain attention for longer periods.

Discuss the difficulties in offering affection or friendship to people you also have to clean up after or whose behavioral symptoms are offensive.

People with dementia decline. As you care for them, you watch this happen. They eventually must move to a different setting, or they die in your care. This means that if you come to care for them, you will have to grieve over and over. Discuss whether you can handle this, whether you want to, and, if so, how you will take care of yourselves.

Ask the group to make a list of things they already do. Use Exhibit 7.4 for more suggestions.

Volunteers

Volunteers have a unique opportunity to bring friendships to people with dementia. Match volunteers with people with dementia over a task (picking and arranging flowers, playing cards, walking). Try pairs of volunteers; they give each other courage. Bringing a pet helps volunteers relate more easily. Like that of the staff, the job of a volunteer is to build a friendship, offering affirmation and acceptance. Volunteers must have training and ongoing support, but they report that the work is rewarding.

Some programs have arranged for noncaregiving staff members to take time as volunteers. Because many people with dementia respond best to short visits, this works well with busy staff members. Gardeners and maintenance people may have something in common with some of the clients. Secretaries and accountants may enjoy brief contact with challenging clients. One program arranged for staff members to visit for three minutes each with one client. This provided much more relationship time for her at little total cost. Three minutes was all the person could tolerate and limited the burden on visiting staff members.

Some programs have involved high school students, troubled teens, or unwed mothers. With care and planning, these programs have worked well.

Before using any volunteer, including your own staff members, have a committed staff and a good program. Volunteers are never "extra help." A staff member must be assigned time to select, train, and support volunteers. Good programs report that running a successful volunteer program uses considerable staff time.

Clinical Experience

Plan and carry out a simple strategy for friendship with one person. If you already relate well to one person, build on this.

Section 7.3. Friendships between People with Dementia

Objective

The student will learn to recognize and facilitate interactions between people with dementia.

Information and Instructions for the Teacher

Friendships between people with dementia are fragile, spontaneous, and often ephemeral. They happen only in settings that will support them, and they dissolve as one person's impairment increases. Staff members in good programs emphasize the importance of all relationships for people with dementia.

Review the content, and teach only those parts of this material that are relevant for your setting.

The concept of such relationships may be unfamiliar to some staff members. They will need guidance to recognize and encourage signs of connections between people. Help them to see the dignity of such connections and never to regard them as "cute."

Connections cannot be forced or arranged. They occur spontaneously, but they can be supported.

Romances are a special type of friendship that can raise ethical concerns, family distress, and staff issues. Know your administration's policy before beginning to teach that material.

Lecture/Discussion Notes to Be Presented to the Class

Ask the group to describe any friendships they have observed between residents. Focus first on relationships that are not romantic or sexual. For example,

> Sitting alone at breakfast, Jem said, "Isn't someone supposed to be . . . someone?" The staff member was rushing to hand out medications and didn't know what he meant, but a few moments later she returned to him, "Are you looking for Meg?" Meg usually sat next to Jem at breakfast. "Meg slept in today."
>
> Two women wandered the halls, hand in hand. Sometimes they tried to help each other with things like putting on sweaters, but both were too impaired to succeed.
>
> Mele was often restless and walked around during sing-alongs. When Jan put out her hand, Mele would brighten and sit down next to Jan.
>
> Bill was too impaired to participate in the sing-along, but when the staff seated him next to Mary, he would hold her hand and jiggle his knee to the rhythm.
>
> Two men seemed to like to sit together and talk, although the staff observed that they were talking about different things.

Teacher: Discuss why such friendships are important.

Some Ways to Facilitate Client Friendships

Friendships will form between people with dementia under the right circumstances, but the staff must enable them. An advantage of day care or residential care is that people with dementia can share companionship with others who do not notice their impairment.

Reduce overall stressors on the unit. Friendships will form only when the people involved are not struggling to make sense of confusion and are not feeling stressed.

Use small groups. Large groups increase overall stress and make it difficult for a person to find her friend. Seat people together at small tables. (Tables for six or eight may be too large.) Small groups reduce the options for finding someone the person likes, but their benefits outweigh this disadvantage. You can help by grouping men together, women together, or people at about the same level of disability. If a person does not "fit" in a group, try placing her in a different group. Make some small groups consistent. With an impaired memory, it takes a long time for a person to recognize others as companions. This is much easier on a small unit. If you have a large unit, consider arranging small groups that are together for longer periods.

Seat a person next to her friend at activities and meals. Friends may not be able to find each other unless you seat them together. Adjust people's schedules so that they do things together.

Friendships are spontaneous. Do not push friendships on people. Instead, reinforce even slight attempts at connection. (Remember how you hated it when your mother tried to push a friendship on you when you were young?) Watch closely how people react after a few days in a stable small group. If someone seems irritated by the others, perhaps this is not the right group for him.

Friendships are not arranged in the bedroom. Well people rarely make friends with "strangers" they find in their bedroom unless they originally chose this person (for example, a spouse). People with dementia will not be accustomed to having—let alone making friends with—a roommate. Bedrooms are private spaces.

Because of the cognitive difficulties people with dementia experience, conversations between them may sound fragmented or tangential to others. For example,

> One man said, "Where is it?"
> Another man answered, "They won't let us."
> "Where did it go?"
> "They don't like us."
> "Where are any?"

Assume that meaning is not as important as the connection between these two people. They are noticing each other and interacting.

Friendships occasionally form between physically ill residents and people with dementia. When this happens, the physically ill person must feel able to withdraw into privacy whenever she needs to. If one person is cognitively well but physically ill, her rights to privacy, comfort, and security of possessions must be considered.

Sometimes two people with dementia argue every time they meet. If either party becomes upset, treat this as a catastrophic reaction and intervene before it escalates. It is more effective to treat conflict as a catastrophic reaction than to assume there are racial or ethnic roots to the dislike. Look for ways to reduce contact.

However, as with people who are well, some quarrelsome relationships are apparently satisfying to those involved. For example,

> Two women were seated at a table. A third was wandering around, hovering as if she wanted to join them. One woman said, "Go away. Can't you see we are busy?" The second woman said, "I don't like any of them." The first woman said, "I said, 'Go away.'" The second said, "Their kind is too pushy."

This is certainly a negative conversation but characteristic of the women involved. It is unclear what anyone was discussing, but being together seemed to have meaning for them because they would sit and talk whenever they found each other. This sort of relationship may be better than no relationship at all. Carefully consider such relationships and intervene only if the conversation escalates. The third woman in this group did not seem bothered by rejection and may not have been aware of it.

Teacher: As a class or in small groups, discuss the following: Describe the bonds you already observe between people with dementia. What meaning do they have for the person with dementia? How could you support them?

Romantic or Sexual Relationships

Romantic and sexual relationships do occur among people with dementia. (See Exhibit 7.5. Also see Section 11.4.) Sexual behaviors are discussed in Lesson 11. It is important to keep family issues and how we cope with them separate from staff members' own feelings. For example, family members may not mind a relationship that some staff members feel is wrong.

It is essential that the facility have a policy regarding intimate relationships between clients. We recommend that the policy be as liberal and flexible as possible. Friendship and love are so rare that denying them seems unreasonable. When partners are separated, even one who is severely impaired will search for the other and grieve. Staff members who have experienced separating a couple can attest to the pain this causes.

Before acting, it is important to know exactly what is occurring. For example,

> In one facility a man and a woman retreated to his room after lunch. Outside the door, staff members could hear her calling, "Help me, help me." Imagining the worst, the staff member opened the door and found him trying to wash her face.

Romantic relationships often make the staff feel uncomfortable. Begin a discussion by talking about intimate relationships in general before focusing on such relationships known to the students.

Exercise 3. Talking about Intimacy

Discuss those of the following that apply to your group:

What is your facility's policy on romantic or sexual relationships?

Do you think affection between people is "cute"? How would you, as an adult, react to your parent saying your romance was "cute"?

Do you think a person who has been married may long for touch and for the presence of someone else in the bed? Ask someone who is divorced and is living alone for the first time how it feels to be in bed alone.

Do you think that people with dementia (or old people) have lost their sexuality or their need for self-esteem, closeness, or touch? Although some people do lose their interest in sex, others, both men and women, do not. Many elderly, cognitively well couples value sex in their relationship.

Do people with dementia have a right to intimacy/romance?

Are you sure you know what is going on between two people? Impaired people may be unable to get undressed or complete the sex act but may enjoy the feelings of cuddling.

When a person does not know he is violating the marriage oath, is this adultery? If a person believes he is with his wife, is this adultery?

Do you have the right to decide these things for someone else?

What aspects of such relationships make you feel uncomfortable?

Consider the following example:

> Jeanette was 82 and cognitively in good health when her husband of 62 years died. Jeanette had been a loyal wife and had strongly disapproved when her children "cheated" in their marriages. Throughout her marriage she vigorously insisted that she couldn't ever love another man. After her husband's death Jeannette found an old friend, then widowed, and fell in love. At 84 she was still herself and completely cognitively well, but she had changed her mind.

Might a person with dementia change her mind, as Jeannette did? Are people with dementia still capable of making here-and-now decisions that involve emotions?

The opinion of the family is important whenever a person with dementia forms a romantic bond with another. It is important that the staff and management not make assumptions about how family members will feel. Many family members accept that their previous relationship has changed or that the impaired person thinks that she is with her old partner. Many families accept these bonds because they want their loved one to be as content as possible. Many families do not feel that this is adultery. Professional staff members, clergy, or support groups can often counsel families who face these issues.

The facility must ask itself who has the right to end a bond that makes two ill (and slowly dying) people happy—facility administrators? staff? Do sons and daughters have the same right as spouses to make this decision?

Exhibit 7.1. About Families

Studies have found that many family caregivers are exhausted, feel guilty, are angry and depressed. One in three families caring for a relative at home is in poor health, and most report three times as many symptoms of stress as others. Most are older and coping with other problems as well, such as the illness or death of spouses, job problems, or the needs of children or grandchildren. Studies show that caregivers lose their relationships, friends, and hobbies. Caregivers often have endured rejection, abuse, and demands from the person with dementia. Families in the United States also bear the majority of the financial costs of care.

Most families use informal strategies (things like doing the caregiving themselves or having others help) for a long time before they turn to day care, home care, or residential or nursing home settings. American families provide 75–85 percent of all care to their elders (they care for many years before resorting to nursing home care). Many care for the entire course of the illness.

The leading reason that people enter nursing homes is that they do not have a family member to care for them or the caregiver has become ill or burned out or has died. (This is one reason that many residents have few visitors—there is no one able to visit.) Complex illness in the person with dementia, serious behavioral symptoms, and inadequate home care and day care resources also contribute to placement. When the primary caregiver is also a wage earner or parenting young children, outside help or placement may be necessary.

There is little evidence that American families or white families tend to dump their relatives in nursing homes more often than other families. In this country the care available for low-income families is often so inadequate that the family must choose between struggling to manage or putting the person in an inadequate setting. In reality the decisions to use placement are complex and painful.

Two sisters, Ethel and Josephine, promised to help each other get through college. Ethel worked, and Jo got her education. Now it was Ethel's turn. Also in the household were Ethel's boyfriend and their baby; the sisters' brother, who had Down syndrome; and the young women's mother, who had a dementia. Ethel's boyfriend was unemployed and therefore the primary caregiver for three people. What should be done when the unemployment office requires that the boyfriend accept paid employment at minimum wage?

Care of people with dementia is an overwhelming burden for families in every country and of any race. In some countries, there are few resources other than caring at home.

The author visited another country where the community leaders explained that it was the custom for "the community to take care of its own." Afterward the author met informally with some women of the community, who were bursting with concerns. In truth, they were overwhelmed. They were trying to transmit their culture to their children, cope with troubled adolescents and unemployed men. Many had taken paid employment to make ends meet. Managing severe behavioral symptoms in their elders, even in the confines of a small cooperative community, was impossible.

As life spans extend, more people live into old age, and there are more elders with dementia. Community and custom everywhere are hard pressed to respond to this need.

Exhibit 7.2. Responding to the Emotional Needs of Families

The chapters of the Alzheimer's Association, education about dementia, support groups, counseling, informative videos, and reading help families find better coping skills. Direct care staff members can manage best by avoiding the use of pop psychology because it does not offer useful interventions. Direct care staff members must be well supported and encouraged to accept the family as they are—like the rest of us. As direct care staff members learn to accept the behaviors of the person with dementia, they may also have to be accepting of the family's limitations.

Try these strategies:

- Do a reality check: Are staff members generalizing or making assumptions based on stereotypes? (See Exhibit 7.1.) The program may be unable to provide the quality care the family wants, and this may be the basis of family complaints. It is understandable that families want the best for the person they care for. It is also understandable that the program may be limited in its ability to provide this.
- Prepare families gradually from the beginning of service for the time when the person must be discharged to a higher level of care. If the care you have provided has been good, it is reasonable for families to resist the change and to grieve for the staff and kind of care they are used to.
- Think of the family in terms of coping skills:

  Instead of viewing the family member as being "in denial," consider that the she is unable to accept the severity of the illness. This may be a way to avoid the grief of losing her partner.

  "Withdrawing" is also a coping skill for people who cannot manage a family history of problems or who cannot face the grief of loss.
- Rather than labeling family problems as "denial," "hostility," and so on, think of families in terms of needs:

  "Needs to be forgiven by a parent, and now it is too late."
  "Needs to be trusted by a parent who always criticized."
  "Needs to turn over care to you and to begin to heal." (But perhaps she cannot do so.)
  "Needs to feel in control of a disease he cannot control."
  "Needs to recognize the severity of the illness."
  "Needs financial resources that are not available."
- Nursing home or residential staff members see different problems with families than do day care and home care staff members. Whereas residential and nursing home care staff members see families who don't visit, home care and adult day care staff members see families who struggle to continue to provide care even when it would be better for everyone to have placed the person sooner.
- Learn to shrug off some criticism. It may be the family's way of staying in control.
- The coping skills the person is using may not be the most effective. Helping families cope better is possible, but change is painful and takes time. In the meantime, caregiving staff members will be more successful if they simply accept the family members as they are and recognize that they cannot quickly change them.
- The person you see and care for has a long family history. The balances a married couple must make (for example, he is the breadwinner and she is the nurturer) no longer work when one of them is ill. In some marriages, couples get along because they do not spend too much time together. The dementia changes this.

(continued)

Exhibit 7.2. *(continued)*

The way parents raised their children, how involved they were with adult children, how much they criticized or trusted their children, what they wanted for their children—all influence how the adult children will cope as caregivers.

- The disease itself changes families. Many caregivers are depressed. Depression often paralyzes the caregiver so that she cannot make any decisions, or it can color her view of the situation so that she makes poor decisions. Depression does not always appear as sadness. It can manifest itself as anger with the ill person or the staff. When home care staff members see families who do not take necessary steps for client care and safety, the problem may be that the caregiver is depressed or overwhelmed. Family members may feel emotionally or physically exhausted, and many become ill. People really can't function when they feel this way. Give simple, direct, concrete suggestions for change. Take small steps. The overburdened caregiver will be unable to make large changes at one time.
- Financial matters alter the way families cope. Caregivers fear being impoverished if they purchase care. Some caregivers keep people with dementia at home long past the time this is wise because they cannot purchase the quality of care they find acceptable. Public resources are limited, and bureaucracies move slowly and have ponderous rules, but the family must decide whether to struggle on at home in order to put a child through college or sustain a struggling family business. Depressed caregivers may unrealistically fear impoverishment.
- Resentment is common among siblings. Second marriages complicate relationships over who will inherit and who will do the work of caregiving.
- Guilt is a powerful motivator. Caregivers may feel guilty about real problems in the family history or over things they could not help. They often feel guilty over their ability to care. Guilt may cause the family member to refuse to give up care or conversely to withdraw.

What is to be done when the staff members know that the person with dementia is at risk? Such situations are best resolved on an individual basis. Often the solutions are less than perfect.

When families act in ways that place the ill person at risk, the first step is to gather the facts and ensure that you have an accurate knowledge of what is going on. Involve the family members. Inform them of your findings and encourage them to participate in a compromise solution. Focus on future care rather than on blaming for previous care.

- Involve the family in care planning. Although time consuming, this will help prevent problems. Instead of a pro forma involvement, ask the family members to spell out their role in care. Negotiate who will do what. Thus, if problems arise, responsibilities will already be in writing in the care plan.
- When serious problems arise between staff members and family members, it is essential that management take the responsibility to spell out the steps the program will take and the consequences. Be honest and direct. Management must set limits that are in the best interests of its staff. Social worker intervention, intervention from the physician, and required counseling for the family member are options.

Exhibit 7.3. Fact Sheet for Long-Distance Family Members Who Cannot Visit Often

Send a box of small individually wrapped items to be opened each day and added to a rummage drawer. Include memory-jogging information: "Remember Spike, your old dog? This is his collar. You used to walk him every day in the woods behind the house."

Try videos of family activities. (This works well with some but not all residents.)

Send tape-recorded messages instead of letters.

Hire a visitor.

Order a special restaurant meal for the resident and a favorite staff member to eat together.

Send a card every day.

If the primary family member does live nearby, be sure to support him.

Call every day at the same time. Don't force conversation. Just say "Hello." A one-minute conversation may be all a confused person can process.

Exhibit 7.4. Helpful Ideas for Interactions

Do a task together.

Make an ADL task time for friendship.

Laugh together.

Sing a few phrases of a person's favorite song.

Hold hands during an activity time.

Smile.

Seat withdrawn people near the nurses' station, and ask all staff members to speak to them often.

Stop as you go down the hall to say "Hello."

Pets can become the friend of an impaired person, or they may be the bridge for staff members or volunteers. Pets are effective at all stages of the person's illness and may reach depressed, mute, or withdrawn people.

Repeat whatever works with the person.

Welcome people when they approach you. If you are rushed, give a quick greeting and then tell the person you have to do something.

Try the following with people who are late in their illness:

- Use touch only.
- Just sit with the person.
- Wait and watch for the faintest response, and respond in turn.
- Sing (your singing skill is not important).
- Share prayer if that was meaningful in the past. Use prayers the person memorized long ago.

Exhibit 7.5. Helping Families Understand Sexual Behaviors

A particularly painful behavioral situation occurs when the ill person mistakes a daughter for a wife and makes advances toward her. This is not incest. Teach families that what is happening is that the person is disoriented. He probably remembers a young spouse who may have resembled a grown daughter. He may not remember either a grown daughter or an older spouse. Support families in accepting that this is not a horrible, incestuous behavior. Daughters can reorient a parent by saying, "I'm not Betty, Dad. I look like her but you cannot touch me that way."

Spouses report that their sexual relationship changes in painful ways. It is important to help spouses place this in perspective. Many spouses find that it is impossible to be a lover and a caretaker. Many report that the ill person may initiate intimacies but instantly forget them, leaving the well partner feeling forgotten and alone. Husbands sometimes report that their wives become less inhibited. They also sometimes worry that they are taking advantage of a wife when the rest of the relationship has changed so drastically. Talking openly with a professional or a support group is helpful. Sometimes a professional may need to discreetly inquire how the intimate side of a marriage is working.

Rarely a person with dementia will become hypersexual and make frequent demands on a spouse. This is a devastating burden for the caregiver. It may be necessary to use medication to reduce this behavior. Placement may be the only compassionate option.

Overhead/Handout 7.1. What People with Dementia Need from Their Families

- Affection, love
- A sense of belonging
- Adequate care and supervision if they are living at home
- Visits
- A way to sustain roles
- To relate to them as they are now
- To take responsibility for their care, safety, and finances
- To relate to the staff so that care is effective

Overhead/Handout 7.2. What Families Need from the Staff

- Good care for the person with dementia
- Good communication with caregiving staff members
- Understanding rather than criticism for their coping strategies
- Information about your program, about the disease, about helpful resources
- Recognition that the families' options are limited
- A balance of control between paid providers and family caregivers

Overhead/Handout 7.3. Strategies to Facilitate Interactions between the Facility and the Family

Give families written information.

Offer a short "welcome" orientation course.

Refer families to support groups.

Ensure that the families know what your program offers, what is expected of them, and what your policies are.

Encourage families to replace valuables.

Be sure that the family agrees with your policy regarding the balancing of safety and freedom.

Know who is responsible for certain tasks—family members? paid caregivers?

Respect and accept the care skills that family members have found to be effective.

Overhead/Handout 7.4. Facilitating Family/Client Relationships When the Person Lives at Home

Teach the family caregiver.

Determine which care techniques work.

Staff members can interpret the meaning of behaviors.

Staff members can be alert to problems of safety.

Staff members can be alert to times when the family caregiver is unable to care.

A staff member can make a referral to therapy and support groups.

Staff members can encourage the caregiver to use the time during paid care for rest and personal recovery.

The home care or day care facility can help the family prepare for residential or nursing home care.

LESSON 8

CARING FOR THE PERSON BY MEETING EMOTIONAL NEEDS

Summary: People with dementia continue to have emotional needs similar to others'. However, the disease and the demands of care make it difficult to meet these needs. Identifying and meeting emotional needs improve the quality of life and reduce behavioral symptoms that result from unmet needs.

Section 8.1. Emotional Needs. Encourages the student to identify and support emotional needs.

Section 8.2. The Changing Profiles as Impairment Increases. Suggests ways in which emotional needs for safety and security, identity and roles, self-esteem, pleasure/comfort/humor, autonomy and independence, control of the situation, competence and mastery of skills and objects, success, social engagement and the need to contribute, affection/friendship/family ties, and spirituality change over the course of the illness.

Using the Sections

Introductory course:

None

Core course:

Section 8.1 optional

Section 8.2 optional

Problems You May Have in Implementing This Lesson

Staffing levels must allow students time to perform these activities without feeling overwhelming pressure. If a setting is not ready for these ideas, the staff may conclude that these things can't be done. You may choose to omit this material if you are still struggling to get staffing levels to a point where basic activities-of-daily-living (ADL) care is done easily. Because meeting emotional needs is not a separate service, such as activities, the staff will have difficulty implementing it in a rigid setting. Address these issues before training the staff members because they will not be able to change the system.

Meeting emotional needs is an intangible. Time spent in this area is usually not documented and may be submerged in a task-based system. Find a way to regularly communicate to the staff the value of time spent meeting emotional needs.

A few people will not have the temperament for this part of the work. If possible, assign people according to their strengths.

When a good team is stressed by change or supervisors, this area will falter before personal care does. Periodic reviews and encouragement are important.

Section 8.1. Emotional Needs

Objective

The student will become sensitive to the emotional needs of people with dementia.

Information and Instructions for the Teacher

The difference between this lesson and Lesson 9 is that this lesson addresses normal emotional needs for safety, identity, self-esteem, pleasure, independence, control, mastery, success, social engagement, ties to others, and spiritual needs. Lesson 9, which at first glance may seem similar, addresses depression and other psychiatric states.

The absence of positive feelings and the presence of feelings of helplessness, hopelessness, loss of self-esteem, anger, and frustration lead to poor quality of life and behavioral symptoms. But experiencing normal, positive emotions no longer happens effortlessly as dementia erodes abilities. The staff must work to create opportunities for positive experiences.

This material has been emphasized in every lesson. You may need to spend no more than 10 minutes on this material, affirming staff successes in this area. If you do this, omit the discussions and use only a few points from the brief lecture before moving on to Section 8.2 and Lesson 9. Use more of the material if your students need additional encouragement and ideas.

Do not teach this lesson if your staff members are too busy or too stressed to carry out the suggestions.

Lecture/Discussion Notes to Be Presented to the Class

All people have emotional needs, such as feeling good about themselves, being liked by others, feeling independent, or feeling safe. People with dementia continue to have these emotional needs, but it is difficult to know just what they need because they cannot talk about it. The loss of feelings such as feeling independent, successful, or proud of oneself contributes to the person's suffering and probably to behavioral symptoms. Instead of experiencing positive feelings, people with dementia probably feel helpless, useless, a failure, lost, and so forth. Consider yourself being in these situations:

- You stand there while someone else bathes and dresses you. You ought to be doing this yourself, but your hands fumble uselessly as she works.
- You usually read the paper while you drank a second cup of coffee, but you can't find the paper, and someone took your cup away before you had a second.
- You sit in a chair in a corridor with a bunch of old people. Surely you are not like them! Eventually you become restless, bored. Your legs seem stiff; you shuffle. Maybe you are growing old.
- Finally you find something useful to do: straightening out the dresser. Then a staff member (or family member) says, "Oh, you're not going to do that again, are you?"
- No one ever visits you. People say your daughter comes every day, but obviously she has abandoned you in this place.
- You are lost, you can't find your way home, you can't find your daughter, and your back aches. Hours and hours pass. You keep trying to tell people you are lost and that something is wrong with your back, but they say, "You're just fine."
- You never spend time joking with a friend, flirting, or laughing.

Experiences such as these happen all day long. One or two probably would not make a difference to a person, but accumulated negative experiences add up to feelings of hopelessness, frustration, sadness, or anger. Such feelings appear to last longer than the memory of the facts that caused them. Most of these experiences are things that the disease, not the staff, causes, but the staff can help.

The disease makes it impossible for the person to find good experiences for herself. Staff members help by *purposely restoring good feelings for the person.* This won't happen automatically even in otherwise good care. And activity time will not solve the problem because people spend a small proportion of their time in activities. Staff members plan to restore positive feelings all day long through both ADLs and activity time.

Because people with dementia have short attention spans and because staff members are busy, most of the task of restoring positive feelings is done during regular tasks and takes little, if any, extra time.

Perhaps you think the person is so ill that these things won't matter. The emotion-processing parts of the brain are different from those parts that remember or that respond. You may be reaching the emotion-processing parts, but the person may have no way of showing that you are helping. Do not expect sudden changes in behavior.

Different people have different emotional needs. Personality, life experience, and culture affect which things are most important to an individual. For example, for one man, control and autonomy have been important all his life. For one woman, being nurturing and having family ties are especially important.

Think back over the previous lessons. As a group, discuss ideas you have learned that will help you *restore* positive feelings. *(Teacher: List these. Use Overhead/Handout 8.1 only if you choose. At this point in the training, students should be able to develop their own ideas.)*

Overhead/Handout 8.1. Restore Positive Feelings

- *Do not make assumptions about abilities.* Very impaired people can succeed at some surprisingly complex things when they are relaxed and free of stress.
- *Avoid being patronizing.* Treat people who have dementia with respect.
- *Protect people from making mistakes,* but *avoid taking away autonomy.*
- *Give the person time to try a task,* then *help when it is clear that she will otherwise fail.*
- *Remember that sometimes the resistance people show is an effort to retain some independence;* saying "I don't want to shower" may be the only independent choice a person still has.
- *Orient people.* Because the aide knew that Mrs. Smith could not remember her name, she always greeted her with "Hi, Mrs. Smith, I'm Betty. I helped you shower yesterday."
- *Try to retain the old details that make a person who he is.* For example,

  Al has always risen early, gotten fully dressed, including a necktie, and drunk a cup of black coffee while reading the business section of the paper. When he watches television, he watches sports. Now he is dressed in a running suit, has coffee with cream handed to him, can't find the paper, and watches the soaps with women. Not only have his memories been lost, but evidence of his basic character has been taken away as well. The staff began dressing him in shirt and tie and took him to a separate room with the other men to watch sports.

- *Consider the person's point of view.*

  One woman sat in the hall most of the day and called out, "Nurse, nurse, help me, help me." The staff members ignored her as they hurried past her. Of course, if they were to respond to her, she wouldn't know what she wanted and would forget their reassurance immediately. But from her *feeling* point of view, she felt, "I need something, I don't know what. All of these people here and no one will help me. I've been abandoned." A smile or a quick hug from all passing staff members helped comfort her, although she still forgot immediately.

- *Remind people so that they aren't made to notice their forgetfulness.*

  Esther rummaged through her purse, pulling out a letter from her daughter, pictures of her grandchildren, and a lucky rabbit's foot. But the disease had taken away her ability to make sense of these items. She said, "I don't know who I belong to." A staff member sat down with her. "This is a letter from your daughter. It says . . . . These are your grandchildren, Robbie, Mark, and Beth. And you have had this lucky rabbit's foot for almost fifty years." Esther seemed relieved. At least somebody knew whom she belonged to. She would forget, of course, but reminders would make her feel less lost.

- *Pointing out successes* is important because the person may be too impaired to notice them himself, but this strategy can backfire and seem patronizing to the person with dementia.

Amy managed to secure the Velcro strap on her shoe. The staff member said, "Great, Amy. That's just great. You're doing so well." Amy refused even to try with her second shoe. Amy sensed that most people could do this easily and felt that the staff member's enthusiasm reflected Amy's general incompetence. A brief, casual comment like "Good" might have worked better.

Mr. James was unexpectedly incontinent of bowel. The staff member said, "Don't feel bad, that can happen to anybody." Mr. James got so angry that he stomped his feet in it. He knew that most people did not have their stool running down their pant legs in the day room. A better approach would have been to take Mr. James away and quietly promise to help him change his clothes. Once he was changed, the staff member could have settled him in the kitchen and said, "Now you can just tease the ladies as you always do. They like it." This would have helped restore his positive identity.

- *Help people save face.*

The staff members knew that Albert was dignified and independent, but he could not cut up his meal. To save him the embarrassment, they cut his food up before they served him.

The staff knew that one woman did not remember people well any more, so as a staff member brought a visitor in, she said, "Here's your daughter, Ann."

A very impaired woman picked up her coffee cup and someone else's. That person was not finished with her coffee. Once she had a cup in each hand, the woman appeared uncertain about what to do next. Seeing the problem, the staff member said, "Here, may I help you with that? [Not just taking the cups away.] Thank you for helping me clear up." As the woman turned away, she handed the cup back to the other person.

- *Acknowledge failures when they occur.* Say something such as, "That did not work out, did it? Would you like a cup of tea and a bit of rest?"

Exercise 1. Discussion of Time and Energy

As a class, discuss these issues: Can you find the emotional resources to do this? Restoring good feelings means trying all day and not seeing dramatic results. You won't earn much praise for this; families may take this kind of care for granted, and regulators don't focus on it. It means trying hard and caring about people along with the rest of your job. Do you want to do this? How can you find the support for yourself? Do you have time to do this? What can you do without taking additional time or emotional strength?

Section 8.2. The Changing Profiles as Impairment Increases

Objective

The student will learn to think about the range of emotional needs people have and how these might change as the disease progresses.

Information and Instructions for the Teacher

This section lists some common emotional needs and how they might change as the disease worsens. The section is based on material from experienced professional caregivers, not on data from studies. Use it to help you think about the needs of people with dementia but not to define emotional stages. To generalize about the emotional needs of so large a group of people with different illnesses and in different stages of their illness would be disastrous.

In addition, staff members can easily misinterpret behavioral symptoms; for example, a man who appears to "tune out" during activities may be assumed not to want to participate or to be too ill to participate. In fact, he may need the stimulation and social interchange but be unable to participate in a complex task or with many people.

The profiles in this section list eleven common emotional needs (Exhibit 8.1) at five levels of impairment (Exhibit 8.2). These are general descriptions of needs that overlap and vary from person to person. There are many other emotional needs, and they also overlap. Each profile is a thumbnail sketch of how emotional needs might change. It can be difficult for staff members to imagine that some needs are retained as the disease progresses. Some are lost. Others change significantly. Encourage your group to think in terms of change.

Use this material for your own reference or for advanced groups. If you use it in the classroom, ask students to discuss their own observations. *This is not a form of staging.*

Lecture/Discussion Notes to Be Presented to the Class

The Person with No Impairment

Safety and Security. The person seeks financial security and security in relationships; he wants appropriate medical care and expects public safety. He may take risks based on the recognition of his own competence.

Identity and Roles. The individual has a strong knowledge of who she is as defined by her history, activities, relationships, character, appearance, and beliefs. The perceptions of others help to shape that identity. The perception of self is not complete until adulthood, but it is essential for successful adult functioning.

Self-Esteem. The individual sees himself as all right, as successful in things that are important to him. He is able to maintain his self-esteem through intrapsychic processes. This may be partially dependent on successes and relationships. Some adults never fully develop self-esteem.

Pleasure, Comfort, Humor. The person may enjoy a range of pleasures including socializing, intimacy, recreation, hobbies, rewards of work, and psychic and emotional comfort. Some pleasures derive from mastery, autonomy, control, and success.

Autonomy and Independence. The individual may perceive himself to be free to make most decisions, to come and go, to do what he wants, to be himself. Or he may see himself as restricted by his job or relationships.

Control of the Situation. The person generally feels in control of life, self, body, job, relationships. She may control others in the family or on the job. She may use strategies such as manipulation to control others.

Competence, Mastery of Skills and Objects. The person is able to master all aspects of life: his job, relationships, communication, the use of objects. He experiences a broader world through television, books, and travel. He may have mastered technical skills, sports, the use of tools, and recreational activities. He may seek training to master other skills.

Success. The person hardly notices routine successes in instrumental activities of daily living (IADLs) and ADLs. Success is valued in relation to the job, personal relationships, hobbies, and sports.

Social Engagement, Need to Contribute. The individual is actively involved with others: friends, family members, and co-workers. The number of close relationships varies with the individual. Many people value some form of altruism or are supportive within the family.

Affection, Friendship, Family Ties. The person needs and establishes bonds of intimacy and love. Ties to the family may be strong, though sometimes troubled. The individual grieves if an intimate relationship is severed.

Spirituality. For some, spiritual life is centered around a formal religion. For others, spirituality is in contemplation, reading, walks in the woods. For many, spiritual life includes altruism. Some will have given little thought to spirituality.

The Person with Subjective or Minimal Impairment, Decreased Job Functioning, Difficulty in New Situations

Safety and Security. The individual may be anxious about future security (care, finances) or may not recognize her need for help. Safety declines in new or stressful situations. She may show poor judgment or be overly cautious.

Identity and Roles. Identity and roles may be threatened on the job but remain intact within the family. The person may feel threatened by a perceived loss of competence, by fear of a dementia, of losing memories, of losing control. Efforts to maintain identity can lead to inappropriate behaviors.

Self-Esteem. The person may be devastated as performance declines. Denial or blame may be used to maintain self-esteem. Feelings that he is worthless may arise from depression.

Pleasure, Comfort, Humor. The person may be able to take pleasure from a full range of activities, or the pleasure may be limited by anxiety or depression. The person may be unable to plan for activities that can still be enjoyed.

Autonomy and Independence. The person is able to retain most autonomy. Driving may need to be restricted. He will have good days and bad.

Control of the Situation. Some people attempt to control the presence of the disease by understanding the illness or making plans. Others maintain control by avoiding issues or blaming others. Some deny the illness.

Competence, Mastery of Skills and Objects. The person will not lose these immediately, but she may be anxious about future losses. Judgment, language skills, and memory will gradually impair the mastery of complex skills.

Success. The individual may perceive herself as less successful in areas that are important to her such as a job. She remains successful in daily life and uses responses appropriate to her defense strategies. Some persons are relieved to retire and reduce the demands on themselves.

Social Engagement, Need to Contribute. The person may narrow his group of friends. He finds some events too tiring or seeks to conceal symptoms, but he maintains most social relationships. Some people may reestablish religious or family ties and may seek to share experiences or accumulated wisdom.

Affection, Friendship, Family Ties. Most relationships remain intact. Stresses of the disease may affect family balance and friendships early.

Spirituality. The loss of the mind implies a change in one's relationship with God and one's humanness. However, familiar religious rituals may give comfort and reassurance. Beliefs may facilitate the acceptance of the illness, or the person may rail against God as a part of the grief process.

The Person Who Has Difficulty with Complex Tasks and Decision Making, Has Some Problems with Communication, Needs Cues and Supervision

Roles and relationships begin to change at this level.

Safety and Security. The person's need for safety may conflict with efforts to maintain autonomy. The lack of judgment affects safe decision making. The individual may resist help or feel unsafe and abandoned.

Identity and Roles. The person begins to redefine himself in light of the changes or may rigidly cling to old roles. Others may question, "Who am I?" or "To whom do I belong?"

Self-Esteem. The individual has increasing difficulty in restoring self-esteem because of memory difficulties, communication problems, and role loss.

Pleasure, Comfort, Humor. The person still needs to be involved in pleasurable events. Some former activities may become stressful or upsetting. Excess disability, anxiety, and depression may prevent pleasure and comfort. Language impairment causes problems understanding puns and jokes.

Autonomy and Independence. Lack of judgment and memory impairment may affect the person's ability to make complex or major decisions. Lack of insight will prevent comprehension of cognitive losses, causing people to resist interventions.

Control of the Situation. Loss of ability causes the frightening experience of losing control. The person may continue to use strategies such as manipulation out of habit. Balance in interpersonal relationships may shift as others assume control.

Competence, Mastery of Skills and Objects. The person loses the mastery of abstract ideas, planning, driving, and job skills and gradually loses the mastery of ADLs. He may fight to retain them, or he may become discouraged.

Success. As insight is lost, the person may perceive herself as continuing to be successful in all areas, despite evidence to the contrary. If insight remains, she may become anxious and depressed as she recognizes her increasing failures. The person may resist being involved because of fear of failure and may prefer passivity.

Social Engagement, Need to Contribute. The disease begins to restrict engagement. Involvement with others narrows as some friends drop away. The person is unable to participate in some former social activities and may resist or grieve as others take over roles and decision making.

Affection, Friendship, Family Ties. The number of close relationships will be reduced, and the person may grieve because of the loss. He will sometimes form new bonds with other impaired people.

Spirituality. Familiar rituals often remain important to the person, although she may be too restless to sit through a service.

The Person Who Is Unable to Do Most ADLs or Needs Increasing Help, Has Significant Difficulty in Communicating, May Be Unable to Initiate Activities, Has Change in Motor Skills and Gait

Relationships at this level depend on outside support.

Safety and Security. Disorientation and cognitive overload trigger overwhelming feelings of insecurity as the person is no longer able to make sense of the environment. The person is sometimes able to perform old, overlearned tasks.

Identity and Roles. As memories are lost and the person has trouble recognizing others, he has difficulty retaining identity. He can continue to be involved only in familiar settings, in familiar roles and tasks, and with familiar tools.

Self-Esteem. The person maintains self-esteem only by having success in simple tasks such as ADLs and other activities and maintaining a good personal appearance.

Pleasure, Comfort, Humor. Some people retain humor but must feel safe and relaxed. A person may not be able to initiate events, but she enjoys them when she is brought to them. For many comfort means not having to try hard but to let oneself be cared for.

Autonomy and Independence. Decision making is limited to immediate issues of daily life, and the person may resist restrictions.

Control of the Situation. The person most frequently feels out of control, and a refusal may be an effort to maintain control.

Competence, Mastery of Skills and Objects. Mastery is limited to daily life tasks. The person will retain the mastery of old, overlearned skills longer. Giving up and being cared for is comforting for some. Others struggle to retain control and competence in ways that result in inappropriate behavior or anger toward caregivers.

Success. Failures can be cumulative and frustrating and can lead to angry outbursts or to refusal to try things.

Social Engagement, Need to Contribute. Loss of ability to recognize relatives increases isolation, as do long periods of nothing to do.

Affection, Friendship, Family Ties. Family bonds are damaged when the person is unable to recognize family members. She may recognize people without recalling the relationship.

Spirituality. Spirituality is probably retained only if rituals are taken to the person through small groups, songs, rituals, and such items as flowers and rosaries.

The Person Who Is Incontinent, Has Almost No Verbal Communication or Comprehension Abilities, Is Not Ambulatory or Needs Assistance, Is Totally Dependent in ADLs

Safety and Security. The person probably needs feelings of physical security. Some are reassured by holding, touch, tone of voice; others are distressed.

Identity and Roles. The extent of loss of self is unclear. Flashes of the old self may be expressed through sudden recognition or smiles.

Self-Esteem. The extent of the loss of self-esteem is unknown. Although little conscious self-esteem may be evident, respectful personal care is important.

Pleasure, Comfort, Humor. The person may enjoy touch, pets, children, affection, and the like and may continue to smile. The person's experience is limited to the here and now.

Autonomy and Independence. The person may be able to express some desires (holding you to get you to stay, rejecting food that is offered, speaking or rejecting touch).

Control of the Situation. Attempts to control are like those mentioned above in "Autonomy and Independence."

Competence, Mastery of Skills and Objects. The person may be able to master the immediate environment such as singing, hugging, holding a pet. Most involvement may be passive.

Success. The person may need small successes such as taking your hand, but comfort and security may be more important.

Social Engagement, Need to Contribute. The person's ability to be involved is very limited, but many people still seem to gain pleasure from children and pets and from affectionate caregivers.

Affection, Friendship, Family Ties. Many people appear to need affection and contact. They may be starved for these.

Spirituality. Touch and familiar songs seem to be important to many people.

This section has listed some of the emotional needs of people with dementia; you will think of others.

Clinical Experience

Select a person you know who has a cognitive impairment. Identify two interventions under each heading that would be effective for this individual. Try these interventions for one week. Did you observe a response? (It may take longer than one week to observe a response, and if the person is experiencing considerable stress, no response may be possible.)

Exhibit 8.1. Common Emotional Needs

Safety and security
Identity and roles
Self-esteem
Pleasure, comfort, humor
Autonomy and independence
Control of the situation
Competence, mastery of skills and objects
Success
Social engagement, need to contribute
Affection, friendship, family ties
Spirituality

Exhibit 8.2. Levels of Impairment

1. No impairment
2. Subjective or minimal impairment: decreased job functioning; difficulty in new situations
3. Difficulty with complex tasks, decision making; some problems with communication; needs cues, supervision; roles and relationships begin to change
4. Unable to do most ADLs or needs increasing help; has significant difficulty in communicating; may be unable to initiate activities; change in motor skills and gait; relationships depend on outside support
5. Incontinent; has almost no verbal communication or comprehension abilities; is not ambulatory or needs assistance; is totally dependent in ADLs

Overhead/Handout 8.1. Restore Positive Feelings

Do not make assumptions about abilities.

Avoid being patronizing: treat people with dementia with respect.

Protect people from making mistakes.

Avoid taking away autonomy.

Try to retain the old details that make a person who she is.

Consider the person's point of view.

Remind people so that they aren't made to notice their forgetfulness.

Point out successes.

Help people save face.

LESSON 9

HELPING THE PERSON BY ADDRESSING MOOD

Summary. Depression is common among people with dementia, and it significantly affects their quality of life, behavioral symptoms, and function. The staff's approach to care is important. This lesson discusses depression and other mental phenomena sometimes observed in people with dementia, including suspiciousness, hallucinations, and delusions.

Section 9.1. Helping People Who Are Depressed. Introduces depression and teaches sensitive and empathetic responses.

Section 9.2. Information about Depression and Other Psychiatric Symptoms. Provides background information about depression, hallucinations, delusions, phobias, and suspiciousness.

Using the Sections

- Introductory course:
  - None
- Core course:
  - Section 9.1 required
- Special audiences:
  - People responsible for diagnosis, assessment, treatment, and referral: entire lesson

Problems You May Have in Implementing This Lesson

There is a shortage of mental health professionals who have expertise in the care of the elderly person or the person with dementia. In addition, funding discourages practice in residential care and nursing homes and for people on Medicare or Medicaid. The biggest problem you will face is in locating the professionals necessary to treat people with depression.

Ideally, the mental health professional will discuss treatment plans with direct care staff members so that they can support mental health interventions. Time and funding for such communication are limited to a few model settings.

Section 9.1. Helping People Who Are Depressed

Objective

Students will learn general principles about depression and be able to feel, empathetically, the appropriateness or inappropriateness of their responses to people who are depressed.

Background

Please read through Section 9.2 before beginning to teach.

Depression is not specific to older, confused people; it is common in people of all ages. In a classroom of 20 students, at least one person is likely to have experienced a depression—her own or that of someone with whom she is close.

Students will have diverse ideas about mental health. Some of these ideas come from other cultures, but widely divergent explanations and treatments for depression are found in the mainstream American culture. Encourage students to express their ideas in the accepting climate of the classroom. Rather than pressing students to give up their ideas, help them accept that, whatever is right for them personally, the techniques of modern psychiatry must be applied to the people they care for.

Contemporary psychiatry is divided over which approaches are helpful for people with dementia. Psychiatric care of people who have both depression and dementia is changing.

Students have personal concerns about depression that they may raise during or after class. Be prepared to do some basic teaching and to refer the student to available resources if necessary. Unfortunately, many people in the community are not receiving appropriate treatment, and there may not be funding for mental health care.

If there is no resource for appropriate treatment of mental health problems for the people with dementia whom your program cares for, limit what you teach to (a) what depression is, (b) how to chart it (to document the need for professional care), and (c) compassionate care.

Information and Instructions for the Teacher

Conduct this section as a discussion, guided by the text. It is not necessary to cover all the material. At a minimum, all students should be able to observe sadness or depression in the people they care for and to make appropriate responses. Empathy for the depressed person is more important than that the direct care provider have technical knowledge about depression. Ask questions that draw out students' opinions and observations. Use discussion as needed. If your students have questions or different attitudes toward depression, use Exhibit 9.1 to guide you, or teach this material as needed. Exercise 1 is optional.

Lecture/Discussion Notes to Be Presented to the Class

Overhead/Handout 9.1. Depression

What is depression? *(Teacher: Ask the students for their definitions of depression.)* Depression is a negative mood, usually sadness, that lasts for two weeks or more.

Depression is common in all people. About one person in four will experience a significant depression at some point in life.

It is even more common in people with dementia.

Depression may be caused by grief over a loss (as when someone you love dies) or when there are specific changes in the chemistry of the brain.

People who are depressed cannot "snap out of it" or "try to think positively."

Depression affects concentration and thinking and therefore can be mistaken for Alzheimer disease. This is tragic when the depression goes untreated so long that the problem cannot be reversed. When depression occurs in the early stages of Alzheimer disease, the person may be depressed because he knows he has the illness or because of changes in the brain. In either case, if the depression is recognized and treated, the person will feel better and have a longer time when he can function well.

Sadness is a common symptom of depression, but some people deny feeling sad. *There are many other indicators of depression.* We will discuss some of these.

Depression is usually treatable.

Overhead/Handout 9.2. Why It Is Important to Understand Depression

Why is depression important?

- It causes suffering.
- It shortens people's life expectancy.
- It causes behavioral symptoms (like anger, restlessness, irritability) that make care more difficult and that upset other clients.
- It causes problems in concentration and memory. When you add depression to the dementia, the person's mental function is much worse than it needs to be. Even younger people with depression often fear they are developing "early Alzheimer disease" because they are aware of the change in their thinking.
- It makes it impossible for people to become involved in the activities that might help them. So they get caught in a downward spiral.
- It affects the body. People lose weight, can't rest at night, move slowly. Such people can die of malnutrition or dehydration.

The biggest reason that understanding depression is important is that we can find ways to reduce suffering, sometimes improve mental function, and treat behavioral symptoms.

Overhead/Handout 9.3. Symptoms of Depression in People with Dementia

How can we tell when people with dementia are depressed? People with dementia may not be able to tell caregivers that they are depressed. Some people will deny depression even when they feel deeply discouraged. Some people deny feeling sad or unhappy and instead complain of various health problems. If there is no real health problem, treating the depression may make them feel better and reduce whimpering and clinging. Never assume depression unless you are sure there is no health problem, however. Sometimes the symptoms of depression include anger or agitation. Diagnosing and treating the depression often helps.

The following list of symptoms was developed to address this problem. Use this list rather than one of the commonly used depression scales designed for people without dementia. These symptoms may look like the behaviors we often see in people with dementia. In part this is because depression is so common in people with dementia. Note that these are all sad, unhappy variations of these behaviors. In addition, weight loss, sleep disturbances, anger, and a personal history of depression provide important clues.

Suspect depression if you observe the presence of any of these symptoms, which you cannot easily alter by attempts to cheer up, console, or reassure the person and which last at least two weeks:

- Negative statements ("Nothing matters"; "I'd rather be dead"; "What's the use?"; "Let me die")
- Repetitive questions ("Where do I go?"; "What do I do?")
- Repetitive statements, calling out for help ("God help me")
- Persistent anger with self or others; easily annoyed (anger at placement, anger at care received, anger at caregiver)
- Self-deprecation ("I am nothing"; "I am of no use to anyone")
- Expressions of what appear to be unrealistic fears (fear of being abandoned, left alone, being with others)
- Recurrent statements that something terrible is about to happen (person believes he is about to die, have a heart attack)
- Repetitive health complaints (persistently seeks medical attention, obsessive concern with body functions)
- Repetitive anxious complaints/concerns not related to health (persistently seeks attention/reassurance regarding schedules, meals, laundry/clothing, relationship issues)
- Unpleasant mood in the morning
- Insomnia/change in usual sleep pattern
- Sad, pained, worried expression (e.g., furrowed brows)

- Crying, tearfulness
- Repetitive physical movements (e.g., pacing, hand wringing, restlessness, fidgeting, picking)
- Withdrawal from activities of interest (e.g., no interest in long-standing activities or being with family/friends)
- Reduced social interaction
- Persistent anger with self or others

Overhead/Handout 9.4. How We Help

Teacher: Use the text, the overhead/handout, and your own experience to guide a discussion.

The first step in treatment is to know that we *can* treat depression in people with dementia, although it is difficult. These people commonly develop side effects from the antidepressants or from drug interactions. Equally challenging, they need an individualized and supportive environment that restores a sense of pride and self-esteem. Not everyone will "get well," but many will improve. Tragically, the mental health providers you need to help you may not be available.

The direct care provider is in the best position to identify a possible depression. Because we often can't ask a person if she feels depressed, we must depend on her behavior.

Clara drifted about, wringing her hands and saying, "Help me, help me. I'm sick." She never stayed still. She left the table after eating only a few bites, drifted in and out of activities, and cried the whole time her husband visited. She lost weight. Her husband said she had had an episode of depression during her change of life.

Clara was placed on a low dose of antidepressant, and the staff began a plan of encouraging her to help clean up after meals (something the staff knew she could succeed at). At first she refused, but as the antidepressant took effect, she began to take pride in being the one to clean up. She was able to stay seated during meals and activities and smiled often. Her dementia did not improve.

Mark refused to get out of bed. He was often awake at 3 A.M., and by the time he got up at 7, he was nasty with staff members. He talked in a rambling way about how the corporation he had worked for had dumped him and was out to get him. The psychiatrist tried two different antidepressants with Mark before he showed any improvement, but when he did, the change was dramatic. He was still confused, but his dementia seemed to be less; he became a cheerful person and played a role in discussion groups.

No one doubted that 80-year-old Burton, who lived with his daughter, was depressed. The problem was treating him. Burton refused to do anything but sit and watch television. His daughter could find no activity that interested him. His family physician treated him with an antidepressant. Burton quickly developed cardiac side effects so severe that he had to be hospitalized. Burton was now seriously medically ill and much more confused than he had been before treatment. In desperation, his daughter, a nurse, consulted another physician. This physician began him on a very low dose of another antidepressant. It took several months, during which the physician, in close contact with the daughter, frequently readjusted the medications, but Burton returned finally to his previous level of health and function and a positive mood.

The next important step is for direct care staff members to report their suspicions. Treatment of depression requires the skills of several people: a mental health expert, activity personnel, and the staff members who provide day-to-day care—and who do most of the relating to the person. It is direct care staff members who provide a friendly, supportive, affectionate climate.

An individualized psychosocial plan is as important as medication. Every lesson in this book provides guidance in creating an effective psychosocial plan.

In addition, use brief but frequent interpersonal activities: touch, a quick hug and smile, a minute of attention. Ask friends to visit one at a time for short periods but to come more often.

- If a person does not want to leave her room, talk with her in her room, and plan simple one-to-one activities in her room.
- Set the person up to succeed; protect the person from even simple failures.
- Avoid complicated tasks; use task breakdown and task analysis.
- Try things and tell other staff members what helps.

- Avoid telling the person he needs to get out and do things. Just make it happen. For example, if the group is singing, sit next to him and hold his hand.
- Avoid long periods of isolation or boredom, but let the person have extra rest if needed. The person who sits and does nothing can slip deeper into gloom. People with dementia often spend long hours doing nothing while their caregivers are busy. At the same time, the depression itself makes it hard for the person to do anything. Try to create a balance the person can tolerate.
- Offer simple, basic pleasures: a bowl of hot, fragrant soup or a hot muffin fresh from the oven. Get people out of doors even in inclement weather. Babies, cats, and dogs are the best therapists known; use them daily.

The administrator brought her golden retriever to work with her. Somehow the dog seemed to know which residents needed her most and would go from one to the next, laying her head in their lap. After a few days the staff noticed smiles and then a tentative hand reaching out for the dog's head. The dog paved the way with people who did not respond to the staff.

- Set simple goals and keep a record. Keep weekly weight records and monitor hydration daily. It is important to know whether the person is beginning to emerge or whether you need to modify your treatment plan.
- The person with dementia who is easily overstressed or who tries to do things and fails will feel even more aware of her failures and her decline when she is depressed. Get the person involved a *tiny step* at a time.
- When activities are childish or are things the person would never want to do, they will make depression worse. Involve children for a childish event. Create moments to bolster self-esteem.
- If antidepressants are used, they may take several weeks to take effect.

In many cases, the person will need antidepressant medication. These are powerful drugs: they can be highly effective or toxic. The treating physician may have to try several different medications in different doses before finding one that treats the depression without too many side effects. It would be unrealistic to expect to hit on the right dose of the right drug the first time. Patience is a big part of the treatment plan. Until the right medication takes effect, the person may be able to tolerate only brief one- to-one activities, and until then the person may be unable to be more involved. Use activities-of-daily-living (ADL) time to interact.

Staff members must monitor recovery and watch for drug side effects. It may take several weeks to see a response. Let everyone (especially the treating physician) know when you see even slight improvement.

Talk of Suicide

Whenever a person (whether that person has a dementia or not) talks of wishing to die or deserving to die, or of thinking of suicide, take him seriously. Listen and acknowledge the person's misery. It's difficult to be with a person who is this miserable. We instinctively want to make the conversation go away or urge the person to feel better, but this leaves the person feeling more lost. Some people think that talking about it makes the person more likely to kill himself, but this is not true. These people are in real pain and need a caring listener. Report such conversations: the person should be seen by a mental health professional. Even a person who is too confused to commit suicide may do herself serious harm.

Some people who are close to death will talk of being ready to die or of being satisfied with life. This is different. Listen in a caring way. Encourage the person to talk about her life.

Some people who are in severe pain seek suicide. Their pain and medication treatment should be reviewed.

Exercise 1. Thinking about Depression

Teacher: This exercise is optional. Use it if your students have no prior training about depression or have varied opinions and ideas about it. Use Exhibit 9.1 to help you.

As a class, discuss the following: Does it seem that most of the people you care for have these symptoms?

How do you think these symptoms should be managed? Do you agree that something can be done to help these people? Do you think that it is "understandable" that people with dementia would be depressed?

Have you or someone you know who does not have a dementia been depressed? How does it feel to watch someone else who is depressed? How does it feel to be depressed? *(Teacher: Make it clear that answering this question is voluntary.)* Sometimes people tell a person who is depressed that if he tries he will feel better. Suppose you felt blue and your family and friends thought you could snap out of it if you tried. Suppose you can't seem to snap out of it and your friends think only weaklings become depressed. In your setting, how would you help depressed clients? How will you manage with limited help from mental health professionals? Use Overhead/Handout 9.4 for ideas to discuss.

Exercise 2. Role Play

Role-play or discuss how the following "dos and don'ts" would make a person feel. Why? Which do you use?

Dos: Psychosocial interventions: Conversations and other activities that work well with people who are depressed and have a dementia, for example:

"What would make you feel better?"

"How does some ice cream [or any treat] sound?"

"Tell me about your mother" (only if the person is grieving over a mother long dead).

"I think we can help."

"How hard that must be for you."

"I'm sorry."

"Let's pray" (only if prayer is meaningful to the person).

Sing an old familiar song and encourage the person to sing with you.

Take a short walk outside (physical exercise helps).

Don'ts: The kinds of things you can say or do that are not comforting, such as:

Avoid the person because she is a pain.

"I had the same problem . . ." and tell the person all about your problem.

"Snap out of it."

"Your daughter wouldn't want you to act like this."

"You should be glad your husband is in heaven now."

Advice: "Here's what you should do."

"Your mother's been dead for years."

"Try not to think about it."

"Oh, you don't really want to die."

Clinical Experience

No clinical experience is recommended unless mental health care is available. If it is, identify one person who meets the criteria for depression and discuss his care plan with the supervising professional. Find out how you can participate in the care.

Section 9.2. Information about Depression and Other Psychiatric Symptoms

Objective

(1) The teacher will acquire the basic information to teach students how to provide caring support to people with depression and dementia, and (2) students responsible for diagnosis, assessment, referral, and treatment will obtain the information needed to recognize possible depression, make referrals and care plans, and supervise direct care staff members. It is not possible in this brief lesson to prepare a person to diagnose or treat depression.

Lecture/Discussion Notes to Be Presented to the Class

Depression in Long-Term Care

Numbers vary, but most experts agree that a high percentage of people with dementia in nursing homes have mental health problems such as depression and anxiety, which are treatable. Yet little effort has been made to identify or treat conditions related to behavioral symptoms and suffering. These individuals with both dementia and mental health problems also increase the burden on the staff.

People with dementia living in other settings also have high rates of depression, anxiety, and other psychiatric disorders and similarly low rates of psychiatric intervention.

Thus, depression, anxiety, and other psychiatric disorders may not be part of the dementia but cause unnecessary suffering that is just as devastating.

In the general population, most people who experience a depressive illness recover. The treatment response rate is lower for people with dementia, but many people with both depression and dementia do improve. There are probably many reasons for this: the pathophysiology of the brain, the presence of physical illnesses that complicate treatment, available geriatric mental health providers, and the challenges of creating an enriching environment for people with dementia. Some programs informally report a much higher response rate than others.

The good news is that it is almost always possible to help these people somewhat within the limitations of the average program. Recognizing the problem, initiating whatever interventions are possible, and training the staff in successful and caring behaviors will alleviate suffering and reduce behavioral symptoms. Intervention programs should never be eliminated because someone does not think this population is responsive to treatment. At the same time, staff members must be supported and encouraged even when they see little change for some people.

Depression from Loss and Grief

Feelings of profound sadness, vulnerability, and frustration are a major source of depression for people with dementia. Supportive treatment is needed. Never assume that it is reasonable for a person to be depressed and therefore limit treatment.

Depression as a Precursor to Alzheimer Disease

Depression is common in the early stages of Alzheimer disease. Its biochemical relationship to dementia is still being studied. However, treatment remains important.

Depression Associated with a Medical Condition

Medical conditions associated with depression include

- Alzheimer disease;
- vascular dementia;
- cancer;
- cardiac disease;
- metabolic and endocrine disorders (hypercalcemia, Cushing disease, Addison disease);
- Parkinson disease;
- stroke;
- other neurological diseases (Huntington disease, multiple sclerosis, brain tumor);
- thyroid disease; and
- tuberculosis, hepatitis, other infectious diseases.

Treatment of the underlying disease, when possible, will usually improve the depression. However, in some cases in which the disease has not been recognized and treated for some time, the depression may not resolve. When the underlying disease cannot be treated, efforts should be made to treat the depression.

> Robert had been diagnosed as having Alzheimer disease. He complained of fatigue and appeared depressed. The home care nurse noticed symptoms of an underactive thyroid. When this was treated, Robert was much less depressed and tired, although he continued to have mild cognitive impairment.

> Marian had an undiagnosed dementia and complained of stomach pain. She called out, "Help me, help me," and moaned. She cried often and refused to participate in activities. She was losing weight. She said she was dying and begged for someone to give her medicine so she could die. Marian was diagnosed as having an inoperable stomach cancer. She was given palliative treatment and analgesics for her pain and an antidepressant. She called out much less frequently, smiled more often, and was affectionate with the staff. When she died four months later, she seemed to be at peace. The staff members also felt peaceful about her death. They were confident that they had alleviated her suffering. They, too, had suffered when she moaned and begged to die.

Depression Triggered by Medication

Medications that may trigger depression include

- psychotropic drugs;
- antihypertensive medications;
- cimetidine;
- cytotoxic agents;
- digitalis;
- immunosuppressive drugs;
- sedatives;
- steroids;
- stimulants;
- alcohol; and
- antianxiolytic agents.

Depression Caused by Biochemical Changes in the Brain

Major depression and bipolar illness are believed to be associated with changes in the neurotransmitters in the brain. They respond well to medication in combination with other therapies. Alzheimer disease and vascular dementia also affect these neurotransmitter systems and thus may trigger depression.

The Use of Psychotropic Medication

The physician selects a medication that she believes best matches the patient's symptoms and history and that has an acceptable side effect profile. This drug is begun at a low dose, which is gradually increased until symptoms resolve or side effects appear. If the first drug tried is not successful, a second or third drug is tried in the same way. The physician monitors this process closely and will require feedback from the family or direct care provider. The patient may take a medication for several weeks before his symptoms go away, and some patients experience unpleasant side effects in the beginning. It is important that the client continue to take the medicine and that the caregiver stay in touch with the physician.

People with dementia are more vulnerable to side effects of these medications than are other people, especially younger people. The recommendation is to start low and go slow. Doses are usually lower than for younger people, and the patient must be watched closely for adverse side effects. The appearance of side effects may be delayed. It can be difficult to reach a therapeutic response without disabling side effects.

Nonpharmacological Interventions

Psychosocial Interventions. Meeting the person's emotional needs is as important as medication and should be part of the treatment plan. Rarely is medication alone successful.

Counseling/Psychotherapy. People who are in the early stages of dementia may benefit from short-term counseling. However, seriously question the usefulness of "talking it through" with people who have no insight or do not remember from one session to the next. These vulnerable people with limited ability to consent can be subtly abused.

Support Groups/Organizations. Support groups help people learn that they are not alone and share information for coping and for obtaining resources. A few programs offer support groups for people in the early stages of their illness and have reported significant success. However, depressed people may need additional supports.

Behavioral Therapies. Behavioral therapy, in which the patient learns to change destructive thinking patterns, is helpful to many people. Because behavioral therapy requires memory and learning, clinicians differ in their opinion of its effectiveness. The choice of treatment is based on the individual patient.

Depression among Caregivers

As many as 90 percent of family caregivers may be depressed, whether the person with dementia is living at home or in a residential care home or nursing home setting. Depressed caregivers need help with their feelings of hopelessness and despair. Occasionally caregiver depression results in a murder-suicide. More often the depressed caregiver is unable to provide proper care or to make wise decisions. The nursing assistant or other staff member may be the only person who observes caregiver depression and should report it. Tell direct care providers what steps they should take when they suspect that a family member is depressed.

Staff Response to Symptoms

Depression and other mood disorders affect the feelings of others around the person. There is an old joke among medical students that if the medical student is depressed after interviewing the patient, the patient is likely to have a diagnosis of depression. In addition, the staff may find symptoms such as hallucinations to be creepy, may avoid people with certain symptoms, or may be bothered by certain behaviors but not by others. *It is more realistic to teach the staff members how to respond to their own feelings than to press them to be perfectly objective.*

- Supervisors should role-model appropriate behaviors.
- A system of trading jobs among staff members when one caregiver is feeling burdened by the mood of a person with dementia is helpful.
- Assign staff members to care for people whose mood or other symptoms do not irritate them unduly.
- Objectify behavioral symptoms such as hallucinations as part of the brain damage.

Tragedies can cause staff members great anxiety; help the staff when a tragedy occurs. For example,

> Mabel was living at home with her husband. He fell ill in the home and died several hours later. Mabel was too impaired to summon help and perhaps to recognize the situation. It was about 30 hours before anyone found Mabel and her dead husband. Her daughter placed her in an excellent facility, and Mabel went through the usual adjustment: she wanted to go home, and she wanted her husband. After a while this stopped, and Mabel settled in comfortably. However, the staff members found this horrible to think about and were certain that Mabel had been traumatized by those hours alone with a dead man.

A realistic appraisal of Mabel's disabilities creates a different picture. She had lost her sense of the passage of time. It would be unlikely that her memory of the incident would include her long hours alone. She may have perceived her husband to be asleep. She may have experienced panic, hunger, and fatigue but may not have associated her feelings with him or his death. She never said that he was dead. We will never know whether she even knew.

Other Behavioral Symptoms

In dementia, even the most straightforward-seeming symptoms can have multiple causes and multiple possible interventions. The best way to treat these problems is to stand in the impaired person's shoes and try to solve the problem. There are many possible reasons for a behavior that at first looks "psychiatric." The most effective intervention may be a nonmedical, low-tech plan.

Do not make assumptions. For example,

> Sharon said she was afraid to go to bed because there was a snake in her bed. This seemed to be an obvious hallucination, and Sharon was treated with a low dose of a neuroleptic. On the neuroleptic Sharon developed Parkinsonian symptoms and drowsiness and still complained about the snakes, so the neuroleptic was discontinued.

There are many reasons why Sharon might report frightening snakes in her bed:

- She has an agnosia and has mistaken the stocking on her bed for a snake.
- She has a language disorder and has called the stocking on her bed a snake.

- She has a visual impairment and has mistaken the stocking for a snake.
- She is hallucinating.
- There is a toy snake in her bed that her young grandson has put there.
- She has had a longstanding phobia of snakes.
- She lived most of her life in a tropical area where a snake in the bed was a real possibility.

After the neuroleptic failed, a creative staff member found a solution. Every night he went to Sharon's room with a gunny sack and returned, holding up the sack and announcing that the snake had been removed. After that, Sharon was able to go to bed easily. (We will never know exactly why this strategy worked.)

Many things that appear to be delusions have other explanations:

- What the person says may be true. There is an old story of a man who insisted that his mother was coming to get him. Nobody believed him until his 90-year-old mother arrived.
- When a person says, "They are trying to kill me," this may not be a delusion. It may be a misinterpretation of the fact that two people have grabbed the person, taken her clothing off, and are trying to drag her into the shower. The treatment intervention will be different from that for a person with delusions, but in either case the patient's terror is the same.
- The person's account may be confused, but the basis for it may be real.
- The person's statement may be wrong, but the facts are correct: "They hurt me" might mean "They took my clothes off." "They robbed me" could mean "I've lost my home."
- It is possible for a person to have no insight into her deficits and no memory of failures. She may still, however, feel vulnerable or inadequate.
- Longstanding mental illness may also cause these symptoms. Older people with schizophrenia often develop a dementia. (The prevalence of schizophrenia is rare. When it occurs, the person's history is usually known.)
- Personality disorders (neurosis) may cause the person to make statements that sound like delusions.

Anxiety and Fears. Anxiety and fears can be specific or vague, real or only in the person's mind. A partial explanation of fears and anxiety is in the brain damage itself—in the accuracy of the person's perception of reality and in a real, if inarticulate, awareness of lost capacities. *Paranoia* is a term used to describe unrealistic fears, but it is not used here because sometimes fears are not unrealistic, just poorly expressed or part of confusion. (See Exhibit 9.2.)

Delusions. Delusions are fixed, false ideas. They are symptoms of many conditions and are common in dementia. Before defining a behavior as delusional, consider whether it is a simple misinterpretation. (See Exhibit 9.3.)

Dysthymic Disorder. Dysthymic disorder is a chronically depressed mood that the person experiences most of the time for two years or more but does not meet the description of major depression. These people often say they are "down in the dumps." Because they have this condition most of the time, they say that they've "always been this way"; their families characterize them the same way. When these people develop a dementia, they may also be depressed, but the depression may be overlooked. Dysthymia responds well to antidepressants. One wife who had endured her grumpy dysthymic husband for 40 years commented, "Now that Wilbur is on an antidepressant, it's strange to hear him singing in the kitchen." Wilbur felt as if, at 68, he had been given a new life.

Hallucinations. Hallucinations are seeing, hearing, smelling, feeling, or tasting things that are not perceived by others. They are symptoms, not diseases, and have many causes. They are not evidence of being crazy. The person cannot control them. Because they produce strong sensory experiences, the person will believe them and usually cannot be talked out of them. Delirium, illness, or medications can cause hallucinations and thus may indicate serious conditions that must be investigated. Sensory deprivation can cause hallucinations. Some people with dementia experience hallucinations as a part of the disease, but other causes must be ruled out first.

People who have other mental illness (schizophrenia or depressive illness) may have hallucinations. However, this should not be considered the cause unless there is a reliable prior history of a long-term mental illness.

Some "hallucinations" are merely misinterpretation of sensory information. The "man" seen outside a window may be a combination of poor eyesight and a moving shrub. However, never overlook the possibility that the person has indeed seen a prowler or that the food actually does taste bad.

Hallucinations usually respond well to medication. However, because of the risk of side effects, avoid using medications unless the hallucination is distressing the person or causing the person to act in a dangerous way. Medication is never used until delirium and other medication reactions have been ruled out.

Lability of Emotional Expression. Occasionally one will see a lability of emotional expression that is based on the neurological damage. These people will reflect the mood of those around them and may shift rapidly from one expression of mood to another. Although this symptom is rare, it is important to be aware of it.

> Bob had experienced a past tragedy. Many years before his illness his brother had committed suicide, and Bob had found the body hanging in the barn. Being a "macho" man, he never spoke of his grief to anyone, even his wife. Now his memory was severely impaired, but he cried frequently. The facility social worker spent two half-hour sessions a week with him, helping him to express his "repressed grief." Bob was unable to express himself verbally beyond "yes" and "no." Bob would weep most of the day after these sessions. After several weeks he showed no improvement in his overall mood.
>
> A psychologist removed Bob to a quiet room to reduce stress and reminded him frequently that he was here to visit him. After chatting quietly a while, the psychologist made a mildly amusing remark. Bob laughed. The psychologist laughed. Bob laughed some more. More conversation revealed that he shifted easily from tears to laughter, following the psychologist's expressed affect. The psychologist recommended that the discussion of sad subjects be stopped and the time spent instead doing things that Bob enjoyed.

It is not always necessary to talk to work through one's grief. This man came from a culture in which talk would have been considered odd. Although we will never know, he may have resolved his feelings in his own way, or he may have talked to another man rather than his wife (the informant). Once the staff members understood this, they recognized the pattern of lability and found that they could cheer Bob up by telling him a joke (usually the same one) and by avoiding cues that would trigger sadness. When he did weep, they would be responsive and comforting for a few minutes and then encourage smiles.

Mania and Hypomania. These are the high moods that alternate with depressed moods in people with bipolar disease. A manic episode is a period of abnormally and persistently elevated, expansive, or irritable mood. Hypomania is a milder variation. They do occur in people with dementia and occasionally account for very active, grandiose behavior or for rage, hostility, and anger. Lithium, which is used to treat these states, is contraindicated in some elderly people, but other drugs are available that work well. It is easy to mistake this agitation for the similar behavior that accompanies some dementia. But the agitation common in dementia responds to reductions in stress levels, while the agitated depression more often responds to medication.

Misinterpretation. People with dementia often misinterpret information. Poor vision or hearing often compounds the problem. The solution to misinterpretations is to cheerfully solve the perceived problem. It may not be harmful to go along with the misinterpretation. Putting a person down always makes things worse. Medication is not effective. (See Exhibit 9.4.)

Obsessions, Compulsions. Obsessions are persistent ideas or impulses. Compulsions are a need to carry out a specific task (such as hand washing), often repetitively. However, the person is aware of the inappropriateness of the behavior. In people with dementia, repetitive ideas or behaviors are usually not obsessions and compulsions, and the person is not aware of the problem. For most people with dementia, repetitive behaviors are usually a combination of perseveration, not remembering having just asked the question, lack of stimulation, fears, anxieties, and misinterpretation. The problem should be treated by treating these phenomena. It is often necessary to tolerate some of this behavior.

Phobias. Phobias are irrational fears of objects or places. This is a symptom with many causes, including dementia. The person cannot control phobias, and they have a powerful effect on behavior. Arguing or explaining will not help. Some phobias, such as fear of snakes or insects, are common. Many people simply avoid snakes or insects. Other phobias, such as a fear of heights, protect us. Occasionally a phobia can endanger the person—for example, the person who is so afraid there are worms in her food that she stops eating. Avoid the stimulus as much as possible, simplify the environment, and enhance sensory cues. Some people will be reassured temporarily by "carrying off the snake" or "vacuuming up all the spiders." Sensory deficits may contribute to some phobias; for example, the "spiders" on the rug may be a pattern in the weave. Accept the person's fears and do not put him down. Reassurance and understanding is important. In severe cases, pharmacotherapy may be helpful.

Tearfulness. Tearfulness may be a response to stress rather than an expression of sorrow. To determine whether the cause of the tearfulness is stress or sorrow, move the person to a quiet place and be kind and supportive. If this works, suspect stress rather than grief. The person may say that she is grieving for her mother. Possibly she is linking her negative feelings to something she can remember as sad. If she does not grieve when she is not stressed, address the stress and then address any expression of grief that remains.

> Callie cried easily and often. The staff members were worried that she was depressed. However, they observed that she usually cried at mealtimes or in the day room when there was a lot of bustle going on. When Callie was with just a few residents and a staff member, she brightened up and sometimes would participate. Callie beamed whenever the facility dog appeared. Callie's tearfulness is an overreaction to the stress of multiple people and activity.

Overhead/Handout 9.5. How We Help

Don't intervene when it is not necessary. When a symptom is not dangerous and is not causing the person distress, consider not treating it. If a person is not bothered by his hallucinations, there is no need to treat them. Tolerate complaints. If a person often accuses the staff of stealing things, support the staff and tolerate the complaint. If a person wants her things arranged in a rigid way, do this for her. If the mirror is upsetting, cover it for a while (but don't cover everyone else's mirror).

Try nonmedication interventions first. Avoid using medications for symptoms that are known not to respond to them.

Don't argue; don't contradict. Arguing and contradicting only increase the confused person's stress and make things worse. You do not have to agree, but you can respond to the person's feelings. "It seems like your things are lost. Let me help you look for them." Or "The movements outside are scary; let me close the curtain for you."

Reassure. Because people with dementia often do not remember things for more than a few minutes, give reassurance over and over. Repeated reassurance is one of the best ways to help an anxious person.

Make success happen. People with dementia fail so much that it colors their whole life. As you do ADLs, look for small, simple ways for them to succeed. "Hold this for me. . . . Thank you."

All suffering is real. Sometimes someone's distress seems to be just fussing about nothing. But when the staff members respond in a caring way, people do better.

> A woman who had taken Valium for many years insisted that it helped her the instant she took it, and, in fact, she responded immediately, although it takes 20–30 minutes for Valium to become effective. This woman is not lying: she is suffering, and the Valium did help her, although not pharmacologically. It helped her because she believed it helped.

Hallucinations and delusions are not "real," but the experience and feelings are real to the person.

Be practical. This manual is filled with practical interventions. Try these first. Consider how the brain damage affects the person's perception of the environment. Consider how life seems to the confused person.

Use personal guarantees. Promise the person that you will not let a scary thing happen or that you will stay with the person through a distressing time. Never violate the person's trust in you. Use this to help people make transitions: "I have to go off shift now, but your new nurse will take care of you." Even when people do not understand your words, they are comforted by your tone and body language.

Write notes. Use signed notes from families or notes explaining what will happen even when the person cannot read these. Make several copies, as some may be lost. Give the note to the person to keep and read it to him frequently. Sometimes a person will know he has a note and offer it to others to read for him.

Accept what you cannot change. Things will never run as planned; weird things will always happen. Learn to be flexible.

One woman was waking in the night and going into other residents' rooms. Sleeping medication was causing her to fall. So one of the night staff members invited her into the nurses' station, gave her a cup of tea and some paper to write on, and let her hang around until she began to get sleepy.

Exhibit 9.1. Understanding Depression

We can do a lot to help people who are depressed, but first we must talk about some of the "myths" concerning depression. These are cruel myths that prevent the person from getting help or understanding. Each one puts an end to our efforts to help. When we use these myths, we write people off. We must replace them with ideas that lead toward helping.

One of the reasons we wish people would try harder to stop being depressed is that it is depressing to be around depressed people. Their misery drags us down. Once we recognize our own reaction, we can look for more successful interventions than telling suffering people to cheer up.

Myth 1. All our patients who act like that have Alzheimer disease. Some symptoms that look like dementia are actually symptoms of depression. Depression behaviors have a negative, sad, lost quality. Distinguishing between dementia and depression is the task of the mental health worker.

Depression appears to have many causes. Certain medications and physical illnesses may trigger depression. Depression may often be an early part of the dementia. Some people have had episodes of depression at other times in their lives. Thus there are many reasons why so many people with dementia are also depressed. Still, there are often ways to help these people.

Myth 2. Anybody who has dementia would be depressed. Never assume that people are really grieving because they have Alzheimer disease, because they had to move into a long-term-care setting, or because a spouse died. In fact, not everyone with dementia is depressed. But even if circumstances are enough to depress people, they should still be treated. It's true that people with dementia do grieve, but normal grieving includes a gradual readjustment and recovery. It can be very difficult to determine whether a person is grieving or is depressed. It is important not to assume that the person is just grieving. Whether the person is grieving or depressed or both, it is important to treat his suffering. Here is an example of a person who was grieving. The staff found a caring way to help him.

Tom came to the nursing home soon after his wife died. He appeared to be deeply depressed. The facility gardener made a point of visiting Tom for a few minutes every day, and soon Tom would smile in greeting. Eventually the gardener coaxed Tom outside to "help." Tom appeared to enjoy this outdoor time. Within a few months, Tom no longer seemed depressed and had found a role for himself as the tomato plant expert. Although Tom was grieving and had to make an enormous adjustment to the nursing home, he showed small signs of adapting.

Not everyone who has a dementia grieves.

A physician was interviewing a man who had Alzheimer disease. This man had been a chemistry professor. The doctor asked several mental status questions, which the man got wrong.

"How did you do with my questions?" the doctor asked.

"Oh, I missed a couple."

"How is your memory?"

"Not too good. I have what's-his-name's disease."

"Now that you are retired, what do you do with your days?"

"Work in the garden. Walk the dog."

"Overall, how would you rate your life now?"

"Life is good."

(*continued*)

Exhibit 9.1. *(continued)*

Although this once very able man knew he had missed simple questions, he was not depressed; he saw his life as good.

Often people with dementia have no awareness of their disability. These people may still be depressed.

While Jane insisted that her memory was fine, she still refused to participate in any activity, even to help with personal grooming, and she always appeared sad.

Myth 3. She's always been like that; she'd feel better if she came to activities and tried a little. If she's always been like that, she may have always been depressed.

Myth 4. There is not much we can do, anyway. It is challenging to treat people with depression and dementia, but many can be helped. The bigger problem is that there are not enough mental health people with skills in treating this dual diagnosis.

Myth 5. People can pull themselves out of it if they try. People who are grieving are doing so for a reason. It would be cruel to ask them to snap out of it. People with a depressive illness have diminished amounts of the neurotransmitters serotonin and norepinephrin in their brain. No one wants to feel this bad: if the person could change, she would. This illness is similar to diabetes in that the person needs a chemical her body is not making for her. When it is replaced by proper medication, the person often feels like her old self.

Myth 6. The medications for depression don't work/are bad for people. Some people think that it is wrong to use drugs to treat depression. This makes about as much sense as saying it is wrong to use insulin to treat diabetes. These are powerful drugs, and they can have serious side effects. This does not mean they should not be used; it just means they must be prescribed by someone knowledgeable about their use in elderly people with a dual diagnosis. When the antidepressants don't work, it may be because the wrong medication was tried or because the medication should have been used differently.

Myth 7. People need to talk about their problems. We now know that depression is caused by many things and not necessarily by something that happened in the past. Sometimes talking helps; sometimes it makes things worse. The psychiatrist or psychologist should take into consideration the person's memory span and language skills.

People with dementia may have problems remembering what they have already talked about and have problems expressing themselves. They may make up things that did not happen to cover their forgetfulness. Thus, talking it out may not be the best plan. Sometimes people with dementia get stuck going over and over the same painful issue. This rumination is not therapeutic.

Exhibit 9.2. How We Help with Anxiety and Suspiciousness

Behavioral Symptom	How We Help
Fear of losing the caregiver (refusing to let the caregiver out of sight even long enough to shower or use the toilet)	For many, the caregiver is the only sure thing in a surreal world. A second person should try to gain the person's trust so that the caregiver can have some respite.
Fear of being alone	The ill person may not be able to locate the caregiver by his voice alone or can't remember where he went. Allow time for adjustment to day care. The staff should meet the person before placement. Use one staff member as a "buddy." Repeat frequently and never lie. Reassure frequently. Give the person a note saying where the caregiver or family member went and when he will return (even if she can't read).
Anxiety about finances, future, health	Provide the person with truthful written information about where her money is. Repeat frequently. Support family. Offer to help find what is lost.
"I'm losing my mind"	If the person asks about her memory, target answer to level of comprehension and insight. If the person has insight and asks questions, answer truthfully and gently. Try: "You are becoming forgetful, but we will always love you." Answer questions about the future in the same way.
Thinks people are talking about him	May be exacerbated by hearing loss; reduce background noise; never talk across the person.
Sees strange men, prowlers	Empathize; take steps to ensure security—look around, lock doors. Assure the person that "Security" has taken appropriate steps.
Anxiety about upcoming events, such as going to the doctor, or being away from home	Avoid telling the person until the last minute; repeat frequently and never lie. Try: "I will not let you make a mistake." If the person wants to go home right after she arrives, she is probably experiencing stress. Simplify the experience, or ask visitors to come to the home.
Vague fear of failure, sense of deficits	Provide frequent reassurance, familiar surroundings. Stress is the most common cause of anxiety: reduce stress. Medication is useful in the treatment of anxiety, but because of the side effects it must be used judiciously.

(continued)

Exhibit 9.2. *(continued)*

Behavioral Symptom	How We Help
Fear of being abandoned or thinks "they" are plotting to place her in a nursing home	Be truthful and reassuring, and tell the person that whatever happens, she will be loved. Do not lie, but try saying something other than "nursing home." Give the person a note of explanation (even if she can't read).

Note: Contributing factors include medication, health problems, pain, disorientation, lack of stimulation, vague sense of vulnerability, real issues.

Exhibit 9.3. How We Help with Delusions

Behavioral Symptom	How We Help
"People are stealing my things"; "People are talking about me"; "My spouse is unfaithful"; "My mother is coming for me"; "I am in danger"; "I must get home to my children"	Always consider that these perceptions may be correct: spouses are unfaithful sometimes; theft does occur. Give the person a note stating exactly where his money is, and read it to him as often as necessary. Establish trust between family and staff. Avoid the use of medication unless the delusion does not respond to other interventions and is extremely distressing to the impaired person. Tolerate, support the family. Unlike in the treatment of other illnesses, going along with the delusion may be successful and harmless. One clinician distracted a client who wanted to go home by getting her to search through her purse for her keys. When the keys could not be found, the clinician "invited" her to stay for dinner, promising to call her daughter after dinner to bring some more keys. Try: "Tell me about your children. How old are they?" Once you have the person's trust, suggest going back to her room so she can show you their pictures. Don't point out that her "babies" are in their sixties. People who believe that they must get home or return to the office must be monitored closely to prevent elopement. Give the person a key and allow her to lock up her room or closet. Keep an extra key. Repeat frequently; do not lie. "I will be right here watching and won't let anyone come in and hurt you." Keep your promise.

Note: Contributing factors include sensory deficits, real events.

Exhibit 9.4. How We Help with Misinterpretations

Behavioral Symptom	How We Help
"Somebody stole my purse/dirty underwear, etc."	This is human nature. If a well person loses her purse, it is likely that she will wonder whether it has been stolen. However, she is able to reality-test: she knows that the people here in the room with her are not thieves; she knows that she has a habit of mislaying her things. The person with dementia no longer knows these things. Offer to help the person with dementia find her purse (and refrain from pointing out that it wasn't stolen).
"There's a man outside!"	Close the curtain or take a quick look outside. Tell people what is happening: "That noise is the dishwasher"; "That tapping outside is the wind."
"There are worms in my soup."	Don't serve this person noodle soup; fish out the "worms" or get another bowl.
"My wife's lover is in the bathroom."	Coat the mirror with glass wax until this phase passes.
"You people are talking about me."	Hearing deficits exacerbate this. Support hearing deficits: include people directly in the conversation ("We're talking about dinner tonight, John. Are you hungry?"). Never talk across the person, and never talk about the person in his presence.

Overhead/Handout 9.1. Depression

Depression is a persistent, negative, unhappy mood that may include anger or irritability.

Depression is common.

Depressed people cannot cheer themselves up.

Depression can be mistaken for Alzheimer disease.

People may deny feeling sad but complain of other things such as feeling sick.

Depression is treatable.

Overhead/Handout 9.2. Why It Is Important to Understand Depression

Depression causes suffering.

Depression shortens people's life expectancy.

Depression causes behavioral symptoms.

Depression adds to problems in concentration and memory.

Depression makes it impossible for people to get involved.

Depression affects the body.

We can find ways to reduce suffering, sometimes improve mental function, and treat behavioral symptoms.

Overhead/Handout 9.3. Symptoms of Depression in People with Dementia

The presence of any symptom that is not easily altered by attempts to cheer up, console, or reassure and that lasts at least two weeks may signal depression.

- Negative statements ("Nothing matters"; "I'd rather be dead"; "What's the use?"; "Let me die")
- Repeats the same question over and over ("Where do I go?"; "What do I do?")
- Repetitive statements calling out for help ("God help me")
- Persistent anger with self or others; easily annoyed (anger at placement, anger at care received, anger at caregiver)
- Self-deprecation ("I am nothing"; "I am of no use to anyone")
- Expressions of what appear to be unrealistic fears (fear of being abandoned, left alone, being with others)
- Recurrent statements that something terrible is about to happen (believes he is about to die or to have a heart attack)
- Repetitive health complaints (persistently seeks medical attention, obsessive concern with body functions)
- Repetitive anxious complaints/concerns not related to health (persistently seeks attention/reassurance regarding schedules, meals, laundry/clothing, relationship issues)
- Unpleasant mood in morning
- Insomnia/change in usual sleep pattern
- Sad, pained, worried expression (e.g., furrowed brows)
- Crying, tearfulness
- Repetitive physical movements (e.g., pacing, hand wringing, restlessness, fidgeting, picking)
- Withdrawal from activities of interest (e.g., no interest in longstanding activities or being with family/friends)
- Reduced social interaction
- Persistent anger with self or others

Overhead/Handout 9.4. How We Help

Use an individualized psychosocial plan.

Use brief but frequent interpersonal activities; take tiny steps.

Set the person up to succeed; protect the person from even simple failures.

Avoid complicated tasks; use task breakdown and task analysis.

Avoid long periods of isolation or boredom.

Set simple goals and keep a record; report changes to the physician.

Be patient.

Overhead/Handout 9.5.
How We Help

Don't intervene when it is not necessary.

Don't argue; don't contradict.

Reassure.

Make successes happen.

All suffering is real.

Be practical.

Use personal guarantees.

Write notes.

Accept what you cannot change.

LESSON 10

RESTORING ENJOYMENT THROUGH ACTIVITIES

Summary: Activities are an essential part of the therapeutic care of people with dementia. In this lesson students will customize an activity program to suit their facility and client needs.

Section 10.1. Making Your Program Work Better. Consists of a series of exercises that allow the team to design a therapeutic activity program.

Section 10.2. Activities and Ideas. Suggests further strategies for success in activities and suggests a range of possible activities.

Using the Sections

Introductory course:
None

Core course:
Section 10.1 required

Special audiences:
Activity staff: Sections 10.1 and 10.2

Problems You May Have in Implementing This Lesson

Activities are sometimes a lower priority for funding than other services. Thus, availability of resources may be a major problem.

As you review the exercises in this lesson, you will observe that it recommends that clients spend considerable time in activities and often in small groups. It calls for collaboration between staff members providing activities of daily living (ADLs) and activity staff members. Implementing some of these recommendations is expensive. (We also suggest many time-neutral activities.)

Programs report that money going toward more and better-trained activity staff members is well spent. It addresses behavioral problems and facilitates getting tasks done. This funding is not being used for "keeping people quiet" or "giving them something to do"; it is an essential part of successful therapeutic dementia care. Nevertheless, adequately funding activity therapy will require continued effort.

In some settings, the staff or regulatory agencies regard activity therapy as less important than nursing care. The expectations of funding and regulatory agencies may conflict with the recommendations made here. Activity therapists may encounter resistance from regulators in several areas. Address regulators' concerns through documentation. Include the specific goal of your chosen activity and why you have not chosen a "traditional" activity. It is against the law to ask nursing home residents to do domestic tasks for the benefit of the facility. Take these steps to demonstrate that a domestic task is therapeutic:

1. State the problem: Mrs. A. has always taken pride in keeping a nice home. She likes to do domestic tasks.
2. State alternatives tried: Mrs. A. is overly stressed and becomes angry in activities and thinks they are childish.
3. State the plan: Mrs. A. will be given towels to fold in a small group of three women. This provides self-esteem, satisfaction, success, and socialization. We will consult with the family before beginning. Adequate staff is available to fold the towels.

Providers may fear liability if the person falls during an activity. It is equally actionable to deny people normal and meaningful activities. Take all possible precautions without unduly restricting the quality of life. A written plan is recommended.

Some regulations hold the staff to a previously posted schedule even when the activity fails. Document in advance the need for residents' freedom of choice.

In some instances, a rigid policy of separation between nursing and activities thwarts improved client care. Make change gradually by training everyone involved and by involving nursing administration and department heads. Discuss as a group in the neutral classroom setting the process for implementation. Also discuss the ways the nursing staff can get people ready for and to an activity on time, if this is an issue.

In response to cost and the general devaluation of activities, some programs have tried to define "activities" as rehabilitative, thus forcing people with dementia into rehabilitative activities that are stressful and unsuccessful.

Some programs have placed increased responsibility for activities on aides. In fact, this lesson recommends blending the tasks of ADL care and activities. However, direct care staff members will resist having tasks added to their responsibilities. In most cases, they already have more work than time. Solving resource problems by shifting work to direct care staff members will always generate resentment. Do not plan for aides or activity staff members to undertake more work. Instead, use time-neutral interventions, or reorganize tasks and responsibilities. Ask basic questions such as: If aides are in the room during activities, what are they doing? Could they interact more therapeutically with the most impaired people in the group? Whose job is bathroom breaks? Involve activity and direct care staff members in all plans for change.

If your program determines that some activity tasks be part of daily care, it may be difficult for the care staff to plan these. The role of planning may remain with the activity therapist. Review Lesson 5. Use Exhibit 10.1.

Section 10.1. Making Your Program Work Better

Objective

The student will develop problem-solving skills to improve the effectiveness of activity therapy. Students will customize activity programs to suit their facility's and client's needs.

Information and Instructions for the Teacher

Activity therapists (not necessarily activity aides if the rest of the direct care staff members complete only the introductory course) should have completed the core course, not just the introductory course. They may choose to read the material that is not taught to the whole class or to work in small groups of colleagues. This lesson should be completed jointly by all members of the class or team, not only by activity staff members.

By this time, your students will have acquired the basic skills of caring for people with dementia. A limited amount of additional basic care information needs to be introduced in this lesson. This lesson is a series of exercises designed to help the students tailor their activity program.

There are many books on activities for people with dementia: the activity staff is cautioned to evaluate them carefully against the philosophy of this text and the criteria in this lesson. Some promote activities that are demeaning or that encourage failure.

All long-term activity plans should be reevaluated frequently as the direct care staff members observe changes in their clients. As stress declines, clients may be able to enjoy more involvement; illness or decline will also require reevaluation.

Each of these exercises will take time. Everyone must do Exercise 1. Select additional exercises for the core course and use others for in-service training. Do the exercises as a whole group if the group is small, or do them in small groups of people who will work together. The exercises can be completed in any order.

Tell the students that this lesson is different from the previous lessons. They have already learned most of the skills they need in caring for people with dementia, and these apply to activities as much as to any other aspect of care. Section 10.1 consists of a series of exercises in which they will work out how to make the best of activity therapy in their program.

If necessary, acknowledge the obstacles to activity therapy that the students will face. Reinforce the goal of finding a better way to care within what is reasonable. Emphasize the therapeutic value of activities. Even when formal recognition of the value of activities is limited, the staff members involved must value their work.

Exercise 1. Implementing Activities

Discussion

Teacher: Conduct the exercise in small groups of staff members who work together in the same program. Discuss each point. How can you implement these things?

Activity therapy is essential to good care. This means that the same commitment from funding, nursing, and other departments must be made to activities as to other services. How well does this work in your program? What can you do that is reasonable and possible?

Activity therapy *restores* positive emotional feelings such as self-esteem and in this way reduces suffering and reduces behavioral symptoms. Activity therapy identifies and uses remaining functions, no matter how impaired the individual. (See Lessons 2, 3, and 5.) When the person is too impaired to have many retained functions, activity therapy finds and restores even small retained functions. This is one reason that we call this activity *therapy.*

Plan activities that meet the guidelines for therapeutic activities. Use Overhead/Handout 10.1 in Exercise 5. Every activity will not meet all these guidelines, but most activities should meet most of them.

Process is as important as the task. How an activity is done is as important as the activity itself. Pay attention to how people, including yourself and other staff members, are behaving. How do you give instructions and involve people? Leaders should be alert to spontaneous behavior: if someone makes paper airplanes out of his coloring book, go for it. All activities are either helpful or harmful. There are no activities or ADL tasks that "don't matter." (See Lesson 5.) Discuss the meaning of process. Consider how an activity is done. How effective is process?

It is all right to repeat successful activities. People with dementia may not remember doing a task before, but they seem reassured by the predictability of repetition. Variety is not necessarily a virtue.

Focus on everyday life, simple pleasures. The routine things well people take for granted restore emotional needs and provide pleasure for those who cannot do these tasks alone.

Activities are therapeutic but rarely restore function. In response to activities being devalued by the system, some programs have tried to make them more like occupational therapy, in which the goal is restorative. This approach is often stressful for the staff and for people with dementia. It is also unsuccessful.

Avoid childishness. If you modify an activity to make it work, the goal is to make the activity feel right to the impaired person and to make it such that the impaired person can comprehend it. Analyze equipment and activities carefully so that they do not convey childishness. Some of the games, coloring books, and "activities" sold for people with dementia clearly convey the nonverbal message that the user is a child or stupid. People with dementia often will cooperate but may be harmed by the message. There are no hard-and-fast rules; however, if a person perceives a task as childish, she will feel demeaned instead of building self-esteem. The challenge is determining what message the individual perceives.

Consider carefully before you ask a person to do a simpler version of a skill or craft she was once good at (embroidery, cabinet making). She may be painfully aware of her deficits.

> For example, consider a brightly colored board for "learning" to lace, zipper, button, and put things in holes. Mr. Jones appears to enjoy it, but this activity has no purpose and closely resembles a toy. How does Mr. Jones, who is a retired businessman, feel about himself in doing this?
>
> Mrs. Smith is stringing large beads. This activity requires fine hand-eye coordination and has little social meaning. It fails with many people with dementia. Yet Mrs. Smith seeks out the activity and likes to display her handwork in her room.

Getting there can be half the fun. The two people an aide escorts to the activity are actually a small group (2:1). The aide can use this time to point out one woman to the other: "Anne, you have on your favorite red dress today. Don't you think it's pretty, Mary?"

Things such as getting washed up for dinner, putting sweaters on to go out, walking to the activity room, and waiting for a visitor are part of the activity. Use them so that they do not increase stress (a rushed or rude escort) and so that they become therapeutic. If you are getting people's sweaters on, remember how much help each needs. Remind people why they are doing this, that they will be back in plenty of time for dinner, and so on.

Restore tasks; do not take them away. People with dementia experience many losses. Use activities to look for ways to restore small tasks, nice experiences, and good feelings.

Both staff members and families inadvertently take things away from the impaired person. "She isn't using that old radio anymore." If it is not distressing her, why take it away? Her feelings of loss may be triggered by its absence.

Look for ways individuals can do more of a task. When you do advance preparation for an activity, consider whether one or two people could help with preparation. Can individuals help you with setup? Hold the dishes? Hold the door?

Make scheduling flexible. Don't expect everybody to do the same thing at the same time. Use parallel programming. Adjust workloads so that direct care staff members can help with some activities.

In a day's schedule, plan some activities that are individual, some in small groups, and some in large groups. Plan some activities that are quiet and some that are active. Let the day progress slowly but not with long intervals of idle time. Give the impaired mind time to catch up but not so much time that people tune out.

Plan continuity between tasks, and remind people where they are and what will happen next.

Stress during an activity or an ADL may spill over into the next event. If a person is upset by the shower, she may need quiet time rather than a group activity next. Conversely, when people return from an activity, they may need to be reoriented to the current ADL.

Who likes a task? When offering a men's group or a ladies' night, consider that some women really like kicking the tires on a car and some men find stacking dishes satisfying. Include people in a group based on what they like, not on their gender.

Be sensitive to the interests and values of ethnic groups. Remember that the experience of African Americans and European, Chinese, Hispanic, and Japanese immigrants in the 1930s–1950s was very different from what it is today.

Try ADLs and instrumental activities of daily living (IADL): do not focus entirely on crafts. Crafts require fine motor control, good vision, an ability to visualize an abstract completed project, and a fairly long attention span. They often do not take advantage of old skills or old roles. They require multiple steps, are often unfamiliar, and offend the generation that values work-related activities. Some people will always like handcrafts, but do not let crafts become the backbone of your program. Review any craft carefully before adding it to your plan.

Of course, you will continue to use crafts and find that some are a valuable complement to your program. Ask yourself what the goals of a craft activity are. Evaluate it with task assessment. Does it require good eye-hand coordination? Will anyone feel that she has failed? Will the person know what she is doing and why? Will the person value the end product? For example, one woman said, "What shall I do with it? Stick it on the refrigerator with my grandchild's art?"

In contrast, ADLs and IADLs are familiar, can be simplified without becoming childish, and recall old skills and feelings. Many of the suggested activities in Section 10.2 are parts of IADLs. (See Lesson 5.) It is these tasks that people have lost, and with that loss, they have lost control of their lives. Make old, familiar tasks that people can no longer do, rather than crafts, the foundation of your program.

Task

Make a plan for changes that can be implemented now, in three months, in six months. Look for small things that can reasonably be accomplished.

Exercise 2. Keeping Clients Involved

Discussion

Teacher: As you teach this, stop frequently to discuss ways these ideas are already being implemented in your program. Ask for examples.

In this lesson, participation in an activity is defined as either doing a task or actively watching others do a task. People who are walking around, appear tuned out, or are too medicated, agitated, or tired to participate are defined here as not being involved in an activity. *(Teacher: These observations are part of a student exercise and do not need to be part of the formal record.)*

Activities and ADLs can be used interchangeably to meet emotional needs. For the person who is too restless to participate in a group, dressing can be planned as a time to provide small successes and social interaction with the staff member. For the person who is upset by an ADL task, an activity can be planned to meet emotional needs, and vice versa. For example,

> One woman found dressing and bathing highly stressful despite the staff's best efforts, but the activity director found that going for a walk with a small group both calmed her and helped use up extra energy. This restored her good feelings about herself and reduced the anxiety that personal care triggered.

> The activity staff could find nothing that one man enjoyed. He was severely impaired and often overwhelmed by the group size. Because grooming is a one-to-one activity, he was less stressed by this, and his aide was able to help him do small things independently, which pleased him.

> Mr. Jones needs some opportunities to control the world around him, but he is so impaired that he must have total care in ADLs. The activity staff can perhaps find some things he can control: sanding, pounding, or raking the garden.

> Lucille seems to have lost much self-esteem. She is too impaired to do the handwork she used to do and becomes angry when asked to do most activities, which she feels are too simple for her. With cueing, however, staff members can help her dress more independently. She also likes to wipe up the lunch tables and feels this is more purposeful than the tasks activities offer.

Walter's participation was watching and tasting during a food preparation activity. He stayed nearby in a rocking chair. The activity staff kept him involved by asking him to taste or smell frequently.

In your program, how will staff members who provide daily care collaborate with staff members who provide activity therapy?

Many of the supportive things that happen do not occur during the planned group activity time. Direct care staff members are already providing brief, spur-of-the-moment ways to stimulate people. Include these in identifying the strengths of your program. For example, one gentleman liked to dance. Staff members began dancing him down the hall whenever they were going his way.

One person often began to hum. Aides would pause a moment to encourage him and to get one or two people to sing along.

Staff members took one or two people outside to look at the sunset.

When someone spilled a glass of water and one woman began to wipe it up, the aide encouraged her rather than taking over.

Events such as these keep people engaged and in touch with the world around them and are as important as the scheduled activities on the activity calendar. For some people you can plan these: "Mary is eager to be helpful. This is important to her sense of self. We will actively encourage her even when her efforts are really not helpful." "Left alone, George begins to tune out quickly. We will try seating him near the nurses' station and speak to him or hug him each time we pass."

People who are in the later stages of the disease can be particularly difficult to plan activities for.

Angie was quite impaired. She was incontinent and rarely spoke. Left alone, she drifted into a doze and became increasingly withdrawn. By the time she was up and dressed, she was often angry. To change this, her caregiver began settling Angie in the chair by her bed and bringing her an adapted cup half full of coffee, so she would not spill it. The caregiver talked to her gently and then checked on her frequently. Once Angie had fully awakened, she went to breakfast in her robe and slippers.

The midmorning activity involved too many people for Angie, so her caregiver bathed her at this time, focusing on sensory stimulation as she did so. Angie napped after lunch, but she loved the sing-along. She was seated next to the piano, which helped her focus, and the staff always commented on her lovely singing voice.

Task

Identify three people who have problems with either ADLs or activities. Determine their activity needs and plan to meet them in the most appropriate setting. Devise a documentation system that justifies your actions. Simple, spontaneous activities will not meet regulatory requirements but will help to improve quality of life and reduce behavioral symptoms.

Exercise 3. Avoiding Obstacles

Discussion

Teacher: This exercise identifies some of the things that prevent people from participating in activities. Stop frequently to discuss people with these problems and ways the group responds.

In general, as a person's mental function declines, she will need a smaller group in order to benefit from the activity. High-functioning people may participate in some activities with 20 people. As they decline, they may tune out or wander away from activities with more than 8 or 10. Very impaired people and people who are highly reactive to stress may respond only in groups of 2 or 3. Restlessness, agitation, tuning out, and walking away are good indicators that a group is too large for the individual.

Small groups are also necessary to facilitate social interactions. People who cannot remember other people or who cannot follow a discussion cannot connect with others in larger groups. In small groups of the same people, they may make friends. People with dementia may not be able to register everyone in a group. This is one reason that families complain that when the whole family visits, "She never even noticed Aunt Claire, who came so far to visit." Divide the family into smaller groups and move Aunt Claire closer.

As people decline, their attention span shortens. Shorter group activities are more effective. When a person becomes restless, it may be time to stop. Plan more frequent but shorter activities.

There is some evidence that people with dementia do not pay attention to events some distance from them. Position people within 7 to 10 feet of the leader and the rest of the group. This may be one reason that people in a large exercise circle do better with several assistants seated around the big circle. Observe whether a person pays attention when closer to you.

Take into account excess disabilities, such as vision or hearing, and short-term "bad days."

Reduce distractions. Begin by counting the distractions in the activity area.

Consider how long an individual can enjoy an activity before he becomes anxious because he needs to use the toilet.

Apathy is often a part of the dementia. Encourage people to participate in activities you know they like, but avoid forced compliance. Because people may lose the ability to initiate getting out of the chair and may not understand what you are suggesting, many will need encouragement. You must know the person to know whether you are forcing her or helping her. When people are not feeling well, their preference may be to sit still. Know when gentle support is enough.

Not everyone likes the activities offered in group living. For some, the only "real" activity is drinking beer and watching sports on television. Some consider leisure activities "wrong." Now is not the time to change these people. Try to find tasks that are modifications of what they have always done.

Stress limits a person's ability to participate in activities. An activity may stress a person one day but not the next. It may stress one person but not another. The impact of stress accumulates as the day progresses. What people can manage in the morning may not be the same as what they can handle later. It is clear that in programs that control stress all day, people with dementia can do more challenging activities, such as group outings.

Task

Review your client list and your current activity calendar. Identify three people who are having problems as a result of one of these factors. Identify three things that can be changed now.

Exercise 4. Life Goes On All the Time

Discussion

Teacher: As you discuss this material, have the group document the amount of time one person known to the group spends active/idle in a 24-hour period.

Nothing goes on in a person's life that doesn't matter. All activity or lack of activity is either beneficial or harmful. The time people spend "tuned out" or doing nothing may be harmful. If people with dementia spend more than an hour at a time unstimulated, doing nothing, or engaged in problem behavioral symptoms, the idle time is probably contributing to dysfunctional behavior that is destructive to the person as well as others.

Because the brain damage prevents planning or initiating even as simple an activity as going to the bathroom (or picking on the nurse), people with dementia spend long periods without stimulation. Even when stimulating events are going on around them, the brain damage may prevent the person from engaging in them; in fact, this may stress the person.

Some of these people seek self-stimulation. This is usually the only activity that they stumble into. It is almost certain to be an activity that the staff members don't want them to do. Eating nonfood, fighting with other residents, scratching oneself, and screaming are extreme examples that may be exacerbated by the absence of stimulation.

Other people tune out. They just sit—through activities, meals, and much else. Look at your group activities. How many people are not listening or watching? The dementia has made it impossible for them to access what is going on. But a hectic pace in which everyone is doing something every minute will be stressful to clients and staff.

The objective is to create a day that moves slowly, at a pace the person can process without experiencing catastrophic reactions; that weaves together rest, ADLs, social interchange, and visits from family; and that strengthens self-esteem and other factors of personhood, physical exercise, and pleasure but does not include long periods of idleness. Increase the amount of the day the person is involved and shorten activity periods. One or two simple tasks may be all that a person can handle at a time, and she may need to rest between them.

Task

Assess the amount of time a persons spends in tasks, activities, and sleep and the amount of idle and negative time.

How much time do people spend asleep?

How much time do they spend in ADLs?

How much time do they spend awake and doing nothing? (This includes sitting in the hall or the activity room out of touch—null behavior.)

How much time do they spend in nonconstructive problem behavioral symptoms? "Yellow zone" or catastrophic reactions?

How much time are they stimulated or involved? (Evidence of being involved or appropriately stimulated includes doing an activity/task, watching actively, eyes following the activity, smiling, tapping out a rhythm to music.)

Consider time on weekends and evenings, as well as time the person is awake at night.

Many programs find that people with dementia are spending a total of 12–14 hours doing nothing. What would happen to a person without dementia if he had nothing to do for this much time?

Identify the periods of null time on your unit. Document the need for additional staff members or other interventions to reduce behavior problems through gentle involvement.

Exercise 5. What Makes a Good Activity?

Discussion: Overhead/Handout 10.1. Guidelines for Therapeutic Activity

Teacher: This is a group discussion of activities. Make copies of a weekly or monthly calendar of activities for your program. Use Overhead/Handout 10.1. By this point in the course, the meaning of these guidelines should be clear.

Activities are intended to be therapeutic. They should meet the emotional and psychological needs of the individuals you care for. Overhead/Handout 10.1 lists guidelines for therapeutic activities. Discuss each one. What does it mean? How does it benefit people with dementia? Every activity you offer will not meet all these criteria, but for activities to be therapeutic rather than just time-filling, the majority of them should meet most of the criteria for most of the people participating.

A good way to judge the therapeutic benefit of an activity is to assess participation. How many people participate in each of the activities on your monthly calendar? Which people? Are there people who do not participate in a particular activity? Are there some people who do not participate in any activity? Is a part of the group present but tuned out?

Is bingo good or bad? What about coloring books? lacing up things? sitting and watching? The answer to which activities are appropriate for people with dementia is not in the activity itself but in how it functions. Test all activities against the guidelines in Overhead/Handout 10.1. (Avoid or modify activities to which many answers are negative.) Most activities can be modified to strengthen them. The following are examples of some activities that succeed and some that fail.

Some groups of elders enjoy bingo; others feel it is socially beneath them. For those who enjoy it, it offers a positive opportunity for a social interchange. Do not take the rules of bingo seriously. If one person fills up a card and claims "bingo," celebrate him. This is a success. Let everyone enjoy his "win," even if he wins constantly. Try larger cards for visually impaired persons, but avoid juvenile versions of the game, which will be new and confusing. For those who enjoy it, bingo meets most of the guidelines; for others, it does not confirm dignity, use old roles, or provide pleasure.

Over several weeks the group was supposed to cut out a large oval, then fringe strips of paper and glue them onto the oval. Then they were to color a picture of a cat and glue it in the middle. No one completed this activity, and few participated at all. Its purpose was not obvious, people did not remember the task from day to day, the object was worthless when completed, and the activity required hand-eye coordination and fine motor skills. In fact, it did not meet any of the guidelines in Overhead/Handout 10.1.

This activity was modified into a one-day valentine-making activity for the high school volunteers. Their photos, taken with residents, were passed around. The task itself was simplified—no cutting, fewer choices—and different styles were suggested to individuals with different abilities. The woman who repeats an activity colored in many small squares; the man who makes paper airplanes made a paper airplane valentine. Modified this way, the activity met most guidelines.

A surveyor faulted sitting on a bench as an activity because people were "not doing anything." Six very impaired residents were sitting outside in the sun watching the cars pass. The leader encouraged them to comment on the cars, and when someone in a car waved and some of the group waved back, this triggered an additional spontaneous activity. Everyone in the group was participating.

The meaning of this activity is obvious, and it is difficult to fail at watching cars. Waving is an old role, and sitting in the sun is dignified. It has only one step and is a social activity.

The leader placed a group of familiar items under a cloth, and participants were supposed to reach under the cloth and identify them by feel. The intended object of this activity was rehabilitation, but the activity failed all the guidelines, and one resident was afraid: "There might be a worm under there."

One group sang while waiting for lunch. Because most members of this group were too impaired to read, words were not handed out and there was no piano. It was a more or less spontaneous activity that an aide with a good voice led to keep people occupied while waiting.

A visitor was once trapped into leading a sing-along. The visitor could neither sing nor play the piano. One resident was recruited and played "How Much Is That Doggie in the Window" several times, but her limited repertoire soon bored the group. Hopelessly, the visitor led off another song. Some family members groped for the right key, and then a few residents joined in. After several songs, one man shouted, "You can't carry a tune in a bucket." Everyone laughed, and laughter at the visitor's tone deafness became the activity. In this example staff members were able to change a failing activity into a successful one by following the mood of the group.

Task

Make copies of the monthly activity calendar for everyone.

How many meet the guidelines?

Can the others be modified or limited to certain groups so that they meet the criteria?

Do they meet the criteria of the previous exercises?

Identify the ways you can strengthen your activity calendar now, and carry these out. Evaluate your success: Are more people participating or actively watching?

Exercise 6. Using the Physical Environment

Discussion

Teacher: There are several excellent texts on the physical environment. Direct care staff members often have little opportunity to change the physical environment; therefore, the teacher is referred to other texts, and little material is covered here.

If a person loses an arm or a leg, he may be fitted with a prosthesis—a highly engineered tool that enables him, to some extent, to do tasks he formerly did. Consider the entire physical environment to be a prosthesis for the person with dementia. Because the person is losing cognitive skills, the physical plant is designed to enable functions. However, just as a rigid, lifelike plastic arm will not be much use for its wearer, some environmental changes will only confuse or fail to help the person with dementia. They must be selected carefully by a person with a professional understanding of cognitive losses. The physical plant can never serve as a substitute for enough staff. It cannot provide either the safety or human engagement that these people must have.

The physical environment must support the staff. If staff members must run the length of the hall or bend over constantly, or if they have no lounge to retreat to when they need a break, they cannot effectively care for people with dementia.

Toilets that are near activity and meal areas are important.

For programs that have the opportunity to remodel or build a new building, the activity and ADL program components should be planned before the plant is designed.

Successful programs report that small spaces work best for small groups.

Ambiance is highly effective in providing cues about what is going on and what behavior is expected. For example, an attractively paneled room, white table cloth, and real china may enable a small group of people with behavioral symptoms to participate appropriately in a "coffee group." The presence of a child legitimizes childish games such as the Hokey Pokey. A salon makes hair care and barbering easier.

Giving medicine in a public area is an "institutional" cue. Pajamalike clothing reinforces a "sick" role. A large room with posters or colored pictures posted provides clues for a classroom for children and no indication that adults should have fun there.

Some programs provide stimulating items in the environment. Do not expect clients to spontaneously notice and respond to these. Point them out as you pass them. This is also helpful for visiting families who are looking for something to do with the client. Some programs have broken up a large space into spaces with many cues—barbershop, bar, ice cream parlor. Use them for real activities.

Our physical environments give us messages about how we should feel. Dentists' offices feel like dental offices and make us feel anxious. Ball parks send the message that it is all right to throw peanuts on the floor. Following are important messages we want the physical environment to communicate. These are all "feeling messages," and they are as important as any other aspect of the environment.

"I must be me because these are my things." Familiar items say something about who we are. As people lose their memory of their history and their recognition of their families, they need their things to help sustain their identity. Loss of identity probably contributes to bizarre behaviors. Personal possessions may also help to orient the person, and they give the staff and visitors something to talk about.

In the home the number of items may overwhelm the person with dementia. Try gathering a few treasured items and putting away clutter. Put away some photos and keep out just the one or two she responds to best.

"This feels like home." Feeling like home has nothing to do with looking like home or being home. Moreover, what feels like home to one person may not to another. One's own home may no longer feel like home. One's own things, friendly people, not too many people, pets, and quiet, familiar music all contribute to feeling like home. If the staff members feel comfortable here, clients may also.

We do different things in different spaces in our home. We also have different relationships with people in different spaces. Only those we are closest to usually enter our bedroom. People we know enter our living room. There are people we talk to in the street or yard that we would not invite into our living room and certainly not into our bedroom.

Nursing homes and residential care settings often blur these distinctions and confuse the person with dementia. All sorts of people may walk into the person's bedroom; there appear to be strangers in night clothes in the living room. Worse, there are far too many people. This contributes to people who wander in search of the "right" place.

Support privacy and arrange settings where you seat the same group of friends together. Perhaps three women can visit and have tea in one woman's room. (This suggestion requires discussion with the regulator and documentation of the fact that a person has the right to invite others into her home.)

"There are things to do here, so I feel useful." Most of us feel more comfortable in settings where we are either useful or doing something. We really do not feel we belong in places where we sit and wait.

"I feel secure here; I won't make a fool of myself." The staff won't let me get lost, not make it to meals or to the bathroom. No one will notice (or at least comment on) my failings.

"This place guides me when I am unsure." Physical cues and helpful staff members take away anxiety that leads to outbursts.

"This place says stop and rest." Can you move chairs or benches to places where people would usually sit and rest? Inside the door after a person has just climbed the front steps? Most of us don't sit and rest in the middle of a long corridor. But people will sit and watch the nurses' station. Put some seating there. Greeting the staff may be an "activity" for some low-functioning people.

"This place says 'Use the toilet.'" To send this message, the toilet must look like a toilet, and it must contrast with the walls and floor so it is visible. Experiment with signage to find out which symbol on the door works best in your facility. One program uses awnings that are visible down the hall. Wastebaskets and outside areas often send toilet cues to men. Try covering the wastebasket. Think about the particular man's habits of urinating outside. You might modify both of these to support continued independent function.

"This place says 'Come outside.'" Sometimes

people with dementia don't use outside areas. Often staff members don't use outside space because it has not been made safe for the confused person. Think about how other people in this age group use outside spaces. Porches might be more familiar than gazebos. Consider temperature and sun as much as surface areas. Divide outside space into smaller areas.

"This place says 'Join the others.'" Observe your clients. Where do they go to join others? Enhance that. In front of the nurses' station is a traditional gathering place. In front of the elevator is another. Instead of discouraging this, make this a nice area.

"This place says 'This is not a door.'" Disguise areas you do not want the person to use.

"This place says 'It smells like dinner.'" The smell of food being prepared is often lost in large facilities, yet it is one way to help people anticipate a good appetite. One husband caring at home heated a garlic clove in the oven and found that his wife ate her TV dinner with gusto.

"There are places to go here." When people don't move themselves, move them. Observe the clients: What invites them to move? Often this is staff members or caregivers.

A good floor plan guides the wandering person into areas where activities are happening and invites her to pause: the meal area (where people are often cooking or having tea), past the toilets, past the bedrooms into a small-group activity, across the garden. In this way, the person is not simply wandering along a "racetrack" design but continually being led to reenter social spaces.

"This place is my private place." This message is essential for people with dementia to function well in their environment. It is equally important for the person being cared for at home whose spouse or adult child has invaded every nook.

"And I enjoy the dog." Home, the place where we belong, includes things that are there just because we like them. Preferring cats or dogs, choosing to watch television rather than being set in front of it, being able to get a cup of coffee at an odd hour are all parts of our identity. The environment must provide them.

Task

Identify the feeling cues that will help your clients feel comfortable. When you identify sensory or cognitive cues such as signs or activity areas, ask yourself what feelings they are likely to evoke for your clients.

Identify the environmental characteristics that are most important for the staff. With the help of the administration, look for reasonable ways to improve these.

Clinical Experience

Teacher: All students should participate. Staff members who will work together should plan together. It may help to include administrators and/or the nursing director/unit director.

Using the characteristics of activities you have just discussed, do the following:

1. Identify the problems in your system that affect activities (e.g., funding, support, values, time). Be as specific as possible. Do not make this a blame or gripe session. Identifying problems should be the first step in a constructive process.
2. Identify the strengths of your program. (Include the new learning acquired in the course.)
3. Identify the things that can be changed now.
4. Identify three things that can be changed within six months.
5. Don't expect to change the world: Can you make change for a few people? Can you plan regular meetings to improve activity director's participation in care planning? Can you review one lesson for ways to introduce activity care into its goals? Can you set aside a short time or a small space for activities for a small group?
6. Begin to implement your plan, and assess how it is working.

Section 10.2. Activities and Ideas

Objective

The student will learn to develop an activity program that meets the needs of the participants.

Information and Instructions for the Teacher

This section presents additional tips for successful activities and a list of activities. Use it as resource material.

Lecture/Discussion Notes to Be Presented to the Class

Adapting Tasks and Activities: Overhead/Handout 10.2. Worksheet: Model of Task Complexity *and* Overhead/Handout 10.3. Sample Worksheets

The following two tools are essential to making activities work:

- *Task breakdown.* You can modify many activities through the use of task breakdown. Individual task breakdown was described in Lesson 5. In addition, you can break tasks down for a group so that each person does one step of the task. Note which person can do each step (remember that actively watching is participation). Get each person started on his task in sequence.
- *Task analysis.* Task analysis allows you to look at any specific task or activity and determine why it is successful or why it causes problems for certain individuals. You can then see how best to modify the task itself so that the person can continue to do it. For each task component (task steps, content elements, and body parts involved), the staff member will analyze four qualities: number, variety, abstractness, and novelty.

Definition of Terms

Task Steps. The task steps are the same as those in task breakdown. For example, in dressing the steps include selecting clothing, planning the order in which to put it on, picking clothing up, lifting feet to put on slacks, and so on.

Content Elements. Content elements are the different items or tools (clothing, soap, cutlery) used in the task.

Body Parts. Body parts are the parts of the body (arms, legs, torso, eyes) that are used in the task.

Number. How many steps, content elements, or body parts are involved in the task? There are many steps in dressing, few steps in sanding or wiping the table. Many content elements are involved in dressing, one or two in sanding or wiping the table. One uses arms, legs, eyes, and torso in dressing, arms and hands in sanding.

Variety. Will the person use the same step over and over, or are the steps different? Will the person use only one item or many? The variety of steps, content elements, and body parts is high for dressing and low for sanding or wiping the table.

Abstractness. Is this a task, item, tool, or body movement that the person must imagine, visualize, or think about? The opposite of abstractness is concreteness. Is the step obvious? Are the items or tools used immediately at hand and visible? Deciding what to have for lunch is abstract because is requires thinking about rather than doing. Craft activities that require visualizing the completed project are abstract. Choosing between hot or cold cereal when both are visible is less abstract.

Novelty. Novelty is the extent to which the task is familiar or unfamiliar (novel, new), the tools used are familiar or unfamiliar, and the movement of the necessary body parts new or an old habit. Dressing is an old, familiar task; the kinds of garments are familiar, and the movement of arms, legs, and so on are old habits. If the person who never wore sweat suits is now being dressed in them, the content elements become novel. If the person always wore skirts, then the movement of body parts to get into pants becomes novel.

Goal. The goal when modifying the activity so that the person can do it more easily is to reduce the number of task steps by breaking them down for the person; reduce the number of items or tools by handing them to the person one at a time, for example; and reduce the number of body parts the person must use (slip-on shoes do not require using fingers and arms).

Reducing variety means changing the task so that the person does or uses the same thing over and over (for example: having the person keep washing one arm while you wash the rest of the body).

Reducing abstractness means making things more obvious for the person—show the object to the person, demonstrate the steps involved. Do not expect the person to anticipate an outing or visit to the doctor until the time comes.

Reducing novelty means avoiding new tasks, new activities, unfamiliar tools or clothing. Using unfamiliar adaptive devices such as canes, walkers, or built-up spoon handles will be too novel for some people.

Suggestions such as these have been made throughout the text. Often, however, specific suggestions will not work for your person or setting. Using this model of task complexity helps you solve unique problems.

Teacher: Discuss the two examples in Overhead/Handout 10.3. Then discuss clients known to the group. It will take some practice for staff to learn to use this valuable tool effectively.

Suggested Activities

Social Activities. Following are examples of social activities; you may come up with others that will work with your group.

- Holidays (keep these low key; remember that these are sad times for some). Try selecting one special event (children coming caroling) rather than trying to create a jovial mood for a long period.
- Coffee groups, tea groups, diet groups (even if no one is on a diet, these are familiar), Hadassa groups, groups of black survivors of segregation.
- Discussion groups. Topic ideas include advice columns such as "Dear Abby" (select and read one letter, ask people to comment); questions such as "Did you like your in-laws when you were young?" or "What did you do at Christmas when you were a child?"; retelling war stories (include WACs). Controversial discussions are often popular: Are the youth today immoral? Are people drifting away from the synagogue? Will we have another Great Depression?
- Bingo (bingo is played by people who like it or who played in the past). There are no rules.

Religious Activities. Be sure the religious symbols and flowers are present and proper solemnity is provided. It is quite common for people with different religious backgrounds to enjoy the services of another faith.

- Singing familiar songs
- Going to church, joining family for special events
- Visits from clergy or other church members (if they know little about dementia, offer to give them some reading materials); private prayer, especially familiar prayers the person memorized in the past
- Praying for others if this has been a lifelong habit. This is a way people can feel useful.

Outings. Remember that people don't always have to get out of the van.

- To a shopping mall
- To get an ice cream cone
- To a park
- To church when the organist practices (less confusion than during a service)
- To ride along in the van or with administrator (a man may feel more like a man riding along to the bank than sitting in the nursing home doing nothing)
- To watch ducks
- "Spur of the moment" ride-alongs

Paid or Volunteer Work. This is a way to keep people connected to the community and to feel useful.

- Folding flyers, preparing garnishes. Break down these tasks so that each person does one step over and over: one person makes fold 1, another makes fold 2, a third staples, and so on. Tell people frequently what they are doing

and why. Ask the recipient to visit the group and thank them.
- Singing for people in a nonambulatory ward

Music, Dance. The pleasure of dancing is often retained until late in the illness; encourage the withdrawn person to tap out a rhythm. If a piano is available, some people will play it independently if they find it. Use music extensively in ADL care. Choose music from the era when those in this age group were young. Sing to a person to help her relax, to get through a difficult task, to draw her out of a blue mood. One person can turn pages of sheet music. Rhythm bands are successful in small groups, and very impaired people will use the instruments.

Outdoor Activities. Being out of doors has many healthful advantages. In climates in which weather is often inclement, use a sun room.

- Sightseeing, walking, raking, sitting, "riding along" for short distances on the bus, picking flowers, sweeping walks
- Sitting in the sun, looking at the stars or moon (good for people who are restless at night; the night air may help them go back to sleep), watching a storm, looking at clouds (ask what they remind people of or what they look like)
- Gardening; using a hose or watering can. Build planting beds with excellent drainage so that people can water as long as they like.
- Pushing a wheelbarrow, pushing a rotary lawnmower. Do not let the gardener pull the weeds out of the cracks in the sidewalk. People with dementia love this task. Set out bedding plants. One program purchased bedding plants at half price at the end of the week. That way if someone pulled them all up, not much was lost.

For some people, it is always "too hot," "too cold," or "too sunny" to be outside. Bundle people up even in warm weather. For those who do not want to go outside, try having them sit inside and look out.

Looking at the Bus or Car. This activity offers several possibilities for both men and women, such as looking under the hood, discussing tires, wiping the car down, and cleaning inside. One couple liked to sit in the back seat and hold hands.

Activities That Use Large Movements

Bowling, shuffleboard, sweeping, and raking are just some of the activities that use large movements.

Activities That Give Immediate Feedback

Certain activities provide immediate feedback. Among these are preparing food, tasting the food, grooming, weeding, and playing with pets.

Personal Care

Activities related to personal care include manicures and pedicures, hair care, and dressing. (Looking good and taking care of clothing are important to men also.)

Domestic Chores

Among the many domestic-chore activities are food preparation, sweeping, folding, wiping up, dusting, and hanging out clothes—some programs have built a clothesline outside. They report that clothes go in and out several times before they dry. Scrubbing potatoes (a good repetitive task), brushing up crumbs, using a manual carpet sweeper, polishing silver or brass (one program installed wood and brass that needed polishing), folding laundry, doing hand washing, mopping, and making beds are some suggested activities. Avoid having these look like "make work." Instead, have people "help" the staff. Consider getting housekeeping staff involved.

Visits from Children and Pets

Visits from Children. Children work with almost everyone, including severely impaired and depressed clients.

One program had a day care facility for children of the staff. Residents could go in and rock babies. Toddlers were taken for rides through the facility.

Another program invited four or five young mothers to bring their 18- to 24-month-old babies for a play group. Very impaired people sat in their reclining chairs in a circle and watched the babies. The babies mostly played with each other but sometimes approached an older person to put a toy in her lap and then take it back. People who almost never appeared active and involved responded to this play group. In some cases a staff member has brought her own young child.

Children under two are most successful. Grade school children can visit in small groups. Teach them what to expect. They will work with a client on a coloring project or singing game. Several programs have used high school students, particularly those who are having problems, as volunteers. Older people with dementia are good listeners and willingly offer love.

Pet and Plant Care. Programs have found that resident dogs, especially the large, gentle breeds, are more successful than cats. A cat needs to be very laid-back. A resident pet must have a real owner who takes responsibility for its care and becomes its leader. Dogs need a leader to focus on. A dog with no specific owner does not function as well.

Rabbits make excellent pets. They like to be held, can be housebroken, and in many areas can live outdoors in an atrium area.

Fish and birds do not approach the ill person and cannot be cuddled, so they may be ignored. Birds that repeatedly produce babies are more successful than purely decorative ones. Parrots can bite. In some communities, organizations or private individuals will bring an assortment of animals to visit. Staff pets may also visit.

Toys

There has been controversy over whether people with dementia should be given dolls, stuffed bears, and the like. The answer is in how the item is treated by the staff. Is it a shared pleasure, or is it evidence that the person is childlike? The same item may communicate either message. Older men may enjoy, with dignity, model trains. Similarly, adults may enjoy a collection of stuffed bears, doll houses, antique cars, or dolls. When the impaired person's interest is addressed in the same way, the items can provide great comfort and reassurance. If the confused person thinks her baby doll is a real child, consider carefully how the staff should handle this, rather than using a policy to decide what to do. In some settings, it clearly is important to the ill person; in others, the staff behavior is patronizing.

Television

People with dementia have difficulty following the dialogue on television, and the rapid cuts may confuse them. A few people may perceive the events on television as real and be afraid of being attacked. Separate these individuals rather than prohibit television for everyone.

Television is not useful as a sitter. Look into a room where people with dementia are watching television. How many of them have tuned out? Try commercial videotapes (musicals work well) or videotapes made by family members. Television and videos will be more successful if staff members or family members join the confused person in watching them. Use selected bits of television programs to start discussions with high-functioning groups.

Activities That Use Old, Overlearned Motor Skills or Repetitive, Rhythmic Tasks

Sanding, rocking, scrubbing potatoes, and brushing lint are examples of such activities. Some people will want to color the same page over and over. Try a pattern design that can be linked into a long chain of successful art.

Activities That Use Old Memories

A person who was about 80 in 2000 was born just after World War I, will remember the depression well, was a young adult during World War II, had sons who fought in the Korean War, and formed adult ideas during the Cold War. Be sure you select films, songs, and other items that suit the ages of your group. The things that today's younger people think are antique and that middle-aged people think are simply "old" were the items of daily life for this group.

Try looking at antiques and old valentines, videos of old TV programs and old movies, old newsreels. Invite the owner of an antique store or a local museum to bring a few items. Remember the special issues for ethnic groups: being black in the 1950s, Martin Luther King, gospel music, the Japanese of this period who survived the internment camps, the invasion of China by the Japanese during World War II. Hispanic families may recall tiny villages, immigration.

Activities to Avoid

- Tasks that require decisions or several steps (crafts that require decisions about which item to select, what step is next)

- Tasks that are new to the person (using modeling clay, finger paints, listening to contemporary music, crafts the person does not usually do)
- Tasks that convey a childish message (childish games, puzzles, or activities that use children's supplies, crayons, colored markers)
- Tasks that depend on lost skills (commonly relying on verbal language when language has been compromised, fine motor skills [e.g., paper folding], judgment)
- Tasks with unpredictable elements
- Tasks that require abstract thought, math, or visualization
- Tasks that encourage "tuning out"

Maintain an Activity Profile and Document Enjoyed Daily Routines

Use these two steps to develop a flexible and ongoing activity plan. Update whenever planned activities fail for as much as a week when the person is not ill.

Know the Individual

Know as much about the individual as the direct care staff members do.

Through observation, keep a record of the individual's approximate attention span and fatigue level.

Be aware of group-size tolerance: the maximum number of people that the person can tolerate in the group.

Note an individual's activity choices/preferences.

Know a person's preferred level of activity: sitting quietly? Laughing and playing a game?

Determine the person's level before illness: sedentary, moderate, active.

Late life can span 20–30 years. Know what the person's interests were shortly before she became ill as well as in the more distant past.

Know whether the person is in pain or depressed, what her best times of the day are.

Exhibit 10.1. Suggestions for Blending Activity and Other Care

Ideally, activity personnel and other staff members cooperate so that all care is therapeutic. There are many ways to do this. The following list offers only a few suggestions.

- Plan therapeutic interventions according to the client's abilities (see Lesson 5). Pleasure, self-esteem, and other emotional needs are met both during activities and during personal care. For example, if the person benefits from a small social group, she will be scheduled for this. If she is too stressed by a group, her direct care provider will try singing with her as care is provided.
- Accept that direct care staff members already have a full schedule. They must be included in planning any change. Do not plan for aides to undertake any more work unless there are trade-offs.
- Find ways to strengthen the policy that all staff members and administration value both activity time and ADL time as therapeutic opportunities to meet emotional needs.
- Try having direct care staff members include 1–5 minutes of activity time in their daily care.
- Try using noncare staff members as volunteers. See Lesson 7.
- Determine whether the activity therapist can change to another activity easily, whether supplies are nearby, whether she can leave the group to get them.

Overhead/Handout 10.1. Guidelines for Therapeutic Activity

Therapeutic activity

- has an obvious purpose and meaning for a person;
- offers a reasonable chance of success;
- reestablishes old roles;
- confirms dignity (it must never be perceived by people as childish or inappropriate to their social status);
- offers pleasure;
- does not reinforce inadequacy or add to anxiety;
- is individualized;
- is voluntary;
- capitalizes on remaining abilities;
- breaks tasks down into steps;
- meets basic human needs for identity, mastery, and self-esteem; and
- encourages social interchange.

Overhead/Handout 10.2. Worksheet: Model of Task Complexity

	Task Components		
Feature	*Task Steps*	*Content Elements*	*Body Parts*
Number			
Variety			
Abstractness			
Novelty			

Source: Weaverdyck 1991.

Overhead/Handout 10.3. Sample Worksheets

Mr. Frank laid out his wife's clothing, in order, and talked her through dressing. Then Mrs. Frank began refusing to get dressed. The home care worker surmised that she was no longer able to manage this level of complexity. For Mrs. Frank, the number and variety of tasks had become too great even though the task was still familiar and concrete. The home worker suggested ways to lower the number and variety of tasks.

	Task Components		
Feature	*Task Steps*	*Content Elements*	*Body Parts*
Number	high	high	high
Variety	high	high	high
Abstractness	low	low	low
Novelty	low	low	low

Jason "tuned out" through most activities. The staff members evaluated the ball toss, which they had thought was quite simple. When they finished the task analysis, they realized that this activity was too complex for this man. Tossing the ball back and forth only between the leader and Jason and using intensive cueing helped him.

	Task Components		
Feature	*Task Steps*	*Content Elements*	*Body Parts*
Number	high: catch, hold, aim, select a person, throw, regain balance	high: ball, 15 people to choose from	high: hands, eyes, legs for balance, torso
Variety	high, as above	high: as above	high: as above
Abstractness	low	high: deciding whom to throw to was too abstract for Jason	low
Novelty	low	high: for a retired farmer, ball toss was novel for Jason	low

LESSON 11

THINKING THROUGH CHALLENGING BEHAVIORS

Summary: The skills for preventing and treating behavioral symptoms have been taught in the previous lessons. This lesson links that material to behavioral symptoms and presents new concepts. Behavioral symptoms are characteristic of dementias and thus cannot be entirely eliminated. However, they can often be modified to reduce the patient's suffering or the burden placed on others. The term *treatment* is used because it implies that, although the underlying disease may not be cured, specific symptoms can be alleviated. Although this lesson was written for staff members, this material is of importance to policy makers, administrators, and planners.

Section 11.1. Facts about Behavioral Symptoms in Dementia. Discusses principles related to behavioral symptoms. Some of these points have been made elsewhere, but it is necessary to reinforce them in planning treatment of behavioral symptoms. This section will be useful for policy makers and planners as well as direct care staff members.

Section 11.2. Strategies for Intervention. Discusses treatment approaches including knowing why the intervention is needed, the six Rs of behavior management, behavior modification, and agenda behavior.

Section 11.3. Addressing Wandering. Discusses intervention strategies—wandering behaviors are used as a model for symptom management.

Section 11.4. Information about Sexual Behaviors. Addresses general principles of managing issues related to the sexual behaviors of people with dementia.

Section 11.5. Behavioral Symptoms in the Acute Care Setting. Offers brief suggestions for coping with behavioral symptoms in acute care. These situations differ significantly from other care of people with dementia because patients in acute care often have delirium. Intervention is different from the care of people with dementia.

Using the Sections

Introductory course:

None

Core course:

Optional review

Section 11.2 required
Section 11.3 required
Special audiences:
People responsible for diagnosis, assessment, referral, and treatment; management: entire lesson, including Sections 11.1 and 11.4
Policy makers, planners, administrators: Section 11.1
Acute care staff members: Sections 11.2, 11.3, and 11.5 required

Problems You May Have in Implementing This Lesson

The resources needed for this lesson are the same as for all the previous lessons: an adequate, well-trained, and well-supported staff. Plant design that supports the staff as well as clients is important. Administrative commitment is essential. None of these resources is ever readily available; however, taking whatever small steps are possible toward understanding the nature of the client's disability and sustaining that person's self-esteem result in small reductions in behavioral symptoms. Use this text as a reference to help in the identification of those steps that are possible for your program.

Behavioral symptoms will never be eliminated completely, and this should not be a goal. In a few people, behavioral symptoms will remain serious or disruptive. The group as a whole, however, will show improvement with good care.

Staff support is a key to reducing behavioral symptoms. Staff members must be able to trade tasks when the needs of one person are exhausting. Staff members must be able to retreat briefly when they are caught in a conflict with a client. The staff must be reminded that the elimination of all "problems" is less the goal than is improving quality of life to the extent possible. Alternatives such as a secure unit and the option of removing the group from an upset client should be in place. Staff support for the home care worker who is alone in the home with a distressed client is more difficult to plan. An effective evaluation, a gradual transition from family to home care worker, a consistent home care worker who knows the client, and emergency backup are necessary.

A change in behavioral symptoms is often gradual, with only slight evidence of change at all. Supervisors can help by pointing out slight changes and ensuring that information is transferred across shifts and across caregivers. In the progressive dementias, behavioral symptoms such as eloping or refusal of care will eventually be lost as the individual declines further.

Treatment is more successful—and more easily measured—when addressed on a unitwide basis than on an individual basis. As stress levels decline and the general ambience of a unit changes, staff members and visitors will feel more comfortable.

A planned case mix reduces the possibility that one or two clients will significantly upset the rest of the group. It also protects the staff from the demands of managing several very difficult clients. For example, one person who is at risk of eloping can be monitored, but even a high concentration of staff members cannot monitor several such people and still provide good care to the rest of the unit. Some facilities are restricted in their freedom to select a suitable new client for a unit. However, the financial costs and risks of a poor case mix often outweigh the costs of holding a bed open briefly.

A major problem in this lesson and others is that policies at all levels define personal care and health care more effectively than they define the vaguer concepts of self-esteem, rights of impaired individuals, or freedom of choice as weighed against safety. At every turn administration is faced with choices and the need to defend them. There are no easy cures for this.

Section 11.4 may be difficult to present to students. Sexuality in elderly and impaired people is a highly emotionally charged issue. Students and teachers may feel awkward with it, and occasional client behaviors are very upsetting. An open and matter-of-fact approach is most successful.

Section 11.1. Facts about Behavioral Symptoms in Dementia

Objective

Students will learn key factors to consider in addressing behavioral symptoms.

Information and Instructions for the Teacher

Students and programs often want to proceed directly to coping with serious behavioral problems. You may be tempted to teach this material before completing the previous lessons. *Do not do this.* The nonmedical skills necessary to manage behavioral symptoms have all been taught in the preceding lessons. This material will not be helpful by itself.

Use the list of concepts in planning care. This information is basic to understanding and approaching behavioral symptoms. Much of it has been presented in previous lessons; however, it is necessary to emphasize it again here in planning treatment of behavioral symptoms.

In teaching the management of behavioral symptoms, reinforce these concepts either as a separate review or as you teach Sections 11.3 and 11.4. Keep this list of issues in mind, and remind students of them as concerns are raised.

Lecture/Discussion Notes to Be Presented to the Class

Concepts

Behavioral symptoms are often complex in cause and result from the interaction of multiple factors. Even when staff members find a cause for a behavioral symptom, the behavior may recur. The staff will then gradually find other factors. Multiple causes make the challenge greater, but the staff need not be discouraged if first efforts do not fully succeed.

In planning care, always keep the goal of a sum of small changes in mind. Programs that achieve a significant reduction in problem behavioral symptoms have found that this allows for success despite limitations in physical plant and occasional staff mistakes.

Staff members are not perfect. Even in the best facilities, they are sometimes tired, irritable, or under stress. They say and do the wrong things. But in settings in which the clients are well supported in sum, clients demonstrate a surprising resilience.

Caregivers find that thinking in terms of increasing positive factors is more successful than focusing on the negatives. Instead of asking, "How can we get him to do that?" good staff members ask, "What can we do to help him enjoy life a little bit?" There is a positive side to everything we have discussed in this course: placing fewer demands on lost skills and supporting retained functions; keeping the person as well as possible; ensuring comfort instead of adding to stress; providing stimulation that the impaired brain can enjoy; and applying these principles through activities of daily living (ADLs), through the use of retained language and nonverbal communication, through sustaining family roles and supporting friendships with staff members and others, by supporting emotional needs and treating depression, and by using activity therapy to restore good feelings.

Behavioral symptoms that are not dangerous or disturbing but appear as apathy, total disengagement, seeming tuned out, sitting with eyes closed, lying in bed awake yet seeming to be unaware, staying in bed asleep more than usual for that person, or making little response to staff care are important indicators of client problems. They may indicate illness, feeling overwhelmed by stimuli, the absence of positive stimuli the impaired brain can understand, or the loss of communication skills. Staff members should take these indicators seriously. For many, the progression of the illness includes apathy, but this does not mean the person does not need appropriate stimulation. Forcing the person to participate against her wishes is not appropriate, but these clients may still respond to gentle, one-on-one touch and sensory stimulation offered at short, frequent intervals.

Some clients respond to illness by becoming sweet and docile and may accept even degrading interpersonal treatment. While this makes their care easier for the staff, it does not meet the client's needs.

Preventing a behavioral symptom is much easier than treating an existing one. It is safer for the client, other clients, and the staff. This makes prevention cost-effective.

The behavioral symptoms will return if the intervention is stopped (except for certain excess disabilities). Just as an amputee will always need a wheelchair, the person with dementia will always need a prosthetic environment. The person will not learn a new response in the absence of the intervention, and the intervention will not "cure" the behavior. To date, many funding sources ignore this reality.

Behavior changes as the disease changes. Some behaviors, such as pacing or repeated questions, will be lost as motor skills or language is lost. This means that annoying behaviors will pass in time. It also means that new behavioral symptoms may arise. Late in the illness, the client may not be able to respond, but a worsening of the illness should not be assumed as the cause without medical confirmation.

Caregivers will not always know how to help the person (for example, they may not be able to understand what the person is asking). Sometimes little can be done for the person. Sometimes limitations of budget or physical plant prevent the caregiver from helping effectively. Administration and supervisors must support caregivers. Caregivers cannot be held responsible for what they cannot do.

There is a role for psychoactive medication in the treatment of problem behavioral symptoms. It is valuable when used as a part of an integrated care approach, but only if someone's safety is in danger should it be used in place of other strategies. Medications are useful in treating symptoms that distress the person with dementia.

Although many behavioral symptoms reflect the distress of the person with dementia, some do not. For example, leaving the facility may be, in the ill person's mind, taking a pleasant walk.

Bizarre symptoms quite often reflect a severely dysfunctional environment. Behaviors such as screaming may be the person's effort at self-stimulation in an environment that provides no stimulation that the impaired person can comprehend. Screaming may also reflect unrecognized pain. Smearing feces is usually an unsuccessful effort to clean oneself. When it is regarded as "regression" or "disgusting," the problem is with staff attitude instead of with the client.

Even when the person has had similar dysfunctional behaviors before developing a dementia, she can no longer voluntarily change them. Treat these behaviors the same way you would treat new behaviors.

Reasons for changing a behavior and the strategy chosen should be charted. Success must be documented and shared. Many staff members dislike charting, and some programs fear documenting failures, but good record keeping tells the staff members they are succeeding and prevents blundering with the next person or situation. Documenting failures narrows the field of interventions that can be tried and often provides clues to success. Administration and regulators need to permit this.

Try focusing on change in the entire unit rather than in one difficult individual. A few individuals may be quite difficult to change, but focusing on reducing behavioral symptoms for the entire unit will reduce stress levels for everyone and improve the quality of life for the staff and residents.

Behavioral symptoms in dementia cannot be completely eliminated. They are a fact of life for many people with dementia. However, many symptoms can be reduced, and the suffering or risk associated with these symptoms is reduced as well. For example:

> At one excellent dementia unit one morning, two people wander aimlessly, several would become angry and resistant if pushed to dress or bathe, and one gentleman has lost his pajama bottoms. The staff sees these not as behavioral problems but as the nature of care. The ambience of the unit is pleasant. Staff members interact frequently with those who wander, avoid pressing people to do a task immediately, and repeatedly replace the pajama bottoms.

Section 11.2. Strategies for Intervention

Objective

The student will learn intervention strategies for treating behavioral symptoms.

Information and Instructions for the Teacher

This section presents five strategies for addressing problem behaviors. The student will use these strategies in addition to, but never in place of, the material taught in Lessons 1–10. These strategies present useful ways of thinking about behavioral symptoms. Teach all or those that meet your group's needs. Use the overheads/handouts, and ask the group to discuss points as you go along. Use examples from your own knowledge or the previous text. Remind the group to use specific descriptions of behaviors rather than vague terms such as "gets upset a lot" or jargon terms such as "acting out" or "resisting care" and to avoid terms that put a value judgment on the behavior.

Lecture/Discussion Notes to Be Presented to the Class

Overhead/Handout 11.1. Know Why You Want to Change a Behavioral Symptom

A first step in addressing a problem behavioral symptom is that the caregivers must know their motives in changing or trying to change another person's behavior. The fact that it is wrong or strange is not sufficient. For example:

> A man who insisted on carrying a purse was admitted to a facility. It was not clear what this behavior implied or why it was important to him, but it made the staff members uncomfortable, so they took away the purse. The man gradually sank into a deep and irreversible depression. Losing his purse was an unnecessary loss.

There are many reasons why a behavioral symptom becomes a problem that needs to be changed:

- *To ensure the safety of the client, the staff, and other clients.* Some behaviors obviously and immediately place someone at risk. Staff members must usually act quickly to stop such behaviors. *Teach staff members how to avoid being hurt.* Environmental modifications can be helpful: secure facilities, stairs that the person cannot access and fall down, safe storage of dangerous items. Prevention of catastrophic reactions will reduce hitting, pinching, and grabbing. The right of the person with dementia to safety must be balanced by the right to quality of life. Although safety is a major concern, management must be careful to not generalize this to a policy that is unnecessarily restrictive, for example:

> Some of the clients in the day care center would wander away if not closely supervised. John, however, liked to sit outside and smoke. He never left the porch. Restricting him from "wandering" would be inappropriate. Closely monitoring him for a change in behavior was more appropriate.

> The residents in one facility were restricted from using the walled garden unsupervised because the facility was afraid they would trip and fall. However, all these residents walked well and none had a history of falling.

> In one facility residents enjoyed sitting outside in the shade of a tree (in a secure garden). The tree was cut down because regulators feared someone would trip over its roots (no one ever had). After that no one wanted to sit outside in the hot sun.

- *To provide for the comfort of others.* Some behavioral symptoms are so distressing to other residents or staff members that they cannot continue. Such behaviors might include masturbating in public, spitting on others, undressing others, or grabbing female staff members' breasts. Efforts to address such behaviors should seek to rechannel or redirect (see below) such activities rather than stop them.

> One woman rolled her skirt up into a wad that exposed her panties. One man kissed (on the cheek) most of the women. Some of them liked it, but a few were upset.

If possible, the staff should find a way to permit such behavior because taking it away may lead to a more distressing behavior. The family purchased some longish ruffled panties for the lady. In the man's case, when he approached the women who did not like to be kissed, staff members diverted him by asking him for a hug.

- *To control behavior that violates others' rights.* Such behaviors can create serious difficulties. Every effort should be made to avoid impairing the self-esteem of either party.
- *To meet quality assurance standards* or community expectations. Marketing, quality assurance, and the opinions of others are legitimate reasons for changing a person's behavior, but when doing so causes unnecessary stress, negotiation is necessary. Family and visitors can be told that patient comfort ranks high among the facility's goals. Documenting alternatives tried and the client's distress may help with regulators. These situations must be evaluated individually. Certainly not everyone should be wandering around in a scruffy nightgown, and no one in a revealing one, but one person may be the exception to standard policy.
- *To control costs.* Cost will always be a factor in the management of behavior, primarily because adequate staffing is necessary to address behaviors and staff members are expensive. Cost is a legitimate reason that some behaviors must be restricted. In facilities where reimbursement rates are low, the potential for excellent care is limited. However, cost is more often an issue of prioritizing. Sometimes facilities with excellent staff levels focus on a hospital-like style of care that uses staff time inappropriately for people with dementia.

Case mix is another way to address this problem. A reasonable staff ratio may be able to handle a case mix including one person who wanders, one who whines, and one who quickly escalates to hitting. The same staff members will not be able to watch six people who wander or six who whine constantly (staff members report this behavior as one of the most stressful).

These issues are usually out of the hands of direct care staff members, but even when budgets are restrictive, creative management can make surprising things happen.

- *To provide relief to the caregiver, family, or staff.* When a family caregiver is providing care, behavioral symptoms sometimes must be stopped so that the caregiver can continue without burning out or becoming exhausted. For example:

Lana was awake much of the night and sorted through the things in her room or the kitchen. Her husband was frantic, and the physician sedated Lana so that the home caregiver could continue.

There are a few people with dementia who drive the staff crazy. The motto might be that these people deserve love too. But so do staff members. Staff members will need good support, the opportunity to trade off so that each one has time away from this person, and a review of case mix that might relieve staff stress.

- *To improve the quality of life for the person with dementia.* Staff members often must decide between what a person seems to want and what is best for him. Think carefully about whether you are making absolutely necessary decisions for a person or unnecessarily inflicting your values and opinions on him. Look for compromises.
- *To make patient care easier.* This, too, is a legitimate goal. Staff resources, both physical and emotional, are limited. There is a limit to the number of times a staff member can walk the length of the hall, backtrack, answer the same question, respond to whining.

Overhead/Handout 11.2. The Six Rs of Good Care

Busy staff members often think only in terms of stopping a behavior. The six Rs are a quick way to review other ways to intervene.

Stopping a behavior or preventing a person from doing it is often the first thing we think of, but many times it is not the most effective. *Restricting* (stopping) a behavior is most appropriate when the behavioral symptom places the person or someone else in danger. When staff members have time to think about ways to intervene, they should consider the other five Rs.

Reconsider a behavior from the point of view of the person who is doing it. Ask, "If I were in his shoes, how would I respond? How must he feel? What is he trying to accomplish?"

Find a way to *rechannel* the energy or emotional need that leads to a behavioral symptom by getting the person involved in another activity that meets his needs. Rechannel restless behaviors into focused activity. Physical activity or interpersonal time often works well. People with a short attention span will respond for only a few minutes, but even this will help.

A man pounded with his coffee mug on the arm of his chair. This behavior became a problem when he broke a cup. A staff member got him a softer item, which rechanneled this perseverative behavior rather than stopping it.

Most perseverative behaviors are responsive to rechanneling.

Redirect people into places or actions that are appropriate. Some behaviors are appropriate when the person is redirected to a private place or into a similar activity. *Remind* a person to wear her robe, or redirect her to eat off of her own plate.

After any tense or angry episode, the person with dementia may appear to have forgotten the incident immediately but may be left with lingering negative feelings. Immediately after such an incident *reassure* the person that she is all right and that you will not reject her. Try saying, "Well, we got in an argument, but we're still friends." This helps to reduce lingering feelings of anxiety that can accumulate into another outburst later.

After any problem behavioral event, *reassess* what happened, what triggered the behavior, what it meant to the person, and how it can be avoided. Try thinking it through by yourself, talking to other staff members, reviewing the chart for previous solutions, or role-playing the event to identify triggers and better interventions.

Use Behavior Modification

Behavior modification is a highly effective method of changing the behavior of animals, children, and other people. Behavior modification requires considerable skill and training and can be harmful.

There are differences of opinion over the effectiveness of behavior modification. Some research shows it to be effective, but other researchers argue that the only behavior that gets modified is that of the staff members. Behavior modification assumes that the person can learn and remember what the response will be to his behavior. These cognitive skills are impaired in people with dementia. Behavior modification, like all interventions, may be more effective with some people with dementia than with others. When you use behavior modification, keep in mind that people with dementia are less likely to learn to respond to behavioral feedback when they are anxious or stressed and that a person's agenda may override the behavioral intervention. For example, if a person feels trapped in a "frightening and strange place," her need to escape will override behavioral efforts.

Avoid behavioral interventions that interfere with treatment. For example, staff members denied friendly conversation to a person who quickly became upset and struck out. This intervention canceled the therapeutic value of interpersonal activity and failed to identify the cause of the person's increased stress.

Avoid negative reinforcement (punishment or ignoring) with people with dementia because their need for self-esteem is so great.

Sometimes the staff and the person with dementia live in different worlds. For example, a naval captain thought he was commanding his crew, but the staff thought he was bossing the other residents. Behavioral modification will not alter his perception. A better plan is to allow him his opinions but protect the others. One person said, "Captain, sir, they are on shore leave."

Use Agenda Behavior

Agenda behavior is a powerful tool. People with dementia often have a reason (agenda) for what they do. Their reason may not make sense to us, but it does make sense to them. This strategy seeks to identify the reason for the person's behavior and honor that reason while redirecting the behavior. Good care always tries to recognize the person's agenda because this helps to sustain personhood and identity.

Examples of agenda behavior include eloping, which may seem to the person that she is going home. Resisting a bath may seem reasonable to the person who thinks she already had a bath.

> In one facility, a man was stopping the staff from entering the facility in the morning. The staff figured out that because he was a retired border guard, he thought the staff members were illegal aliens. He was only doing his job. Giving the staff false "green cards" to show him solved the problem.

> One man tried repeatedly to leave a locked facility and eventually took the door off the hinges. The staff put him in a reclining chair with the tray across his lap. However, he slid out of the chair and eloped again. This time, the staff restrained him in the chair with a Posey restraint. They discovered him going down the hall with the chair tied (by the Posey) to his back. In this case, trying to stop the behavior was unsuccessful, despite strong measures. This man had his own agenda for leaving: he had to get back to his job.

Being with Someone

Sometimes what the person with dementia really needs is someone to just be with him without taking any specific action. Human beings find comfort in the presence of another. When a person is ill, stressed, or late in his illness, a shared presence is especially comforting. In many cultures, members of the community simply sit with women in labor, the ill, and the dying. But simply being with a person with dementia is difficult for most of us. We want to do something. Often in the late stages of the dementia or when a person is distressed, there is nothing we can do. Do not underestimate the importance of simply being with a person and taking no action beyond sharing your presence.

> One woman was either restless or tuned out most of the time. The staff tried many ways to reach her without success. Finally, one staff member found time to sit quietly with her or walk with her for two or three minutes occasionally. The staff felt strongly that this simple approach was comforting for her.

Section 11.3. Addressing Wandering

Objective

The student will learn how to implement interventions taught in the previous sections and previous lessons when the behavioral symptom is complex and has multiple causes. Wandering behaviors are used as an expanded case example.

Information and Instructions for the Teacher

In this section, wandering will be used as an example behavior in discussing the intervention concepts covered in this text. Wandering is a difficult behavior to manage. It does not respond well to medications and has many different causes. It is very common. Discuss wandering by using the strategies you have taught previously: Ask your group to select individuals known to them and to consider what causes this behavioral symptom in this individual; is it part of a catastrophic reaction? Is it a response to excess disability? Is it a result of brain damage? When can it be simply accommodated? Is it the result of multiple causes? Is psychoactive medication a reasonable approach? Can the six Rs help? When is safety an issue? Is it agenda behavior? Teach the text as a discussion or break the group into small groups to discuss individuals known to them. When the cause of an individual's wandering is unclear, try role play or try videotaping the behavior and reviewing the video in class.

Lecture/Discussion Notes to Be Presented to the Class

Describe the behavior in more detail. Exactly what is the person doing? Is it idle wandering? agitated wandering? an effort to elope? an invasion of others' space? Each type has its own probable causes and intervention strategies. Use Overhead/Handout 4.7 to gather more information about the behavior.

Idle wandering is often caused by lack of appropriate stimulation or a need to be moving around. Can you provide other stimulation that the person can understand without being unduly stressed? Can you provide time outdoors in a secure setting, outdoor tasks, walks? When idle wandering is not caused by long periods without stimulation, is there any need to intervene?

Agitated wandering is often part of a catastrophic reaction—often to a prolonged level of excessive stress. Can you reduce the stress? Restless wandering is often a part of the illness. When it is not an indication of too much stress, is there any reason to intervene?

Eloping (leaving the facility) is a normal behavior in well people. For the person with dementia, this continues to feel like a normal behavior; for the staff, this behavior places the person at risk. Successful interventions allow the person to maintain his agenda without danger. They include distractions and white lies. Reminding people to check that they have their car keys, enough money, or a purse often distracts them.

> One strong man was determined to climb the fence. The staff member told him this was "against the law." This reminder deterred him for a few minutes (long enough to get help). On one occasion the cook saw him setting a chair beside the fence. She dashed out and sat in it, thanking him profusely. His natural courtesy kept him from tossing the cook.

There is regulatory policy, as well as continuing debate, regarding secure facilities. There are also buzzers, bells, bracelets, and tracking devices that can help. In planning and regulating security, several facts must be considered.

- People who cannot plan for themselves need a secure setting.
- Increased staff, smaller unit size, and case mix can make it easier for the staff to constantly keep track of a few people with a tendency to elope.
- Despite all these strategies, people who are determined to leave a facility may well succeed. No security device is a substitute for human supervision.
- Treating wandering people with medication may result in a person still determined to leave but who is additionally unsteady on her feet.

- It is absurd to expect staff members to provide loving care and ADLs and cope with the constant anxiety that a person may leave, fall, or be injured. The needs of staff members must be considered in planning interventions.
- Have a plan in advance to respond if a person leaves the facility. Who coordinates communication between searchers? Who stays with the other residents? When will you call family? police? It is often successful to send one person out to simply walk along with the client without making any effort to get the person to return. This protects the person while she unwinds. If necessary, the staffer can walk along a few steps behind the person. Then a second staff member can "accidentally meet" the two and invite them both back for a treat.
- People who enter other people's space are causing a problem not for themselves but for others. Monitoring this behavior with adequate staffing and smaller unit size is the least intrusive intervention. Personal items may be secured in a person's room. "Out of order" signs sometimes help.
- A desire to leave is often triggered by observing others, visitors or part of the group who are getting ready to go out. Exiting through a cloak room that is not visible from the unit is helpful. This is a particular problem for day care, where some clients leave earlier than others.
- Review Lesson 2. Wandering behaviors are often triggered by the behavior of others or the sight of a door.
- People who wander and who are living at home present a different set of issues. The family caregiver must have respite from the constant demand of monitoring the person.

Section 11.4. Information about Sexual Behaviors

Objective

The student will learn to think about sexual behaviors in terms of the needs of the person with dementia.

Information and Instructions for the Teacher

This section is targeted to the staff responsible for diagnosis, assessment, referral, and treatment, who can teach it to direct care staff members as needed. (Also see Section 7.3.)

Lecture/Discussion Notes to Be Presented to the Class

Sexual issues trigger greater anxiety in both teachers and direct care staff members than do other issues. Many people are uncomfortable with sexuality in people who are disabled or elderly (or both). In fact, many people are uncomfortable with their own sexuality. A basic task for the teacher is to make these behaviors as routine as other problems. Role-model a calm, matter-of-fact approach, but avoid reprimanding staff members who giggle or have biases. A relaxed role model allows students to leave their tensions behind.

When faced with sexual behaviors, everyone has strong values: staff, educators, administrators, and families. These values must be articulated openly and policies set if care is to be successful. Even when a facility has stated policies, staff members often act quickly based on their unspoken values. Staff members must know when their personal values are in conflict with those of the resident or the facility. Policy needs to be flexible enough to adapt to a new problem, and staff members need to know clearly how policy is to be enacted in day-to-day life on the unit.

Even though our society is drenched in sexual images, studies have found that many adults lack basic information about sexual behavior and even what the terms mean. Be sure your students know what you are talking about and that people with dementia have the same needs as others for affection and self-esteem and may seek to fulfill these through sexual behaviors. Both men and women may also continue lifelong sexual behaviors, including masturbation.

The key to approaching sexual behaviors is the same as the approach to all other care: consider the person and her feelings and needs first.

> A nun with dementia began aggressively approaching other women in the facility. The combination of the three factors—sex, nuns, and lesbian behavior—plus the distress of the target residents was extremely stressful to the nursing sisters. The mother superior put the issue in a new perspective when she pointed out that this woman had spent her life trying to conceal her impulses and praying that God would take them from her. Then she developed the only disease that would give away her secret and keep her from controlling her impulses. When the situation was put into the new perspective of the nun's suffering, the staff members were able to find sensitive ways to cope with the practicalities. Giving the ill person more affection and more tasks that supported her self-esteem plus redirecting her when she approached others worked wonders.

The general principle of response is to meet the ill person's need for affection and self-esteem. For many people, sexual remarks or flirtatious touching reinforce self-esteem and have always been a part of their self-esteem ("I'm still a man"). As other opportunities for self-esteem are lost, sexual behaviors become more important. Sexual touching may be the only way that a person with dementia can find to initiate affection. Although this may seem counterintuitive, increased friendly touch and building self-esteem help reduce unwelcome approaches. But, staff members ask, won't this encourage the person? Staff members can give a man a hug across the shoulders and at the same time say, "John, you cannot touch me there. That is for my husband only." This is orientation plus friendship.

Behaviors That Only Appear Sexual

Sometimes behavioral symptoms are incorrectly identified as sexual. People who experience itching in the genital area or discomfort from incontinence wear may appear to be masturbating. Determine first whether the behavioral symptom is actually the result of some other issue.

Some odd behaviors are sometimes regarded as sexual. One woman who entered the facility preferred to wear men's underwear. (Some men like women's underwear also.) Although this is unusual, it does not indicate sexual deviancy. It is also harmless. Forcing a change will only increase the person's feeling of dislocation and increase stress.

Often people are simply longing for touch. Most married people are accustomed to a full night with someone else in the same bed. People with dementia may climb into another client's bed to fulfill an old habit and to seek personal contact. Viewing this behavior as sexual complicates the solution. Treat it as a need for affection and touch and as disorientation. One aide solved a problem by lying down with a resident until the resident fell asleep.

Sexual Approaches to Staff Members

A few clients will touch staff members on the buttocks or breasts, proposition them, or make sexual remarks. Of course, this is offensive for the staff. The best staff members find ways to reduce such behavior while recognizing that it is not personal. The person who approaches the staff members is likely to be disoriented to person or place or seeking self-esteem. *Teach staff members to reorient the person and support self-esteem in nonsexual activities.*

> One man developed an erection while being given personal care. He suggested the caregiver have sex with him. She declined. He looked down at his erect penis and said, "It's a shame to waste it."

Sexual arousal during care is a physiological, involuntary response. Staff members can find ways for the person to save face. This staff member said, "You're a nice man, but I have a husband and so I cannot do this." Confusion can sometimes be prevented through careful orientation; say, "Hello, I'm Ann. Can I help you wash down below with this sponge?" or "Step in here so we can help you in private."

It is reasonable to ask the staff to be understanding of the nature of sexual approaches from people with dementia, but do not expect the staff to accept sexual abuse as "a part of the job." These issues are stressful for staff members. They need support and constructive, positive feedback.

Flirtatious Staff Members

Most people use flirtatious behavior in daily life. Sometimes flirting works, and sometimes it sends confusing messages to people with dementia. Avoid blaming staff members for flirting as a cause of inappropriate behavior. Consider this example:

> Although female staff members were careful to be friendly and cheerful but never to use "flirtatious" behavior, a male staff member often flirted with women residents with excellent results. He would say, "I bet you have all the men at your feet" or "You're sure a pretty lady."

Is this "sexist," a difference in personal style, or a response to the attitudes of individual clients?

The solution is for the staff members to be aware of their own personal styles and to modify these to fit the needs of the individual resident. Staff behavior that supports one client may give confusing messages to another. Feedback from the care team, focused on one staff member's interaction with one client, is the most successful intervention.

Sexual Activity between Clients

This is a challenging issue involving family values, staff feelings, and facility policy. The staff member must begin by answering the following question:

Is your response consistent with your overall policies of client quality of life? Sometimes, under the fierce pressures from outside, facilities forget that the client's need for or right to touch, affection, or sexual partners is part of the overall issue of life quality.

Masturbation is the easiest to address. This is a normal behavior for some people of both sexes and of all ages. It affects no one but the individual. The easiest solution is to reorient the person to a private place.

When two residents engage in intimacies, the first step is to ask yourself what exactly they are doing. Hand holding and hugs may need a different response than intercourse. Sometimes people who are found in bed together are merely cuddling. They may have too much apraxia to take their clothes off or perform the sex act.

> Tom and Amy clearly felt a deep affection for each other. They sought each other out. Staff members helped them to sit together. They often wandered together, holding hands. One day Tom was observed trying to put his hand on Amy's breast, but he had a severe apraxia and usually missed the mark. Amy gently lifted his hand and placed it squarely on her breast. The two sat that way for a long time.

Sometimes staff anxiety confuses things. Encourage staff members to determine whether the activity is safe. Both men and women have fragile skin that can tear. Check carefully for skin tears in genital areas. Two people sharing a nursing home bed for whatever reason are at risk of falling out of bed. Consider how to address this.

Never pull two people apart if you find them engaged in a sexual activity. You can injure them badly. Close the door and decide what to do next time.

The staff must decide whether the behavior is consensual or whether one person is taking advantage of a passive and impaired person.

> One man frequently persuaded passive women to meet his needs. He had always been a dominant, commanding person, and the women he chose were confused and docile and had a history of complying with the demands of their husbands. Deciding whether these women were acting voluntarily or needed protection was difficult.

A few people have a consensual sexual relationship. Staff values, facility policy, and family wishes must be considered. Facility policy must be preplanned and consistent with overall goals. Staff members need help to accept that others may have the right to exercise values the staff members do not share.

Exercise 1. Talking about Sexual Issues

Staff members are often uncomfortable discussing these issues. A board game exercise is an effective way to bring these issues into a discussion.

Use or make a game board such as a Parcheesi board on which pawns are moved according to a roll of the dice. Make a set of cards that say, "What would you do if . . . ?" On every turn the player rolls the dice and moves her pawn. She then turns over one card and answers the question. Make up questions that meet the needs of your group. Be sure that the questions are at a level acceptable for the group. Use the information in this section for ideas and to teach appropriate responses to situations. Expect embarrassment and giggles. This is an effective way to make open communication fun.

Ideas for "What would you do if . . . ?" include the following:

- You found a couple in bed.
- You found a man in his room fondling himself.
- Two people are holding hands.
- One person says another client is her husband.

Section 11.5. Behavioral Symptoms in the Acute Care Setting

Objective

The student will learn to respond to the special needs of people with dementia and an acute illness, which often includes delirium.

Lecture/Discussion Notes to Be Presented to the Class

One woman entering the hospital was extremely difficult. She shouted, bit, kicked the staff members, fought off care, and repeatedly got out of her restraints. "You are trying to kill me. I see bad men. Is the train coming? Why are all these people standing around?" One staff member attempted to covertly monitor this woman by peeking through the hospital curtain. The woman immediately saw this and accused the staff member of spying on her. By the end of the night shift, the staff members were frustrated and exhausted. That afternoon when the family and the physician visited, the woman appeared perfectly cognitively well.

Refer to Lessons 1 and 3. Anyone sick enough to need hospital care or to have recently been in the hospital is almost certain to have a delirium in addition to his usual cognitive level. This is important because delirium presents a whole new ball game for patient management. The strategies used for dementia are not enough. Delirium characteristically fluctuates over hours or days and is usually worse in the evening and at night. This explains why people may be "fine with their family" or great on the day shift. Delirium presents the odd combination of hypervigilance with severe confusion. Such people are supersensitive to staff behavior and environmental events and sounds.

Delirium commonly includes hallucinations, delusions, and paranoia. It is important to know that these behaviors will not necessarily remain once the acute cause of the delirium is treated.

Behavioral interventions such as reinforcement are futile and should be avoided. Do not argue or explain (avoid saying "I'm only trying to help you"). Staff members may be accused of assault or be subjected to racial slurs. Don't laugh or be defensive. Ignore these behaviors.

Because of the hypervigilance, delirious people can be highly perceptive of staff mood (and staff members often feel stressed, frustrated, or angry). The most successful staff members reveal only calmness and a sense of being in control. This is not easy to do, but it can come with practice.

The best responses are simple and similar to "I understand," "OK," "You're doing great," "I'm almost done." It often helps to invoke the doctor's authority: "The doctor said you have to have this." Accept delusions and hallucinations as real to the impaired person. Do not contradict them. Use very simple instructions: "Hold my hand," "Drink this." Avoid "Don't do that" because it will trigger outbursts. Often these people are as much terrified as angry.

Antipsychotic medication or physical restraints may be necessary, but staff members and physicians must recognize that they usually are counterproductive: medication compounds confusion, and restraints frighten the person and increase suspiciousness. The best solution may be for the staff to help family members stagger their visits and to come at the patient's worst times. Friends and trained volunteers can be recruited to supplement this one-to-one reassuring presence.

Patients like this must be in private rooms. Much of the staff's time is spent trying to protect the other sick people in the room, a task resulting in much frustration. In the above case, treatments were canceled the next day for two patients because they were exhausted after a night of no sleep and uproar. This is expensive for the hospital. In addition, a severely upset person can easily harm other vulnerable people.

Overhead/Handout 11.1. Know Why You Want to Change a Behavioral Symptom

To ensure the safety of the client, staff members, other clients

To provide for the comfort of others

To control behavior that violates the rights of others

To meet quality assurance standards or community expectations

To control costs

To provide relief to the caregiver, family, or staff

To improve quality of life for the person with dementia

To make patient care easier

Overhead/Handout 11.2.
The Six Rs of Good Care

Restrict

Reconsider

Rechannel

Redirect

Reassure

Reassess

LESSON 12

A PLAN AND A CELEBRATION

Summary: The purpose of this lesson is to firmly establish a transfer of information to the workplace and to confirm commitment to this task. It consists of two parts: the development of a realistic plan to implement new learning in the workplace, and a celebration of the completion of the course including the presentation of certificates.

Section 12.1. Making a Plan. Helps students make a plan for implementing new learning in their work setting. The success of this implemented plan will be evaluated at intervals.

Section 12.2. Celebrating New Skills. Discusses celebrating the completion of the course and the presentation of student diplomas.

Using the Sections

Introductory course:
- Section 12.1 recommended
- Section 12.2 required

Core course:
- Section 12.1 required
- Section 12.2 required

Problems You May Have in Implementing This Lesson

Time is your biggest enemy in this lesson. At this point, you may feel pressed to finish the training. There may be issues you have not had time to address, or there may be pressure to get the students back into the workplace. *Do not skip this lesson.* Like the keystone in an arch, this lesson holds together all of everyone's efforts and makes possible the evaluation of the training.

This lesson should culminate the introductory course as well as the core course.

Section 12.1. Making a Plan

Objective

The student will learn to make a realistic plan for the implementation of new learning in the workplace.

Background

Throughout the course, students have been asked to apply new knowledge in their clinical setting through the clinical experience exercises. In this section, students are asked to make a plan that they will implement over time to make change in the workplace. This is essential. Without actually making change, the training is pointless, and students will perceive their efforts as meaningless. If training is to be of any use in the workplace, the student must be committed to it. This final lesson—both sections—is designed to cement that commitment.

This plan also provides an informal basis for measuring the success of training. (See Chapter IV.)

Information and Instructions for the Teacher

Ask the students to make a plan for implementing new learning in the workplace following the instructions in Overhead/Handout 12.1. Have the students work in small groups that will work together in the workplace. If the students will not return together to a workplace, have them work in small groups with similar interests or plans. Academic students in training should make a plan for the type of site in which they expect to work or teach.

A representative from management should be present in the classroom during the development of the plan. The administrator or management representative is to consult with students about what can be accomplished and to negotiate compromises when needed. Implementation of new learning is ultimately the responsibility of management. The presence of a management representative is needed to assist in developing a plan and to endorse it.

Management will need to be honest wth students about fiscal realities. If there is no budget to hire more staff members, students need to know this. However, management must be willing to work with students for a compromise solution.

Keep copies of the students' plans. At stated intervals, the students and teacher can review the plans and identify their successes. Plans can be revised during the year. If possible, the teacher can revisit the training site and meet with the students to review their plans, identify their successes (which often exceed their expectations), and reinforce the concepts and values included in the training. This process serves as an informal evaluation of the training. It allows management, teachers, and former students to recognize their successes and make modifications.

Lecture/Discussion Notes to Be Presented to the Class

Overhead/Handout 12.1. Making a Plan

The plan must include the following aspects:

- *Be realistic.* Suggest things that can actually be accomplished. As we have stressed throughout this course, these may be small or simple changes. Students should not try to create an ideal care setting when that is not financially possible or when there are other serious obstacles.
- *Be concrete.* The plan should state specifically what students will do and should not contain vague terms such as "improve quality of life."
- *Address quality-of-life issues* such as reduction of stress, reduction of excess disability, support of remaining functions, and meeting emotional needs.
- *Address physical care issues.* Unless physical care issues are not currently being met in the program, the plan may be limited to ways that quality of life can be improved through existing physical care procedures.
- *Contain things that can be implemented now,* things that can be implemented in three months, and things that can be planned for implementation within a year.

- *Be simple.* Emphasize again the importance of small, simple changes. These are easier to implement, and there is a high probability that staff members will see changes in their clients.
- *Focus on a unitwide approach.* Previous clinical experience exercises have focused on making change for one client. However, at this point, the student must consider the functioning of the unit as a whole. Home care students may make a plan for their caseload or continue to focus on one person.
- *Take into account those who were not trained.* The tasks and expectations of those who were not trained will affect the success of a plan for change. Will the final plan be simple enough that it does not involve untrained staff, or will part of the plan be to arrange training for others? Home care students must plan for family caregivers.

Students should use as reference in making this plan (a) their clinical experience exercises throughout the course, (b) the course outline used for this class, and (c) their notes. Where clinical experience exercises have presented problems, the plan should recognize and respond to this.

The plan may be simple with few changes if that is realistic for the setting. Students should not (and do not have the time to) draft a large planning document. This is a straightforward, directly implementable plan.

Although the plan may contain strategies for the care of individual clients, it should (in a group setting) focus on the care in the total unit. In home care, it may focus on strategies that will be used in most home visits.

The plan should take into account the reactions of those in the workplace who have not been trained. Will they be trained later? Will they resist or resent the new approaches?

Section 12.2. Celebrating New Skills

Objective

The student's commitment to new skills will be reinforced.

Information and Instructions for the Teacher

Plans for a celebration and certificates must be made well in advance. (See Chapter I.)

Students in this course have been asked to invest far more than their time. They have been asked to work, contribute their ideas and values, and change deeply held concepts. A celebration confirms for students that their efforts are valued by leadership. If this step is ignored, it conveys to the students that their commitment is not valued and therefore that the hard work of implementation will not be valued either.

Hold a presentation of certificates by management. This can be as formal or informal as the program chooses, but the commitment and presence of leadership are vital.

Following the presentation of certificates, hold a party. Again, this can be formal or informal and of any style. The class can be involved in the planning. Client families, clients, and students' families may be invited. Some students have arranged an off-site barbeque that children can attend; some have included program clients. In any case, leadership representatives must be present.

Lecture/Discussion Notes to Be Presented to the Class

There is no specific lecture for this section. Make brief comments on the success of the course and its effect on the program. Use this time to celebrate the students' effort and gains.

Overhead/Handout 12.1. Making a Plan

The plan must

- be realistic;
- be concrete;
- address quality-of-life issues;
- address physical care needs;
- include things that can be implemented now and at intervals in the future;
- use what you have learned in this course;
- be simple;
- focus on a unitwide approach; and
- take into account those who were not trained.

PART THREE

ADDITIONAL INFORMATION FOR EDUCATORS

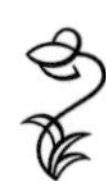

CHAPTER IV

EVALUATING YOUR TRAINING

This chapter discusses methods of evaluating your training. Evaluation and planning are complementary activities. Evaluation tells you whether you have done what you planned to do and how to plan what you will do next. There is no one right form of evaluation, and no evaluation approach is perfect. Select an evaluation method based on what you wish to learn about your training and on the time and cost of the evaluation process. Plan the evaluation as a part of planning the course. A retrospective evaluation will tell you little about your success.

An evaluation motivates the entire system. It tells the system, including the teacher and students, whether they have accomplished anything or simply wasted time. An evaluation is an important part of seeking funding for further training. Evaluating care approaches helps to justify seeking waivers for care methods. An evaluation tells the facility and the teacher how to improve the next training session. Perhaps most important, the evaluation places a measured value on the students' and teacher's efforts at change. When training is not evaluated, the implication is that it is not valued.

Although most people believe that staff training improves the quality of client care, you may not be able to prove this. There are many variables in the quality of care (staff, administration, plant, families, the clients themselves, client physical health), and it is difficult to be sure that changes are due entirely to the training. The fact that different people respond to different interventions further complicates the picture. Decreases in problem behaviors and clients who seem less stressed may be obvious; unless you are conducting a formal research evaluation, your own documentation is sufficient. Following are the pros and cons of some possible ways to evaluate your course.

Types of Evaluation

There are many types of evaluation. You are probably familiar with *evaluations of research studies* (often published in professional journals). Although such studies can be simple, they must be carefully designed in order to allow for the many variables in dementia care. *Evaluations of learning* (examinations) are necessary to meet academic and licensure requirements. These should be developed by the educator. The student objectives at the beginning of each section of each lesson provide a starting point.

Training programs often use a *course evaluation* that asks the student to react to statements such as "How helpful was this information?" or "How helpful were the handouts?" This kind of evaluation tells you what the student thought of the course and whether the environment and materials were useful, but it provides no information about how effectively students will apply the new skills in the work setting.

Another type of evaluation is a *test of student knowledge* (tests, quizzes, papers). These are similar to academic examinations and licensure qualifications. When tests of knowledge are given before and after a course, they tell how much of the student's knowledge was acquired in the course. Tests of knowledge reinforce new learning. Preparing for the test, reviewing the test with the teacher, and discussing the answers help fix the information in the students' minds. However, as discussed in Chapter II, students who are not accustomed to classroom learning or whose written language skills are limited may be sufficiently anxious that they do poorly on tests.

Tests of knowledge do not measure the clinical usefulness of the training. Students with extensive knowledge may be unable to implement their knowledge for many reasons.

Many instruments are available to *measure client behavior and function*. A well-designed instrument will provide a good assessment of the impact of your training. Client behavior and function should be measured before and after the course to determine change. Select an instrument with established reliability and validity, one that is sensitive to subtle change, uses specific terms rather than general terms such as *agitation*, does not measure staff perception of change (which is different from real change), and includes questions about small changes and positive quality-of-life change. Client change may continue for several weeks after the end of a course: a pretest, post test, and test after six weeks to three months are preferred. Such measures of client behavior and function are limited by the accuracy and quality of the test instrument and changes in client health. They are time-consuming and may require the expertise of an outside researcher.

People with dementia will change some behavioral symptoms in response to care, but little except medications, including drugs that directly affect the dementia, will change other behavioral symptoms. Not all clients will change uniformly, and different programs may observe different responses. It is important to know what is possible and what is not. The kind of interventions described in this book will not cure diseases such as Alzheimer's or alter the progression of the underlying neurological damage.

The interventions described in this book reduce stress, help people use what cognitive function remains, and help them experience more positive feelings. Fortunately, this may be enough to reduce agitation, anger, combativeness and many other problematic symptoms. Exhibit IV.1 lists client changes that are somewhat more responsive to the kinds of interventions described in this book. Symptoms such as memory loss and problems with using language and motor skills will usually not improve significantly. Activities such as walking, eating, and dressing require complex, multiple skills. They will respond somewhat when stress is reduced, but the basic neurological disability will remain. Other symptoms such as restlessness, irritability, and some types of wandering are influenced by stress, disorientation, the environment, and caregiver behavior. These can be expected to decline with improved care. In identifying gains, remember that null behavior (being tuned out or being passive) may be a way of coping that is not in the client's best interests.

Coons and Mace (1996) developed a measure of *unitwide quality of life*. This approach helps to balance out idiosyncratic client variability, including ongoing client decline. It can be used as a pretest/posttest measure of quality of life. This instrument has had limited testing for validity and reliability; however, it is a useful measure for assessing the impact of training on the entire unit.

Informal but Effective Measures of Course Success

In most cases, a different approach to evaluation will provide more useful information. You may choose to use some of the assessment tools and some of these informal but effective measures of the successful transfer of information to the workplace.

A *quick test of new intervention tools* given at the end of the course asks the student to list three things that he has learned that he can put into practice immediately. Students should be instructed to list specific things that can actually be implemented even if these are quite small or seemingly "insignificant" changes. This test is useful after short courses and seminars, can be used to meet continuing education requirements for short seminars, and helps the student connect learning with planning interventions. The student may be able to follow through to assess whether he was able to implement his ideas. This approach measures the student's grasp of the concept of making realistic and effective changes as covered in the course. It does not measure the amount of change that occurs. It is not useful for students not currently providing or supervising care and does not cover the full range of material taught.

A *facility's long- and short-term goals* provide an assessment tool. Chapter I recommends that administration, educators, or others set goals before the training. Goals may be in any area: cost, family satisfaction, and so on, as well as change in staff or client

Exhibit IV.1. Symptoms of Cognitive Impairment and Their Response to Changes in Care

Little or No Change	Partial Change	Highly Responsive to Environmental Change
Memory impairment	Walking	Restlessness
Aphasia (problems with language)	Eating	Agitation
Apraxia (problems with motor skills)	Dressing	Wandering
Agnosia (problems recognizing things)	Household tasks	Anger
Impaired learning	Coping with money	Crying
Scores on MMSE	Bathing	Combativeness
	Continence	Screaming
		Social inappropriateness
		Weight loss
		Sleep disturbance
		Anxiety
		Withdrawal
		Apathy

Note: Function may also decline in the presence of delirium.
Source: Adapted from U.S. Congress (1987).

behavior. Lesson 1 recommends that students set goals for the course. Student goals may be a mixture of personal (obtain my certificate), task-oriented (get through my work faster), and care-oriented (help my clients feel better).

After completion of the course, the extent to which these goals have been met provides a useful evaluation of the course. The same group of people who set the goals should determine whether they have been met. When students are reviewing their goals, make copies of the goals drafted in Lesson 1 and hand these out. A Likert scale is helpful in rating the extent to which goals have been met.

Because implementation takes time, the goals should be reviewed at six weeks after training and three months after training. These later reviews will help to determine how well the new skills are retained. Questions that may be considered include: Did the course meet your goals and program needs? Did the course result in changes in client function or behavior (or both)? If you plan to offer training again, should you modify the course content, scheduling, or environment, or should you change your target students? Is follow-up teaching needed? Were there unexpected gains? What was the response of staff members who did not participate in training? If there were negative changes, what response is needed? What was the impact on clients who do not have a dementia but who share space with those who do?

Change is not always where you look for it. For example, although you may see no change in a person during the time he is in day care, his family may report that he sleeps better.

The effectiveness of this type of evaluation depends on the clarity of the original goals. It does not measure the change in client function or behavior: it measures the opinion of those reviewing the goals. It is not a measure of student knowledge, although if students have not acquired new skills, they will not see changes in their clients.

The strength of this kind of evaluation is that it is relatively quick and unambiguous. It gives positive feedback to planners and educators and, most important, shows the students that they have accomplished their goals. The presence and review of goals give direction and relevance to the training. This kind of evaluation is useful even when the students are not working in a care setting.

You may want to *assess the experience of untrained staff members.* Staff members who do not participate in the training will have opinions about the training, may be affected positively or negatively by the training, and can have a significant impact on the implementation of the training. You may design a questionnaire or simply meet and talk with staff members in small groups. Do they see their colleagues' training as useful to the entire system and to their work? Did they feel it was a "waste of time" or "added to their own workload"? How do they react to their colleagues' suggestions for change? Do they welcome these ideas? What information survived this transfer of knowledge? Do they want the training? In what ways do they think the training would help them? Query both direct care staff members and supervisors who did not receive the training and staff members who do not provide direct care (such as kitchen staff, housekeeping).

Lesson 12 asks teams of students who will work together, their teacher, and a representative from administration to *develop a realistic plan to implement improved dementia care* in the facility. This is both an excellent teaching tool and an effective assessment instrument. It provides ongoing feedback to leadership and to the newly trained staff. It allows for ongoing adaptation as the plans are carried out. It allows the student to define the changes that she can make and involves the student in making change.

Immediate, short-term, and long-term plans for change are defined. At preestablished intervals, the team will meet to determine the extent to which the plan is on course or needs adjustment.

This is a working tool, not a research tool. There are many uncontrolled variables in the process of change that are not controlled for in this evaluation. Change in client base and change in administration or in supervisors can interfere with implementation. However, in practice, this tool appears to most effectively, without investment in a research design, indicate the success with which new knowledge is applied in caregiving. It has all the advantages of a review of goals but has the added advantage of being an active tool in the process of implementation.

Whichever forms of evaluation you select, do evaluate your course. Use the findings of your evaluation to justify funding; to provide feedback to administration, supervisors, and students; to justify change to regulators; to document cost-effectiveness and staff retention; and to promote the excellence of your program. Evaluation is important: use it.

CHAPTER V

MAKING THE BEST USE OF CHARTING AND INFORMATION-BASED SYSTEMS

The long-term management of dementia requires an information system that helps caregivers connect behavioral symptoms with causes and that facilitates exchange between staff members. Interventions vary with each individual, symptoms often have multiple causation, and patients require fine-tuning of multiple strategies, including medical treatment, psychosocial interventions, and environmental supports. This chapter discusses ways to make key information readily available to all staff members involved in care. The material presented is written for clinical application only. It does not teach the use of assessment for meeting standards, diagnosis, research, or other purposes and does not replace a battery of assessment tools. This material is used in patient care.

Problems You May Have in Implementing This Material

Many problems arise in developing an information system, including the following:

Staff members who provide direct care may prefer caregiving to charting. They may resist, postpone, or avoid paperwork.

In some settings, patients' records do not facilitate good long-term clinical care.

It is the nature of systems to resist change, and changing record-keeping practices can involve outside agencies, the head office, or surveyors. The organization of charts is often mandated. Changing charts so that they are more useful may be akin to trying to move a graveyard. Adding more charting to existing cumbersome systems only adds burdens for the staff.

Computerized systems are often unfamiliar to staff members and *are only as good as their program design.*

Considering Your System

As you evaluate your record-keeping and charting system, consider these questions:

- How accurate and current is it?
- Can you quickly identify patterns and relationships? For example, spotting multiple causation in a fragile individual is almost impossible without effective documentation. This is one reason that some people seem "impossible to help."

  As you read through this manual, you will learn many possible causes for each symptom, but trying each possibility would be time-consuming and discouraging. Staff members tend to make generalizations ("noise upsets everyone" or "sundowning is caused by fatigue"), but records must show individual causes and relationships (e.g., this person's behavioral symptoms worsen when several of her physical symptoms converge).

  Many behavioral symptoms occur infrequently or only a few times a week, making relationships hard to spot. Can you highlight possible causes so they are easier to find?
- Where is the key information? How much time will staff members spend flipping through the chart, asking others for more information, paging through the log, sorting through old information? Does your charting help the staff

identify priorities for individuals? Can you quickly pull out the most important issues for this person's care?

- Does the documentation define the problem with specificity and in detail?
- Are you documenting the person's strengths?
- Are you getting the information to the people who use it? How much and what kind of information do staff members tend to remember rather than record? Staff members often know that one person needs a different kind of approach than another person does or just how to get a difficult person to cooperate, but is this information recorded? Is it available and shared with all caregivers?
- Do those who use the records know how to get the most out of them? Do staff members make good use of existing charts and logs? Will the day shift know about early signs of illness noticed by the night shift? Will those on the day shift know that their efforts paid off on the second shift with less "sundowning"? Do physicians and other therapists have the information they need? Do they pass along what they know?
- Review the assumptions that are made about who needs to know what kind of information. Do supervisors assume that aides do not need to know certain things? Do aides assume that supervisors do not need or want to know certain things?
- How do you handle people with dementia who come with inadequate information?
- Is information transfer between staff and families effective?
- Do you already have too much information? Should you get some things out of the way so that you can see the forest instead of the trees?
- If you use a computerized system, does it work for you?

Helping the Caregiving Staff Use an Information System

Information is useful only to the extent that it is used. Review how your staff members now use the information in charts and logs. Use the classroom to help the staff try out new ways to use information. Make change gradually.

- Accept the fact that direct care people may never read or write out more than a small amount of information. Make what they do read eye-catching, short, and to the point. Give up the fight to persuade them to read and write more. Verbally pass on the information from medical reports, tests, and so on—e.g., "I reviewed Maria's record. She is having severe difficulty understanding, which she conceals by smiling and nodding and pretending she understands. We may be overestimating her comprehension. This may help explain her frustration."
- Avoid making additional demands on staff time. Provide time dedicated to charting, reporting, and looking for information.
- Try making changes in charting with just one or two clients, or select just one bit of information to highlight. Use the classroom to create teamwork and to convince people of the need for information by asking them to use information in their clinical work.
- Match methods of transfer to people's styles. (For example, will the physician provide more detail if she dictates her notes? Will aides talk at report or staff meetings with more ease than writing things down?)
- Mandating better charting or new forms usually does not work.
- Reward compliance, and point out the ways that the new approach helps in care.
- Focus on getting information to those who need it.
- Help shifts communicate well with each other.
- Use an informal daily walk round to identify successes and needs and to teach staff members.
- Use information posters.
- Avoid taking up staff meetings with business and policy. Use staff meetings for informal role modeling and teaching. Staff meetings should be relaxed and should encourage participation and problem solving. Try addressing a function or behavioral symptom in one person. Give direct care staff members time to describe what they observe. Use one case to generalize to others.

Direct care staff members often dislike charting and see no use for it. Exhibit V.1 is an exercise de-

Exhibit V.1. Exercise to Introduce Staff Members to the Usefulness of Charted Information

Information and Instructions for the Teacher

The *teaching goal* of this exercise is to introduce direct care staff members to the usefulness of information. It gives these staff members a fuller sense of participation in the data-gathering process.

There are several variations on this exercise. Select one that is relevant (e.g., information needed on new clients, information that must be passed on to the next shift, information from one home care worker to another, information from the physician). Modify the notes below to change the exercise. The example given is for a recent admission.

By involving direct care staff members, we increase their investment in using information and encourage them to think critically about how they can care better. Traditionally, supervisors and others decide what information is needed based on their broader knowledge; however, in this exercise, leave the process of selecting what they need to know and shaping questions in the hands of direct care staff members.

Plan in advance to use the finished product the group designs or to integrate it into existing documents. If you cannot use the product, do not do the exercise. Not using the students' work reinforces a "why bother?" mentality. You may introduce student products into your program on a 90-day trial basis with a plan to revise the document after it has been field-tested.

Be realistic: if staff members complain that they do not have time to read things, trying to talk them into reading will not improve information transfer. Whether they have time or not, they don't think they do, so look for a different approach. Treat "Nobody ever told us that" the same way. If staff members don't think they were told, communication is failing; find another way.

To the extent possible, include direct care staff members in the effort to find better communication tools and hold them responsible for living with their ideas. This may be an ongoing project. Follow up.

For a Recent Admission

In advance, select one client who is of concern to your group. Gather all the information that was obtained on this person in the first month of admission. This might include a referral, medical report, social work notes, psychological testing, clinical notes from first few days of admission, letter from family, Resident Assessment Instrument, and so on. Omit confidential and financial information. Depending on the setting, you may need to block out the client and family names. Make copies of the information you have obtained. If no one client is known to your entire class, use a sample client, with false identifying data.

Lecture/Discussion Notes to Be Presented to the Class

Step 1. Staff members often ignore much of the information in charts or assume it is someone else's responsibility. They may have a limited idea of what information is available or how it is organized. The purpose of this step is to teach the staff members that the chart contains information that is useful to them in daily care. Staff members may never have time or skills to read a chart in search of information, but if they know information is there, they know they can ask for it.

Pass out the materials about the client. If they include too much information for the group to read quickly, walk the group through the materials so that they know what is included and explain why this is useful. Entry-level staff members may have no idea how documenting medications or bowel movements can help with care. Keep this exercise lighthearted and enjoyable. The size and opacity of many charts are grounds for humor, and humor helps people retain information.

(*continued*)

Exhibit V.1. *(continued)*

Focus on the information this chart provided at the time of admission. Discuss and list on a flip chart:

- What information was most useful when this person was admitted?
- What information is here that the class did not know?
- What information that they did not know (or was not available) when the person was admitted would have helped staff members with this person?
- How can this information be made more useful for caregiving staff members? Talk about better ways to convey information to the staff. For example, if the staff members say they do not have time to read the chart, ask them to think of a better way to pass on information: displaying a poster about the new person in the staff room? Would they read this? Who would make it? A presentation in the morning report? How would this work? What about the afternoon shift?

Step 2. Ask the class, "The day a new person walks into our program, what do you need to know about her to care for her and to help her adjust?" Let your students lead this discussion. Do not assemble an exhaustive list. Seek to identify key information. If the group generates many ideas, prioritize these. Remind the staff members that the program will implement this list on a trial basis. Whatever they list, they will have to read or listen to.

Some information other groups have listed:

- Name the person uses
- The people the person is likely to talk about
- Names and relationships of people who will be visiting and of people the person with dementia may ask for
- Specific techniques for daily routines
- What works best to calm the person when she becomes upset
- Other care "tricks"
- Whether the person will need time alone, time to rest
- Whether the person is at risk for falls
- What words or cues the person uses or understands for important things
- What things upset the person or should be avoided

Step 3. Prepare a list or questionnaire. Put together a short list of information that must be gathered and communicated at the time of admission. (If the members of your group have had little experience with a task like this, they will need a person with experience in diagnosis, assessment, referral, or treatment to assist them.)

Step 4. Use the new data in the program for a time-limited trial. This will involve obtaining the approval of the administration, the admitting social worker, and perhaps others. Plan how and when the information will be given to caregiving staff. At the end of the trial period, meet with everyone involved and decide whether the new data were useful, how the data need to be modified, and whether to continue using the data. This process should be handled as much as possible by the caregiving staff members. These are "their" data, and decisions about the data should not be unilaterally made by the administration, nursing, or social work staff.

signed to give direct care staff members insight into the value of record keeping and charting.

Improving Data Bases and Addressing System Resistance to Change

Sometimes long-term-care charts fail to facilitate problem solving. They are modeled after acute care charting, and necessary information may not be entered or may be scattered throughout the chart. The emphasis is on medical issues; behavioral symptoms may not be charted or may be impossible to link to cause. In some charts, even diagnosis is buried in several places: the admitting diagnosis (e.g., senile dementia), subsequent findings (e.g., complaints of back pain), lab reports (e.g., anemia), medication given (e.g., a prescribed laxative implies constipation), other (a hard-to-understand neuropsychological report filed in the back of the chart). Behavioral symptoms may be recorded in a daily log. Staff members can easily waste an hour paging through logs and charts looking for causes of behavioral problems.

It is unlikely that programs will be able to abruptly change the way records are handled. If a program did rewrite the charting process, more problems might be introduced into the system. Adding new forms and new data can make the system even more cumbersome. In most cases, programs are stuck with the record-keeping/charting/log-keeping system they have. Nevertheless, you can make some improvements:

- Before implementing even minor changes, obtain approval from management and regulators. Present your case in a way that shows the benefits to management and regulators (lower staff time costs; ease of review). Propose that the change be on a trial basis, to be reviewed or eliminated at a preset date.
- Negotiate agreement from affected departments (nursing; social work).
- Start slowly, with only a few clients, and make only small changes.
- Regularly solicit feedback from those involved.
- Consider how accurate and timely your information is. Is information transfer slow, does it not reach the staff in a timely way, or is it vague or incomplete? Although making improvements here may not be easy, regulators and administrators are likely to approve them.
- Look for a way to collect all diagnoses in one place, summarize all treatments in one place, summarize all symptoms in one place. See Exhibit V.2.
- Look for a way to highlight changes in client health, behavior, complaints, and so on. Exhibit V.3 describes a method of graphing relationships between behavioral symptoms and other factors.
- Ask yourself whether you are documenting the most important issues in the patient logs. (For example, one facility documented bowel function for all patients but included no information about stumbling or other indicators of potential falls.)

Exhibit V.4 is a compilation of items that other programs have suggested as useful. Do not use this list as it stands: it requests too much information to be useful. Use it to jog your memory as you compose your own database.

Programs find that documenting the interventions that they have tried with an individual helps define what will work. This often means documenting failures as well as successes. Exhibit V.5 describes this process.

Exhibit V.6 lists 18 questions that help assess the caregiving situation.

Chapter VI describes the process of interviewing a person with dementia and how to make the best use of two common instruments, the Mini-Mental State Examination and the Minimum Data Set.

Computers

Computerizing the charts is an ideal way to maintain clinical data. A good computer program can show you, almost instantly, the relationship over time between any selected factors: behavior and health status, behavior and environmental factors, and so on. However, to make this work, (1) the computer program must be written for this kind of care, (2) the data have to be entered (which is no more time-consuming than entering them in a log), (3) the direct care staff members and their supervisors must know how to use the computer program to obtain the in-

Exhibit V.2. Short List of Essential Information

This list of items must be in a form that the staff can find and use easily. To be effective, a summary sheet must

- put frequently used information together in one place;
- be short;
- be available;
- be current; and
- be written in terms all staff members can use.

Entries must trigger a further review of the chart; full information cannot be recorded on this short document.

Programs suggest that it is useful to jot new information directly on the sheet so that it stays current without having to be frequently recopied. Obtain this information from the most current Resident Assessment Instrument, the client's medical information, and the most recent caregiver.

If possible, involve students or caregiving staff members in designing this instrument. Following is an example of such a list. Adapt it to meet your needs. You may want to include material from Exhibit V.1.

Summary of Health and Quality of Life

1. Primary dementia diagnosis

2. Other medical diagnoses (include "minor" diagnoses); drug sensitivities

3. Psychiatric diagnoses

4. Oral/dental problems
   Make this functional information (e.g., "needs dentures to eat" or "has sore gums").

5. Visual/auditory impairments
   Use functional information (e.g., "can hear in quiet room," "peripheral vision best").

6. Factors that come and go for this person (e.g., usually cooperative but can be stubborn about baths)

7. Factors that contribute to increased confusion, behavior problems, or delirium (e.g., urinary tract infections trigger irritability; becomes restless in large groups)

8. Significant abnormalities on physical/neurological examination
   List only the clinical implications of the neurological report here: Is the person likely to fall? Is the person on too much neuroleptic medication? Will the person need time to get started moving?
   Potential neurological findings that are clinically relevant include gait and posture (tandem gait, arm swing, en bloc turning, standing on one leg); abnormal movements (benign tremor, myoclonus, dyskinesia, etc.); Parkinsonism (tremor, cogwheel rigidity, bradykinesia, loss or reduction in postural balance, etc.); cranial nerve function.

9. Medication summary
   Taking any dementia drug?
   Taking any other medications that may affect cognitive function? may cause drowsiness? falls? (antihypertensives, cardiovascular; e.g., anginal, antiarrhythmic, sedative-hypnotic, antidepressant, tranquilizer, antipsychotic, insulin, thyroid, anticonvulsants, any anticholinergic drug)

(*continued*)

Exhibit V.2. *(continued)*

Taking any drug for which a diagnosis and care plan are not clearly given? (These often include over-the-counter pain relievers and laxatives.)

Total number of medications taken. Include topical and over-the-counter drugs.

This information is also on the Resident Assessment Inventory. Its usefulness here is to allow physicians and nurses to glance at the total list to identify possible causes of excess disability.

10. Psychosocial factors

    Give functional, specific answers. Imagine that you are telling a newcomer how to work with this person. Get some of this information from families of new clients (for example, may miss family pet, words used for specific needs). Keep it current.

11. Communication

    Expressive (able to express self)
    Receptive (able to understand)
    Nonverbal (list important behaviors/gestures; e.g., pacing means he needs to use the toilet)

12. Desire to be independent/desire to be comforted or reassured (e.g., "likes to feel independent" or "needs a lot of reassurance to complete a task" or "comfort is primary goal")

13. Sensitivity to failure/put-downs, need for success (e.g., "often feels she is being put down" or "needs reassurance that you won't let her mess up")

14. Worries

    Things the person worries about (e.g., "worries about her children"). What helps? Do white lies work better than explanations?

15. Things that are stressful

    List a few specific things that upset the person.

16. First signs of stress (e.g., becomes restless or tearful, begins pacing, starts fidgeting)

17. Steps to avoid stress (e.g., what would you tell a newcomer to avoid?)

18. Steps to take when the person is overly stressed

    What to do when staff members notice signs of stress or when the person becomes upset.

    Items 21 and 22 are things all staff members need to know to divert a person or to help him through a task comfortably.

19. Things the person is able to do

20. Things the person enjoys (sing to her while you work, giving hugs)

21. Ways the person enjoys others (likes to sit near the group; likes to walk; best in small groups)

22. Ways to help the family

    Identify specific things the caregiving staff members can suggest, like "try taking him for a walk" or "she will enjoy you more if you visit one at a time."

Exhibit V.3. Using Diagrams or Graphs

A diagram or graph provides a visual way to find a relationship between behavioral symptoms and interventions. On one axis, use graded, specific descriptions of behavioral symptoms, such as "no behavioral symptom observed," "slightly grouchy if approached," "begins to get restless, refuses needed ADL," "threatens to hit," "strikes out, physically aggressive." On the other axis, use time. Diagram an individual's behavioral symptoms. Note what is occurring at the times when behavioral symptoms increase. Examples:

> A man who is living at home is receiving haloperidol as needed. Staff members are not sure how much the drug is helping. They made a graph showing time on one axis and behavioral symptoms of irritability on the other. They marked the times the haloperidol was administered on the graph. This showed that the medication helped some but was being given too late to stop outbursts. They were able to show the caregiver that by giving the drug about an hour before expected agitation, serious outbursts could be avoided.
>
> A woman's behavior ranged from being cooperative to hitting. By charting her symptoms for a week using day/time as one axis and behavioral level as the other, staff members observed that her symptoms became worse shortly before meals. Giving her a snack between meals helped her without affecting her appetite.

formation they need, and (4) the program must be user-friendly or people won't try to use it. Many computer programs do not meet these standards.

Using the Results of Neuropsychological Tests

An increasing number of people with dementia are being given neuropsychological tests. These tests are used to make a diagnosis and to differentiate among the various dementias. The results of neuropsychological tests also have the potential to provide the caregivers with insight into function and behavior. Tests identify spared and impaired areas of function in more detail than observation alone. They often describe deficits that are disabling but not easily identified by other means.

> Only if we in some sense understand what the world is like to demented persons can we maintain the personal concern and tolerance that these very demanding people require. Because neuropsychological assessment can document the limitation in patients' capacities to perceive, remember, comprehend, and manipulate the world around them, assessment enhances our appreciation of the difficulties patients face. Periodic identification of the spared and impaired abilities during the disease course may be of considerable importance to patients and their care givers in planning the patient's daily routines. (Cronin-Golomb, Corkin, and Roen 1993, p. 132)

This individualized understanding of multiple lost and retained functions and of the impaired person's perception of the surrounding world is a primary concept of this text.

Unfortunately, this potential is not always realized. The skill of the neuropsychologist is essential to making the data meaningful. The neuropsychologist may lack knowledge of clinical applications or may not be reimbursed for this effort. The job of interpreting these data may be given to the physician, whose training did not prepare him for the clinical value of this material.

Obtaining this information may be a process of educating the neuropsychologist, physician, or even the reimbursement source. The insight provided by neuropsychological findings is so valuable in managing behaviors and facilitating function that you should aggressively press for them whenever you know that testing has been done.

Skilled neuropsychologists can usually conduct testing in ways that do not exhaust or upset the impaired person.

Exhibit V.4. Detailed Questions for an Information Base

Use this compilation to jog your memory. Many items repeat other sources, and many you will not need. What information do you need in each area? Which areas do you not need? How informed are direct care providers and professionals in each of these areas for each person with dementia in your care?

Personal History

Birthplace, date, early childhood, parents, schooling, early values learned (Example: Harriet was born on a farm just before World War I. She never knew her father because he died in that war. Her mother was a laundress, and the family lived in poverty. Harriet learned to work hard and to save, values she still holds.)
Does the person believe that his parents/spouse/siblings are living?
Occupation, employment, second (postretirement) career
Religion, religious practice
Name and address of clergy
Does the person desire to continue religious practice? If so, how will this be achieved?
Lifestyle in late life (Consider both postretirement years and the year immediately before placement.)
Who does the person live with? (Include everyone.) Include pets.
Who provided care?
Financial experience: lifelong history of affluence or poverty
Cultural background, ethnic group/values
To what socioeconomic status is the person accustomed? (Is she accustomed to servants? Did she have a room of her own? Did she usually stay indoors? live in a high crime area?)
Volunteerism, hobbies (Consider postretirement years and the year immediately before placement separately.)
Is there a pattern of gradual withdrawal or ongoing energetic dedication, participation, and so on?
Does the person enjoy pets? Important past or current pets.

Personal Information

Is the person right-handed or left-handed?
What does the person prefer to be called?
What are the person's remaining strengths or abilities?
Does the person value privacy?
What are her favorite foods? treats? disliked foods, medical or religious dietary restrictions, vegetarian? snacks preferred?
Are there any unsafe activities? eating unsafe things? going out alone? fall risk? need supervision at which times? tries to cook?
Likes to be hugged/gives hugs. Does not like to be touched.
Grumpy in the morning/more upset in evening. Early riser, late riser; goes to bed early/late?
Who are the people the person may ask for, and when will they visit?

Lifestyle in the Past Few Months

Consider lifestyle after retirement and lifestyle in the prior year separately. (There are 20 years between retirement at 65 and age 85—time for many changes in interests, health, and abilities. Although it is important to know what interests the person has always enjoyed, her activities in the past year may be more relevant to care.)

(continued)

Exhibit V.4. *(continued)*

What does she do with her day? Obtain a schedule of routines, bedtime, arising time, mealtimes, frequency of baths, pastimes.
Does the person enjoy holidays?

Medical/Physical Status

Premorbid medical history
Dementia diagnosis
Stage of illness
Prior illnesses, surgeries
Current illnesses, surgeries
Prior episodes of delirium
Mental status, current MMSE
Presence of delirium
Complaints of pain, probable pain due to medical history
Wears glasses, dentures, hearing aid
    Has but refuses to wear? Needs?
Needs visual, oral, or auditory testing
Other sensory deficits
Current medications, medical reason for
Skin conditions
History of alcohol abuse? tobacco use? use of other recreational drugs?

Emotional Health History

Obtain a description of the person's personality before he became ill, preferably from more than one person.
Prior psychological defense mechanisms?
Had illness with mental symptoms in past?
Prior history of depression, familial history of depression?
Presence of depression, needs work-up for depression? other mood disorder?
What are the person's prior/present sexual needs/interests?
What losses/bereavement experiences has the person experienced? When? Is the person still grieving?
Suspiciousness? What helps?

Records

What evaluations exist for this person?
Prior MMSE scores
    Assessment of cognitive function/specific problem areas
Neurological assessment
Neuropsychological evaluation
Assessment of motor functions
Have ADL assessments and cognitive assessment been completed?
Are "Do Not Resuscitate" documents included?

Health Attitude History

How has this person responded to physical illness and to illness with mental symptoms in past?

(continued)

Exhibit V.4. *(continued)*

How has the family historically responded to illness, and what is the patient's and family's attitude toward the dementia?

Functional Level

ADL function
    Assessment complete?
Identify those parts of the ADL that the person can do/can sometimes do/tries to do and the ways the caregiver helps the person do what she still can; which tasks will need to be done for the person/how best to do these?
What cues does the caregiver use? Step-by-step description of cueing from caregiver? Situations or things to avoid.
Does she prefer bath/shower?
How are dressing/grooming accomplished? Provide details/strategies/preferences.
Constipation? Incontinence? Leaking? What is the best way to help the person?
How well does the person walk? Does she need a walker or wheelchair?
Can the person get into and out of a chair independently?
Does the person fall? Under what circumstances?
How is night waking handled? Waking at night to toilet?
List behavioral symptoms
    What triggers?
    Strategies for intervention
    Do these vary through the day? occur at certain times?

Assessment of Communication Skills/Limitations

What language does the person speak?
What do commonly used words mean?
How does the person use nonverbal communication?
Words, terms that are helpful to use?
What words does the person use for fear, worry, pain, need to toilet?
What is the person likely to be talking about?

Assessment of Stress

What were the person's prior ways of coping with stress?
What things upset or stress the person now?
What triggers stress?
How has the caregiver managed these?
What are the early warning signs of stress for this person?
In the recent past, what things has this person found satisfying, comforting, reassuring, calming?

Quality of Life

Activities enjoyed/disliked
    What songs does the person know/like?
Interests to be sustained
Safety/security needs

(continued)

Exhibit V.4. *(continued)*

Identity needs
Self-esteem needs
Pleasure/comfort needs
Need for autonomy
Need for control/mastery/success
Spiritual needs
Level of engagement
What is the person's current attitude toward/awareness of her illness?
What are her personal values?
What kind of care does she want?
What life goals/unfinished business does he have?
What are person's own concerns now (whether reasonable or not)?
What things or issues hold special emotional importance for the person now?

Friends/Psychosocial Needs

Informal support network; will it remain in place after placement?
Have friends remained in contact with the person? Who are they? Will they visit? How can these friendships be strengthened?
Was the person highly social, a loner, usually had only a few friends?

Personal Family History

Primary and secondary caregivers
  Caregiving roles in recent past, roles after admission?
Responsible family's ability to make decisions, plan, learn, adjust to change?
Relevant family history/family conflicts
Marriages, divorces
  Is the spouse living? What is spousal role in relationship now?
  Of other family members?
Children, siblings, other family members, and significant others
  Who are living/deceased, living at distance?
  What is their role/relationship with client now?
(Many families are not nuclear. Divorced spouses may remain close and support each other. Partners may be gay; partners may be unmarried but living together. There may be stepchildren, half siblings, foster relatives, unrelated close companions.)
  Who provides daily care?
  Who will be visiting?
  How does the person feel about these individuals?
  Does he recognize them?
  What are past and current relationships? (Relationships and values change over the years and with increasing dependence.)
  What are the expectations of family members for care?
  Are there family conflicts?
  Do close family members suffer from serious illness, unemployment, depression, other problems that directly affect their relationship with this person?

(continued)

Exhibit V.4. *(continued)*

Are there family members who are not involved in decisions or care?
What are the family dynamics around illness?
How has the family coped with crisis in the past?

Photos of Person/Others/Pet

Be sure these are labeled with at least a name and some explanation.
Be sure they are large enough for the person to see.

Familiar/Treasured Items

Be sure these are labeled with at least a name and some explanation.
Use an engraver to label items.
Replace jewelry (rings) with paste copies.
Anchoring items with "Quake-Hold" or "Blu Tac" reduces the risk that they will be lost.
Plate rack shelves can hold personal possessions out of reach of others.

Personal Items

Eyeglasses, dentures, hearing aid, ambulation aids, braces? Are these labeled? Are they listed in the chart?

Exhibit V.5. Interventions Tried

There are many reasons to document, at least as notes, the interventions you have tried for specific areas. Staff frustration is reduced when each person does not have to reinvent the solutions. When a strategy works, even part of the time, others need to know this. If a strategy often fails or further distresses the person, others need to know this also.

As a person relaxes in a low-stress environment, new interventions may begin to work. As a person's disease progresses or when the person develops excess disabilities, old strategies may fail.

Documenting interventions is essential to demonstrate to regulators that conventional strategies have not been successful before less traditional interventions will be approved. Make simple notes that include

- specific problem symptom;
- date;
- intervention tried;
- success/failure/partial success;
- staff member;
- what task assessment or task breakdown staff members have tried and whether it helped.

Notes may be as simple as:

"Luke shouts and may hit when being bathed.
June 3: aide Beth offered him an ice cream cone, and Luke took his bath calmly.
June 12: aide Anne tried this, and Luke did not understand and became angry."

A review of such notes may indicate that Beth is generally better with Luke, that his ability to understand varies a lot, and so on.

These records help to give staff members feedback when they succeed.

Exhibit V.6. Assessing the Caregiving Situation

This is not an information-gathering instrument or an assessment tool; it is a problem-solving exercise that helps the caregiving staff narrow down and identify causes of difficulty with ADLs, IADLs, and activities. It can be modified to meet the needs of individual programs. Answering these questions will also help programs organize their arguments in requests for waivers or justification of a care strategy. This material is a review of issues discussed in the lessons.

How does this person's brain damage make it difficult for her to do things? What things?

This question addresses Lesson 2.

- For example, if the person doesn't seem to be able to start things, can the caregiver get her started? Will she then be able to continue on her own?
- If the person tends to get stuck doing the same thing over and over, can the caregiver get her started washing one leg while the caregiver washes the rest of her?

Can the person hear you? See well enough to do a task?

This question and the next recall Lesson 3.

- For example, can the person hear in a noisy area like the dining room or in the shower?
- Might the person be confused by bright light coming in the window or by the dimness of the closet?
- Could the person wear his hearing aid and glasses in the shower?

Is the person feeling well? in pain?

- For example, stiff arthritic joints can hurt when you manipulate them. Dental problems may lead to eating problems. If a person abruptly (over a few hours or days) has more difficulty with or resistance to an ADL, this should trigger a search for excess disability.
- Frequent requests to be toileted are rarely attention seeking; check for urinary retention.

Is what you are saying/doing registering?

- Is the person paying attention?

What awareness does the person have of his abilities/limitations?

Insight varies from "none" through "sometimes" through "about some things" to "most of the time except about one thing." It is not an either/or concept. Observe and listen for clues to partial insight into specific tasks. Insight declines as the disease progresses and must be reevaluated frequently. Evaluating insight is particularly important in evaluating the person's ability to continue independent living. For example,

> Mr. Leone denies any problems with his memory but reports that "they" won't let him drive any more because he is "too old." He makes no effort to drive since his license was revoked. Is this partial insight adequate to keep him safe?

How safe is this activity?

Safety means different things to different people, and it varies from day to day in the same person. A person may be able to prepare a simple meal some days but not others. Whenever safety is discussed, issues of values and quality of life are also being discussed. Be aware of this as decisions are made about what is safe for a person.

(continued)

Exhibit V.6. *(continued)*

Can you make this situation safer?

Using your knowledge of brain function, retained abilities, sensory function, the specific physical environment, and the support system, can you brainstorm ways to make specific situations safer? The goal usually is to find little adjustments and small changes that help.

Is doing this important to the person? What is the person's agenda? Can you fit what you want into her agenda?

This is discussed in Lesson 11.

In every instance, no matter how impaired the person is, we must consider the importance and meaning of the activity for the person with dementia. Whether or not we can honor the person's wishes, trying to understand how the person feels about the activity helps get the job done. It is important to recognize when the person's agenda is different from that of the caregivers. Consider the person's need for independence, control, and self-esteem. What caregiving tasks are done because they help the caregiver or provide safety but do not meet the person's agenda?

What parts of this task does the person like to do or can the person do?

Resistance to tasks often occurs because the person has a feeling of "being done to" rather than of "doing"; of being controlled rather than controlling. When you assess this area, you are looking for ways to restore positive feelings in order to gain the person's cooperation. A high-functioning person can do many things but may do them slowly or sloppily. You may have to search for the things a more impaired person can do. Here are some suggestions for people who are quite impaired.

- Hold a washcloth over her eyes to keep the shampoo out (with lots of reminders).
- Hold the pillow while you make the bed.
- Hold a towel around his waist for privacy while you wash underneath it.
- Walk to the dining room slowly.

How is this situation affecting the caregiver or caregivers?

Whether the caregiver is the family member or a staff member, her frustration, satisfaction, sense of haste, or disgust is a factor in accomplishing the task. People with dementia are sensitive to our feelings and may respond to how we are being affected. For example:

> Cathy complained, said she was ill, plucked at people's sleeves, and called out, "Help me." She did things the staff members thought were manipulative. Even the most caring staff members were frustrated with her. Good care for Cathy will mean helping her caregivers cope.

What are your strengths and weaknesses?

Some staff members are patient; some are jolly; some have an air of authority. Sometimes staff members are tired, are annoyed, or don't like this work. Knowing yourself will help you find ways to get a job done. Good staff members trade off their skills. If one staff member cannot gain cooperation, maybe another can. For example:

- Estelle is patient. She can shower people who resist care from everyone else.
- Rebecca has a wonderful sense of humor and can get difficult people smiling.

(continued)

Exhibit V.6. *(continued)*

- Jake has authority. When all else fails, he will come out of his office and tell a client what must be done. "Who says?" asked the client. "I do," Jake said, "and I'm the boss." (Use authoritarian approaches as infrequently as possible: like everyone else, people with dementia will rebel against too much authority.)

What will the physical environment support?

Look around and use common sense. What needs to be done to make it easier to do the task in this space?

What things have you tried, and what can you try?

Can what has been tried before be modified so that it will work?

When you tried something that did not work, what did that teach you about the person/situation? If you tried something that worked once and then failed, what does that tell you?

Have others been successful? How?

Always check whether somebody (including family caregivers) has been able to do this task, and if so, find out what he did.

Is this task absolutely necessary?

If the person with dementia resists a task strongly, assess whether it is absolutely necessary, can be done later, can be done a different way, can be done by someone else. Who thinks it is necessary?

When is it best to just do the task?

For some people and at some points in the disease, being passively cared for is desired. Struggling to see, hear, or understand the task may not be appropriate for the person who is physically ill, exhausted, or in the later stages of the illness. For these people, gentle caregiving is best.

Can you wait out the problem?

If the behavioral symptom is not life threatening and if the caregiver (including staff members) is supported, perhaps you need to do nothing in response to some problems.

> John had always been a controlling, difficult man. He called the staff members by insulting names and treated them as servants. There was little to be done to change him except to give him neuroleptics, which had serious side effects for John. With understanding and a lot of support from their superiors, the staff members were able to accept this behavior.

As the disease progresses, problems change. Many problem behaviors go away as the person becomes less able to engage in them.

Can you work with, rather than against, specific disabilities?

For example, if a person tends to grasp things, give her something to hold. This keeps her hands busy while the caregiver gets the job done. If a person paces, give her sandwiches instead of trying to get her to sit down to a meal.

Use an old social skill.

> One family installed a new but simple lock. Because it was new, the person with dementia was unable to figure out how to operate it.

CHAPTER VI

USING ASSESSMENT INSTRUMENTS

This chapter discusses (1) the selection of published client assessment instruments, (2) instruments for determining the stage of a dementia, and (3) how to interview a person with dementia. It describes how to use the Mini-Mental State Examination (MMSE) and the Minimum Data Set (MDS) as *clinical tools* to identify the spared and retained functions discussed throughout the lessons.

Selecting Published Assessment Instruments

Many excellent assessment instruments are available. Each has strengths and weaknesses. The use of some assessment instruments is mandated. Others are selected for a specific purpose: to identify the stage of the illness; to identify spared and impaired functions; to measure behavioral symptoms or skills involved in activities of daily living (ADLs) or in instrumental activities of daily living (IADLs); for use in diagnosis; or as a research tool. In selecting an instrument, ask yourself how well it will fit your program's needs. Never accept an instrument simply because it was recommended for other programs like it. Assessment instruments that are useful for one purpose may be useless or misleading for another. For example, some ADL assessment tools work well for physically disabled people but do not reveal the cognitive disabilities of people with dementia.

Before selecting an instrument, consider the following:

- What do you want to accomplish with this instrument? Assessment instruments have specific uses. Choose one designed for the task you wish to accomplish. There are no ideal instruments to guide clinical interventions. We suggest two here, but their uses are limited. There is no substitute for good clinical skills.
- Is it practical to use? Will your staff be able to use it? How long does it take to administer once you get used to it? How frequently must it be repeated? Is the investment of time and personnel worth the information you gain from the instrument?
- Is the instrument based on the best research available? For example, checklists designed to predict the risk of falls, incontinence, or concurrent illness should be based on studies that have identified the most common risk factors. (Some checklists omit one or more common causes of falls or waste time recording causes of falls that rarely occur.)
- Does the test actually measure what you are trying to measure? Some tests give misleading results. For example, if you use a questionnaire to measure memory and the person has a severe language impairment, you will find out what the person can't say or can't understand, not what she cannot remember. Questionnaires that ask nurses to assess behavioral symptoms tell you what the nurse perceives; however, some nurses are more accepting or tend to overlook certain behaviors. Such an instrument measures the nurse's opinion (which is important) but may not accurately measure the person's function.
- If different staff members obtain different results from a test, the test is useless. The best way to ensure that assessment instruments do not introduce this kind of error is to use in-

struments whose reliability and validity have been studied. The higher the reliability coefficient, the more confident you can be that the test will provide consistent information; thus, a reliability of .89 means the test will provide consistent information more of the time than a test with a reliability of .56. Avoid cutting and pasting to make your own instruments from instruments for which validity and reliability have been established. Using part of test A and part of test B may yield less than using either of them in their entirety.

- Do the terms in the instrument ask the questions in the best way? Terms such as *wandering* and *agitation* mean different things to different people. An instrument that lists only "wandering" will not help you identify individual reasons for wandering or whether the problem is walking the halls or leaving the facility. Specific wording such as "seemingly purposeless wandering" and "trying to go home" better describes specific behaviors. Avoid questionnaires that express behaviors in a pejorative way: "inappropriate sexual behavior" is vague and places a social value on a behavior that might be acceptable if the person did it in private.
- Has the instrument taken into consideration the way people answer questions? A check-off questionnaire is quick and easy but can miss important information. A take-home form allows families to spend more time with it, think things over, and look for information, but families may forget to bring it back. Yet completing a questionnaire may be overwhelming to a stressed family at the time of admission.
- Avoid instruments that use jargon. For example, if a person likes to do things in a set order and to keep her possessions just so, this may be a way that she makes her world manageable and comfortable. Losing these routines may make her anxious. Labeling this behavior as obsessive-compulsive disorder may be inaccurate and misses the importance of the behavior for the person.
- Observation of the person's behavior may affect the significance of the assessment. The data written down on a form are only a small part of the information gathered. Was the person with dementia tired or restless while completing this interview? Did the family members hesitate or roll their eyes when asked certain questions? Did the assessor pick up changes in odor? skin tone? apathy? If the person with dementia ended the interview, what happened?
- Staff time usually influences who will do an assessment, but other factors should be considered as well. Does the person completing the instrument know the client? Is he a good observer? Is he encouraged to record additional observations about the person or the setting? Is the interviewer slow and gentle? Will she wait for the confused person to think? Is she an orderly thinker who does not fill in for the person? Does the staff communicate well with her? Questions asked by a rushed person or one who is easily misunderstood will affect the responses of the person with dementia.
- Sometimes a nurse assessor instead of a unit staff member completes the MDS. There are good reasons for this, but it seriously limits the instrument's clinical usefulness. The staff members responsible for care are aware of trends that an outsider may miss, and the clinical director gets information secondhand from the assessment.

Assessing the Stages of Dementia

Being able to define the stage of a person's illness has many advantages: providers might use staging to determine whether a person will fit into their program, as a part of care planing, or to determine costs of care. Researchers need people in the same stages, and families want to know where they stand and what to expect. Staging, then, is a valuable and commonly used tool. However, it is important to understand what staging can and cannot do.

There are many different staging instruments. Some have three stages, others five, and still others nine. Some instruments define the early stages better than others; some define the late stages better. Some use neurological symptoms, others use ADLs, and some even include behaviors. Some are very specific; others are open and vague. Because different instruments are in common use, what you mean by a stage may be different from what someone else means.

Staging terms are an artificial description of a gradual process. Because Alzheimer disease and some of the other dementias progress gradually, there is no clear-cut line between one stage and another.

People with uncommon dementias may not fit into the stages because the symptom pattern is different for different diseases. Incontinence, for example, usually occurs late in Alzheimer disease but may appear early in normal pressure hydrocephalus. Categorizing people by stage when the disease is not known can lead to misdiagnosis and inappropriate treatment.

Most of the time, certain disabilities emerge in a general order in all people with Alzheimer disease. This observation makes staging possible. However, certain symptoms may occur prematurely if the person has an excess disability, is not receiving good medical care, or is stressed. If these symptoms are regarded as evidence of the onset of the next stage, the potential for treatment is overlooked. For example, incontinence usually marks a later stage of Alzheimer disease. When it occurs early in the disease, it indicates a need for intervention or a review of the diagnosis.

When staging is used to plan a case mix, other factors may be more important: for example, the severity or nature of behavior problems or the presence of certain concurrent illnesses.

Problematic behavioral symptoms may occur at various stages as the result of the care given, the environment, excess disability, or the specific disease. Thus, they can be misleading when used to define stages.

Individuals vary widely. A particular disability cannot always be predicted by the stage of the individual's illness.

Each person must be assessed individually. Both strengths and symptoms may be overlooked when quick assumptions are made by staging the person's disability.

Interviewing the Person with Dementia

In many situations it is important to interview the person with dementia. Do not assume that people who are awake and alert but cognitively impaired cannot provide useful information. It is possible to conduct short interviews with most people with dementia without upsetting them. Interviews may be formal or informal. They may include exploring the presence of pain, unidentified emotional needs, likes/dislikes, and so on; assessing mood or mental illness; or conducting an MMSE. Do not be hesitant to interview people; if things go badly, just stop.

Verbal interviews become more challenging as the individual's language skills decline. Review Lesson 6. Simplify questions, and observe nonverbal communication closely.

Plan ahead: interview at the person's best time of day. Avoid testing when the person is experiencing excess disability. If the person is upset or not feeling well, postpone the interview. Minimize the impact of medications by testing before the administration of the next dose.

Provide for your own total concentration. Plan a time when you will not be interrupted. Do not attempt to interview someone while you are watching what is going on in the room or when other staff members or residents may interrupt you. If you must carry a beeper or cell phone, turn it off.

Allow plenty of time. Do not rush the person either before or during the interview. People with dementia need extra time to think. Hurrying a person to the interview will spill over into restlessness or impaired concentration during the interview.

Because people with dementia often tire easily, consider breaking up the interview with rests or a snack. Break up long interviews over several days.

Avoid interviewing where others can eavesdrop or participate, even if you know they will not remember the conversation. If the person is worried about why you want to go into her room to talk, consider talking where she feels comfortable.

Chat briefly about something the person might be able to respond to. For example, "How are you feeling today?" or "It's a beautiful day today."

Ask questions directly: "How is your memory (or mood) today? . . . Good. May I ask you some questions to see how your memory is working?" People rarely say no once you have had the courtesy to ask. Agreeing to be questioned puts them in control. If someone does say no, do not test her then. Try later.

If the person has difficulty focusing or concentrating, find something to do with him that puts him at ease. Do some simple activity such as shelling peas or taking a walk—something that does not upset the person or take much of your attention. Walk with people who are too restless to sit for an interview. If the person becomes distracted during the interview, bring her gently back to the point.

Your approach should be matter of fact and nonjudgmental. Show genuine interest in this person. Smile. Make eye contact. Make it clear that you are enjoying this person.

If the person become upset, it may be due to fatigue, restlessness, or stress. If the person becomes angry or restless during the interview, stop. Try later.

Stress from any cause is likely to limit the person's ability to do well on the test. Physical needs (pain, hunger, need to toilet), noise, distractions, not perceiving the interviewer as a kind, helpful person, feeling rushed, needing to move about, upsetting experiences in the hours before the test all contribute to stress, which will reduce interview performance.

Go slowly to avoid stressing the person. Offer positive but vague feedback to each response: "You are very helpful"; "I really appreciate this"; "You've had a very interesting life"; "We're doing very well."

You may want to conduct some interviews several times. For example, if you are trying to localize pain for a person, have a brief chat about it several times during the day. If you receive approximately the same answer each time, the answer is more likely to be correct.

Staff members often worry that a person with dementia will be upset by tests of mental function because she becomes aware of her deficits. Most people with dementia lack this insight and will not realize that they continue to make mistakes. If you make the test situation a time for enjoyable social interchange, they will enjoy the process and the individual attention. They will not remember or add up their errors.

If a person expresses concern about mistakes and if you are concerned and gentle, it likely that the person will be grateful for your concern and help with something that has been worrying her. If the testing does upset someone, acknowledge her feelings. Never trivialize or deny these feelings. However, a simple rather than extended answer usually helps: "Yes, you are starting to forget things. That can be upsetting." Try giving a truthful but indirect answer: "Actually, we're doing well" or "You're doing well."

Pay attention to how the person behaves in the interview. Is the person able to focus on you and on one question at a time? If not, consider delirium. Is the person suspicious? Are the first few words the person says targeted to answering the question but then followed by rambling remarks? If so, alert caregivers to focus on the first few words a person says because they are more likely to have meaning.

Does the person answer "I don't know" to your questions? Suspect depression. People with a dementia are more likely to try to answer, but this is not a hard-and-fast rule.

Is the person making up answers? Alert caregivers that the person may supply confusing information. Is the person restless? Can you find out why?

Avoid making excuses for the person's mistakes. Don't say, "Oh, well, you don't really need to know what city you are in" or "Most of us are no good at math." Instead, make a positive response: "That's good" or "OK, now . . ." (and move on to the next question).

Some people try to conceal their memory loss. They may refuse to let you test them, but they are more likely to give answers such as, "I already know all that" or "Young lady, how dare you ask me such things!" Score these as not answered. Say something nice about the person or gently make a joke. Try, "I know you do, but I have to fill out these forms. Would you just help me do that?" Try introducing questions with, "I know you know this, but . . ."

Don't skip questions because you know the person can't answer them.

In general, it is better to test people outright in a kind and empathetic manner than to try to infer information from indirect questions. The latter will quickly make people suspicious. Never try to trick the person into answering questions. Even people who do not remember can have feelings of trust or mistrust.

Ask questions about mental experience only when clinical observation indicates the need. Some questions about mental experiences such as hallucinations or depression may seem difficult to ask. However, you can ask even a very confused person these questions. If you do so in a caring way, people will feel reassured that you are concerned for them. Directly ask about spirits or mood. Ask or find out from the caregiver whether mood varies from morning to evening. Your goal is to appreciate the mental life of the individual, not to judge it.

Professional expertise is needed to evaluate mood or mental illness. However, you can ask informal questions effectively. If either you or the client is not comfortable, stop the interview and have a professional complete it. Never deny the reality of feelings by saying something such as "It can't be that bad" or "You don't really believe people are spying on you from Mars." Ask questions like the following, and make nonjudgmental responses that neither confirm nor deny the person's feelings:

"Are you happy?"
"Do you feel that things are hopeless?" (Reassure honestly, try: "That is painful. Even so, perhaps things will get better.")
"Do you ever feel that you are a worthless person?" ("I think you are special because . . .")
"Do you feel that things are going badly for you?"
"Are some people out to get you?" (suspiciousness)
"Are they taking your things?"
"Do you hear people talking about you?" "Can you tell me what it sounds like?" (hallucinations)
"Do you see things that frighten you?" "Can you describe them?"
"Do things ever seem so bad that you have thought of killing yourself?"
"Do you ever have thoughts you can't put out of your mind?" (obsessions)
"Are you afraid of . . . ?"

Ask people to describe these things. Listen. Respond empathetically. "I'm sorry you feel that way" or "That must be very frightening." Don't respond, "I sometimes think I'm hearing things too." Listen and take a person's concerns seriously, without trivializing them.

It is unlikely that you will "set a person off." If the person does become upset, offer to stay with her until she feels better. If she becomes upset with you, ask someone else to stay with her. Talking about suicide does not make a person more likely to attempt suicide. You will have to infer from clinical observations symptoms such as hallucinations in people with limited verbal ability, but be cautious. The person you think is hearing voices may be listening to the ringing in his ears.

Do not assume you know the answer or assume you understood. If you are not sure, ask the person, or note that you were unsure. The object in interviews is to understand the person. Do not let yourself judge, rescue, demean, brush aside, "band-aid," cure, or treat. Do the hardest thing—just being with the person as one human with another.

Watch for the beginnings of irritability or restlessness, and stop the questioning if necessary. Never push to complete an interview at the risk of upsetting the person. End the interview in a friendly way, and try to finish it another time.

Clearly state that you are finished, and thank the person for the help. Tell her what she is going to be doing next (for example, "I'll walk back to your room with you").

Recording

Record your impressions right away. Recording is as important as testing. Write down each score or answer as you go, as it's easy to forget. Staff members sometimes feel shy about writing things down in front of a person. This rarely bothers a person, but if she asks, show her what you are writing.

Don't cheat on the person's behalf when scoring. It is easy to say, "She almost got it right" or "I think she knew the answer." If you did not complete the interview, note why: Was the person unable to pay attention? Did he get angry? wander away? Could he not hear you? Were you unable to understand the person? This information may be of more use than the final score.

Never dismiss details that don't fit or that don't make sense to you. Record observations: Could you hardly wake a person to interview him? Was the person tired or restless? Was the person suspicious? Did he answer in a flat monotone with little affect? Is this person comfortable? Is she tense? Is she able to focus on you? Is she drifting off? Can she remain still? Does she seem driven? What can you elicit? a smile? What is interesting about this person?

Write down your own knowledge of the person. If you know that the person can usually do the task, note this: "She usually or spontaneously can do this."

Communicate your findings to the direct care

staff promptly. For example, "I got answers but I had to wait a long time for each answer. Try waiting to give her time." "He's very impaired, but he's a whiz at math. You can probably get him to joke around with numbers in order to get him through morning ADLs."

The Mini-Mental State Examination

This instrument is internationally accepted as the benchmark test of cognitive impairment. It is useful in diagnosis, documentation of the progress of the illness in individuals, research, drug studies, epidemiology, staging, and other areas. Its reliability, validity, and widespread use make it one of the most useful tools available. Versions adapted for other languages and cultures are available. The MMSE is quick to administer and can be done by a trained layperson.

The MMSE tests specific cognitive skills (orientation, registration, attention, calculation, recall, language, and spatial perception). This allows the caregiver to identify individual areas of strength and weakness.

The MMSE has been shown to relate to the density of plaques and tangles in the brain and has been correlated to stages of the illness; performance has been correlated to computerized tomography.

Although various articles have attempted to standardize this test, we will use the test as originally proposed by Folstein, Folstein, and McHugh (1975).

Of the many uses of the MMSE, two are discussed here: (1) identification of cognitive impairment and documentation of change and (2) identification of spared and impaired areas of function.

Identification of Cognitive Impairment and Documentation of Change

The MMSE documents the presence of cognitive impairment. By itself it does not *diagnose* Alzheimer disease or *discriminate* between dementia, delirium, and lifelong mental retardation. It screens for *difficulty in mental functioning,* which can be followed by diagnosis. Once a diagnosis is made, if the MMSE is given at intervals, it will document changes in function. In addition, because this instrument is so widely used, many clients will have earlier MMSEs in their records for comparison.

The MMSE will not reliably identify the earliest stages of dementia. And at some point in the illness, individuals will score a 0 on the MMSE. It will not discriminate between "0" and "worse than 0." Thus, this test will not show a difference between severe and more severe dementia.

Identification of Spared and Impaired Areas of Function

People with cognitive impairment may present in a socially appropriate way, which can mislead caregivers into overlooking disabilities. Other people with cognitive impairment are so disabled that caregivers don't notice remaining abilities. The MMSE will roughly identify strengths and weaknesses in these people. While it is not a substitute for neuropsychological testing, it can be helpful in identifying strengths and weaknesses in clinical care as well. Because it is a rough estimate, however, and you might be in error, always assume that the person may have strengths you did not identify.

The instructions that follow are to be used only to encourage the caregiver to think in terms of an individual's strengths and weaknesses. A total score provides a valid measure of function. When individual items are used as suggested, they provide only an estimate of an individual's specific areas of spared and impaired function. When the MMSE is used this way, we might observe from it that one person's short-term memory is so impaired that we tend to overlook other abilities he has retained, or that another can still do many things but her loss of the use of language is severe. For example:

> Henry was a happy man who loved to tell jokes. Caregivers laughed but did not understand a word he said. He was incontinent and very disabled, could do none of the craft-type activities, and needed a lot of direction. Staff members were sure that Henry would score a 0 on the MMSE. They did not want to embarrass him by asking him to do the diagram on the test. But he was thoroughly enjoying the attention during the interview, so the interviewer handed him the diagram. He said, "interlocking pentagrams," and copied it correctly. This question tests knowledge of spatial relationships. Henry might be able to set the table because he could still understand the relationship between

> table space and place mats, between placing the knives and placing the spoons. With some help getting started, Henry soon had "his" job and became an important part of meal preparation.

This is a real case. However, this pattern of spared function is rare. It is used as an example only.

Instructions

The MMSE is easy to use. The following instructions are designed to facilitate the clinical use of the instrument. Before beginning the test, make the person comfortable and establish rapport. During the test, praise success.

Administering the MMSE and Applying Its Findings in Care

Follow the general instructions (given earlier in this chapter) on how to interview. The MMSE is on p. 364, and a page you can photocopy for the patient is on p. 365. Ask the interview questions as they are written. You may repeat questions if you are not sure the person heard you or was focused. You may also offer reassurances as you go along. Ask all the questions and sum the scores. The discussion corresponds to and explains each part of the instrument.

ORIENTATION (10 points: score 1 point for each correct answer)

This test item determines the person's knowledge of place and time. Ask one item at a time. You can substitute appropriate places for *hospital* and *floor.*

How to use this information: If the person has problems in orientation, try gently telling her where she is, but if she does not retain this, caregivers may find that repeated reorientation may only frustrate both the person and the caregivers. It is not necessary to provide people with orientation that they will not immediately need: the town, the date, the weather if they are not going outside. It is usually more helpful to orient these people about *immediate* issues. "This is the dining room. This is your lunch," " This is your room," "I am your daughter."

When a person is partially oriented, look for ways to support retention of that information: signs, cues, reminders, a pocket card with an address or telephone number, daily trips outside to check the weather.

If the person firmly believes he is in some other place or time, be sure caregivers know this. The person will act on his assumption, and reorientation may upset him. For example:

> Alice had no idea where she was and did not seem to mind as long as she was kindly cared for. Alice became upset if she thought her son or daughter had forgotten her. Reassuring her was the only orientation she needed.

> Jorge insisted that it was 1972 and he was in Mexico. Jorge periodically set out "for the mountains." The staff members found that he was more comfortable when they diverted him into preparations for his trip than when they tried to convince him he was in a northern state in winter.

People with problems in orientation may be confused when they leave a place (the unit, the house) and when they return. This can lead to catastrophic reactions. Tell the person where she is, who is taking care of her, and what is happening as she leaves and *reorient her on her return.*

REGISTRATION (score 1 point for each word recalled; for example, three words recalled = 3 points, one word recalled = 1 point)

Name three common objects, such as *car, nickel,* and *pony.* Take about one second to say each. Then ask the person to name all three after you have said them. Give one point for each successful recall. If the person does not recall all three, repeat them and ask him to name them. Record the number of trials. If the person's recall has not improved, stop after five trials.

It is wise to select three words that you can remember and stick to them; otherwise the day may come when neither you nor the client can recall the three words. (If this happens, have a good laugh with your client.) This part of the MMSE measures whether the person takes in information (registers it). If information is not registered, it will not be recalled.

How to use this information: People who do not register information will not remember instructions or information for even a few minutes. People with problems in registering information may not know things they have been told many times: that their children are visiting, when they will have a meal, why you are leading them somewhere, or that you just reassured them. These people will need a lot of help. Do not confuse their awareness of some things with their inability to register information. Some individuals will remember one or two but not all the named items. This tells you that they will be able to register (briefly retain) information if it is simple and brief enough. Staff members can explore exactly how much an individual retains.

ATTENTION AND CALCULATION (score 1 point for each successful subtraction or each letter correct in "world")

Ask the person to subtract 7 from 100. Then ask her to subtract 7 from that number and so forth until she has subtracted 7 from the previous number five times. Do not give her the correct number. Say, "OK, now subtract 7 from that."

Alternatively, ask the person to spell *world* backward.

We suggest you use both tasks and record the higher score. The two tasks in this item test whether the individual can hold one thought in mind long enough to finish the task or completely express an idea.

How to use this information: People who cannot do these tasks may not be able to focus on simple activities. They may forget what they are doing partway through a task. The staff will find that frequent reminders as a task is carried out, reducing distractions, reminders combined with reassurance, and patience help. Have the person rely on old, overlearned motor behaviors. Try to reduce background sources of stress, anxiety, or confusion. When the person was partially successful at the test, observation in the care setting will help identify things that help the person function.

RECALL (score 1 point for each word successfully recalled)

This item tests the person's ability to hold information in memory briefly even though a distractor (the attention and calculation question) may have diverted him. Recall is possible only if registration was successful. If the person registered one or two items, look for recall of those.

How to use this information: People with problems in recall may not know what you told them earlier, what they did earlier, that their family visited, or even that they just finished eating. Recall is not the same as long-term memory, to which the person may still have access. Some people who cannot recall information may make things up. This is not lying and should not be treated as such. The brain is just "filling a gap," and the person probably believes what she said.

People who have problems in recall will need many reminders and lots of patience. People with problems in registration and recall have not just forgotten what they were told; the brain behaves as if the person had never been told. Thus, even if a staff member has told the person the same thing every five minutes, each hearing is the first hearing for the impaired person.

Failures in memory and recall often happen within a minute or two of giving the person information. By the time you have gotten the person out of her chair, she may have forgotten where you were taking her. People with problems in registration and recall must depend on the caregiver for basic information about where they are and what is happening. Their ability to recall reassurance is only fleeting. This requires that they have a high level of trust in caregivers whom they often do not recognize.

Use multiple cues, many frequent reminders, reassurance. (If a person is still anxious after being told several times what is happening, try saying, "I'll take care of you.") For many people, remembering and knowing what is happening may not be important. It is not necessary to keep reminding such people if affection and comfort meet their needs. It is not necessary that they remember a family visit if they had a good time during the visit.

If the person can recall only one or two items, she may be able to remember simple, one-step information. Frequent reminders and cueing may help these people significantly.

Note whether the person remembers the first or last word if only one is recalled. This pattern may appear in daily routines as well.

If a person does not register or recall well, he will not recall that he is making errors on the MMSE if you provide cues that he is doing well.

Intrusion errors must not be counted as recall. Some individuals will produce the registration words in answer to later questions even though they gave no evidence of registering or recalling them in the first place. This indicates that inappropriate information is presenting itself in the individual's thinking. Sometimes these individuals will interrupt a task and revert to an earlier behavior. If intrusion errors occur, they may explain odd things the individual does.

LANGUAGE (9 points total; scoring of individual points is indicated on the instrument form)

Each of these six tasks tests for a different language skill. For the first task, point to your pencil and then your watch. Ask the person to name each.

How to use this information: If the person can make his intent generally understood but cannot answer these two questions, consider that he may be having difficulty finding names of things in general. Staff members can help by supplying the word when they know what it is, by not frustrating the person by asking for names. Some people sound articulate, and it is not until you find difficulty with these two questions that you realize the person is developing problems in communication. It is important to assess further whether the person is having more difficulty than you suspected.

Some people will be able to describe a watch and pencil or tell you what they are for, but they will not be able to name them. This is a strength that the staff can use: if the person cannot tell you something, ask him to describe it.

Ask the person to repeat after you, "No ifs, ands, or buts." The person must repeat this phrase exactly, including all three s's. Failure here indicates problems in expressing oneself and in understanding. Missing a common phrase indicates difficulties with language (aphasia). Note whether the person has any hearing loss.

How to use this information: Failure in any of these three questions indicates that the person has significant difficulty expressing his needs and concerns. If he has difficulty here, he probably will be unable to name his pain, his fears, his desires. This does not mean these feelings do not exist.

Hand the person a sheet of paper and ask her: "Take this paper in your right hand, fold the paper in half, and put the paper on the floor." Give all three steps at once and do not prompt the person.

How to use this information: This is a three-stage command and tests how much information the person can process at one time. The person's ability to do none, one, two, or all three of the steps reflects how much she will be able to do in daily life. If a person can do only one step, she is likely to need one-step instructions in ADLs (for example, "Take this towel." "Now, dry your face.") Sometimes you will find that the person can do more than the staff expects. Note whether the person retains the first or last bit of the command. In combination with registration and recall, you now have a picture of how much information a person can process and act on.

Show the person the statement "Close your eyes." Ask the person: "Read the words on this page and then do what it says." If you recopy the statement, be sure it is large and easy to read. Observe closely whether the person reads the words and whether he closes his eyes. Do not verbally prompt him.

How to use this information: The people who fail to do what the instructions say may be unable to follow instructions even though their registration and recall are intact.

Some people will be able to read the words aloud but will not close their eyes. The ability to register, or read, information and the ability to act on it are separate skills. It is important that the caregivers understand this. These people may read their name on their door but still be unable to find their room. Do not expect such people to follow instructions. Protect them: they may not obey exit signs, follow reminders to take their pills, or eat their lunch.

Staff members and families report conversations like these:

"Stay here while I go to the kitchen."
You return and the person has gone outside.
"What did I tell you to do?"
"You said to stay here."

"The soap is right here, Margaret."
Nothing happens.
"Margaret, did you hear me?"
"You said the soap is right here."

Such conversations can drive families and staff members crazy but in fact indicate the complexity of the brain deficits the person is experiencing.

Next ask the person: "Write a sentence." The

sentence must have a subject and a verb and make sense.

This question further examines the ability to follow instructions and use language. It will also show changes in the person's handwriting, which may be the first evidence of apraxia.

Hand the person the picture of interlocking pentagons. Ask the person: "Now copy the design that you see printed on the page." The result must be two five-sided figures with the intersection forming a four-sided figure. The original drawing should have five equal sides in each pentagram. If the person complains that she cannot draw, reassure her that you are not testing her drawing ability. Allow time. Some people get stuck repeating the same part of the sentence-writing task or copying the design. When you are sure that this is what is happening, you may interrupt the task.

How to use this information: This task tests the individual's ability to plan and carry out coordinated movement and to comprehend spatial relationships—that is, to perceive all the components of a group (place settings at a table or individuals in a room). People who have difficulty with this test may fail to pay any attention to some of the obvious elements of a group around them. For example, they may ignore some of the foods on their plate, some of the items in an activity, or even some but not all of their visitors. Laying out all their clothing at once may upset them, but laying out one or two pieces at a time may help. If a person ignores some members of the family, tension may be reduced by explaining this phenomenon to them.

This task will also show problems holding and using a pen correctly, which is evidence of inability to carry out an overlearned motor skill.

Both the interlocking pentagrams and the sentence writing will reveal perseverative behavior—when the person gets stuck repeating a word or line. People with this problem will repeat a word or phrase, repeat an activity (wiping, wadding skirt, pounding). Try interrupting these behaviors with a motor action—give the person something else to hold, or ask the person to sing if the perseveration is verbal. These people may enjoy repetitive tasks such as dusting or sweeping.

Level of consciousness: At the bottom of the form, record your assessment of the person's level of consciousness.

None of these questions provides final answers. They are clues. Compare them with what caregivers observe. The individual's abilities will vary somewhat from day to day. Retest the person later if you are uncertain of your findings.

Scoring

The possible total score is 30. Subtract from 30 the total of all points missed to obtain the final score. A higher score indicates higher functioning. Consider a score above 24 to be normal.

Level of consciousness is assessed along a continuum. If the person was not fully awake, a low score may indicate delirium.

Patient________________________
Examiner_______________________
Date___________________________

"MINI-MENTAL STATE" EXAMINATION

Maximum Score	Score	
		ORIENTATION
5	( )	What is the (year) (season) (date) (day) (month)?
5	( )	Where are we: (state) (county) (town) (hospital) (floor)?
		REGISTRATION
3	( )	Name 3 objects, taking 1 second to say each. Then ask the patient to repeat all 3 after you have said them. Give 1 point for each correct answer. Then repeat them until he learns all 3. Count trials and record. Trials ________
		ATTENTION AND CALCULATION
5	( )	Serial 7's. Give 1 point for each correct answer. Stop after 5 answers. Alternatively, spell *world* backward.
		RECALL
3	( )	Ask for the 3 objects repeated above. Give 1 point for each correct answer.
		LANGUAGE
9	( )	Name a pencil and a watch (2 points, 1 for each item named)
		Repeat the following: "No ifs, ands, or buts" (1 point)
		Follow a 3-stage command: Take a paper in your right hand, fold it in half, and put the paper on the floor (3 points, 1 for each step completed)
		Read and obey the following: CLOSE YOUR EYES (1 point)
		Write a sentence (1 point)
		Copy design (1 point)
	____	TOTAL SCORE

ASSESS Level of consciousness along a continuum

Alert Drowsy Stupor Coma

Source: Folstein, Folstein, and McHugh 1975.

CLOSE YOUR EYES

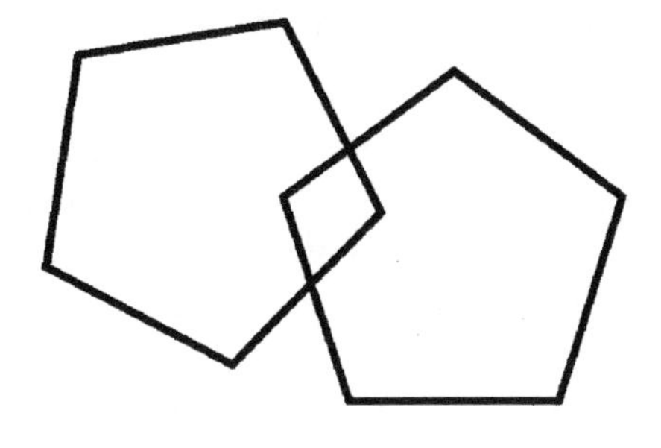

The Minimum Data Set

The Minimum Data Set is the questionnaire portion of the Resident Assessment Instrument (RAI). It was developed by a committee of experts for the U.S. government's Centers for Medicare and Medicaid Services. This instrument is required for residents of nursing homes who receive either Medicaid or Medicare. It identifies change in function and behavior and links this to care plans and interventions.

Because of its link to regulation, the MDS has had more than its share of negative criticism, yet few instruments have been as carefully designed and extensively tested. It is short and consolidates considerable material in one place.

Beyond its mandated and research uses, any program (residential care, nursing home care, day care, home care) will find the MDS, or selected sections of it, a valuable and succinct clinical tool to identify and address problems that arise in function and behavior and to monitor patient change. *This text discusses only clinical uses of the MDS.*

For clinical use, subscales can be used independently or informally at any time a clinical review seems appropriate. When subscales are used in this way, staff members can quickly assess a specific area. For example, a resident seems to caregivers to be "not herself" this morning. A nurse or trained staff member may quickly run through the items in the delirium subscale to help decide what is happening with the person.

This instrument provides an overview or minimum database. Use other materials, in particular the Resident Assessment Protocols (RAPs) section of the RAI, to supplement it. Extensive material on the use of this instrument is available.

For clinical use, the instrument, or sections of it, should be completed by staff members who work with the client.

Instructions are provided in the Resident Assessment Instrument User's Manual. It is full of valuable clinical information.

The RAPs show you how to use the findings from this instrument to help the person. Use them each time you trigger a RAP.

Using the Minimum Data Set in Routine Clinical Care

This discussion is limited to the *nonregulatory clinical application* of the MDS and RAPs only.

Section A: Background Information at Admission

This includes basic information about the person that the direct care staff must know in order to provide care. This is a *minimum* level of information. Chapter V recommends additional information.

Section B: Cognitive Patterns

This section is a quick screen for dementia and delirium. If you have positive findings in this section, review the RAPs. This instrument identifies a cognitive problem but does not specify a dementia or Alzheimer disease. Positive findings in this section should trigger a more thorough investigation of the cognitive problem.

In the screen for delirium (Section B.5), staff members may point out that "all our patients are like this." The key here is the phrase "when a–f have changed within the past 7 days." This *change* is the hallmark of delirium. Use this section informally any time staff members observe change in any of these six areas and when staff members suspect increased confusion.

Section C: Communication/Hearing *and* Section D: Visual Patterns

Caregiving staff members must know the patient's status in each entry in these sections. Review these sections when you observe a decline in function or a worsening of behavioral symptoms. Such a review is the first step in identifying common causes of excess disability. Most common among visual disabilities are macular degeneration, cataracts, glaucoma, and diabetic retinopathy. Also common are inappropriate medication for eye diseases, inappropriate use of visual appliances, and a need for environmental modification. Most common among communication difficulties are hearing impairments, vision impairments, delirium, infections, medications, medical status of ear, use of appliance, asthma, stroke, chronic obstructive pulmonary disease (COPD), and *the opportunity to communicate.*

Section E: Mood and Behavior Patterns

Other assessment instruments rely on verbal questions and answers to identify depression. The authors of this instrument, recognizing that people with cognitive difficulties may not be able to process verbal questions, have selected indicators of depression that do not depend on comprehending questions and verbalizing answers (Section E1.2.3). This section will indicate whether further investigation of depression is needed.

Section F: Psychosocial Well-being

This is an essential starting point for understanding the person you are working with. Staff members must know the *current* status of these issues. The questions lead directly to further evaluation and intervention.

Section G: Physical Functioning and Structural Problems *and* Section H: Continence

All caregiving staff members must know the patient's current status regarding each of these issues. For example, if night staff members do not know a person's limitations regarding range of motion, they might position a person or change her incontinence clothing in a way that causes her pain and prevents sleep or triggers an angry outburst. Programs other than nursing homes will need to modify the language of the instrument slightly (for example, "how resident moves to and returns from off unit locations" may be modified to "how client moves to and returns from different areas").

Section I: Disease Diagnosis

This section pulls together the medical conditions that affect ADL status, cognitive status (including delirium), nursing care, and risk of death. It helps identify causes of excess disability and provides justification for all interventions (for example, all medications, physical therapy).

Section J: Health Conditions

Like disease diagnosis, these factors profoundly influence all care and indicate excess disability. This information provides clinical information such as how much energy and ability the person has to participate in care. In addition to identifying the need for prompt medical care, problem conditions indicate whether the staff should encourage a person to do more for herself or should provide supportive, nondemanding care.

Section K: Oral/Nutritional *and* Section L: Oral/Dental Status

In addition to indicating a need for dental care, these factors are common causes of excess disablility. Staff members cannot assist in feeding people with dementia without this information.

Section M: Skin Condition

This section triggers nursing interventions. In addition, staff members must know what hurts a person during care and whether the person is insensitive to pain or pressure.

Section N: Activity Pursuit Patterns

Unfortunately, in the urgency of addressing the multiple needs of complex patients, this section is often answered more mechanically than individually. However, an accurate assessment of activity preferences, skills, and function is essential for quality of life and subsequently improvement in problematic behavioral symptoms. This section should be completed with a sound knowledge of the individual and kept current.

Section O: Medications

Nursing supervision must keep in mind the potential of any medication to trigger excess disability. To be of any use, this material must be updated more often than the mandated 90 days. Medication changes are frequent in this group of people; side effects are frequent, and they may not occur as quickly in older, disabled people as in other populations.

Section P: Special Treatments and Procedures

These factors profoundly affect care and help identify excess disability.

REFERENCES AND RESOURCES

References

American Psychiatric Association. 2000. *Diagnostic and Statistical Manual of Mental Disorders.* 4th ed., text revision. Washington, D.C.: American Psychiatric Association.

Brawley, E. C. 1997. *Designing for Alzheimer's Disease: Strategies for Creating Better Care Environments.* New York: John Wiley & Sons.

Coons, D. H. 1991. *Specialized Dementia Care Units.* Baltimore: Johns Hopkins University Press.

Coons, D. H., and N. L. Mace. 1996. *Quality of Life in Long-Term Care.* New York: Haworth Press.

Cronin-Golomb, A., S. Corkin, and T. J. Roen. 1993. "Neuropsychological Assessment of Dementia." In P. J. Whitehouse (ed.), *Dementia.* Philadelphia: F. A. Davis.

Dowling, J. R. 1995. *Keeping Busy: A Handbook of Activities for Persons with Dementia.* Baltimore: Johns Hopkins University Press.

Ekman, P., and W. V. Friesen. 1975. *Unmasking the Face: A Guide to Recognizing Emotions from Facial Clues.* Palo Alto, Calif.: Consulting Psychologists Press.

Folstein, M. F., S. E. Folstein, and P. R. McHugh. 1975. "'Mini-Mental State': A Practical Method for Grading the Cognitive State of Patients for the Clinician." *Journal of Psychiatric Research* 12(3):189–98.

Gibran, Kahlil. [1923] 1970. *The Prophet.* New York: Knopf.

Hellen, C. R. 1992. *Alzheimer's Disease: Activity-Focused Care.* Boston: Andover Medical Publishers.

Lezak, M. D. 1983. *Neuropsychological Assessment.* New York: Oxford University Press.

Lidz, C. W., L. Fischer, and R. M. Arnold. 1992. *The Erosion of Autonomy in Long-Term Care.* New York: Oxford University Press.

Mace, N. L. (ed.). 1991. *Dementia Care: Patient, Family, and Community.* Baltimore: Johns Hopkins University Press.

Mace, N. L., and P. V. Rabins. 1991. *The Thirty-Six-Hour Day: A Family Guide to Caring for Persons with Alzheimer Disease, Related Dementia Illnesses, and Memory Loss in Later Life.* 3rd ed. Baltimore: Johns Hopkins University Press.

Morris, J. N., L. A. Lipsitz, K. Murphy, and P. Belleveille-Taylor. 1997. *Quality Care in the Nursing Home.* St. Louis: Mosby.

Rabins, P. V., C. G. Lyketsos, and C. Steele. 1999. *Practical Dementia Care.* New York: Oxford University Press.

Rader, J. 1995. *Individualized Dementia Care.* New York: Springer.

U.S. Congress, Office of Technology Assessment. 1987. *Losing a Million Minds: Confronting the Tragedy of Alzheimer's Disease and Other Dementias.* OTA-BA-323. Washington, D.C.: Government Printing Office.

U.S. Government, Department of Health and Human Services, Centers for Medicare and Medicaid Services. 2002. *Revised Long Term Care Facility Resident Assessment Instrument User's Manual for the Minimum Data Set Version 2.0.* www.cms.hhs.gov.

Warner, M. L. 1998. *Alzheimer's Proofing Your Home.* West Lafayette, Ind.: Purdue University Press.

Weaverdyck, S. 1991. "Intervention-Based Neuropsychological Assessment." In N. L. Mace (ed.), *Dementia Care: Patient, Family, and Community.* Baltimore: Johns Hopkins University Press.

Whitehouse, P. J. (ed.). 1993. *Dementia.* Philadelphia: F. A. Davis.

Zgola, J. M. 1987. *Doing Things: A Guide to Programming Activities for Persons with Alzheimer's Disease and Related Disorders.* Baltimore: Johns Hopkins University Press.

———. 1999. *Care That Works: A Relationship Approach to Persons with Dementia.* Baltimore: Johns Hopkins University Press.

Resources

Alzheimer's Association, Chicago, Illinois (www.alz.org).

Benjamin B. Green-Field Library and Resource Center, Alzheimer's Association, Chicago, Illinois.

Dover Publications, Inc., 31 East Second Street, Mineola, New York 11501-3582 (www.doverpublications.com).

INDEX

Exhibits are indicated by the letter *e* following the page number; overheads/handouts are indicated by the letter *h*.

ABOUT THE AUTHORS

NANCY L. MACE is the coauthor of *The 36-Hour Day* and editor of *Dementia Care.* She was formerly a consultant to the Office of Technology Assessment, U.S. Congress. She has been a coordinator of the Sir James McCusker Training Programs in Perth, Australia, and an assistant in psychiatry at the Johns Hopkins University School of Medicine in Baltimore, Maryland.

DOROTHY H. COONS is the editor of *Specialized Dementia Care Units.* She is a consultant to Alzheimer's care units. She was formerly director of the Alzheimer's Disease Project on Subjective Experiences of Families and director of Alzheimer's Environmental Interventions at the Institute of Gerontology of the University of Michigan at Ann Arbor.

SHELLY E. WEAVERDYCK is assistant research scientist and dementia specialist at the Turner Geriatric Outpatient Clinic of the University of Michigan at Ann Arbor. She is director of the Alzheimer's Research Project at Eastern Michigan University and a consultant in geriatrics and long-term care.